WOMEN IN THE WAR ZONE

Other books edited by Anne Powell:

A Deep Cry: First World War Soldier Poets Killed in France and Flanders
(Palladour, 1993; Sutton Publishing, 1998)

The Fierce Light: The Battle of the Somme July – November 1916
(Palladour, 1996; Sutton Publishing 2006)

Shadows of War: British Women's Poetry of the Second World War
(Sutton Publishing, 1999)

WOMEN IN THE WAR ZONE

Hospital Service in the First World War

ANNE POWELL

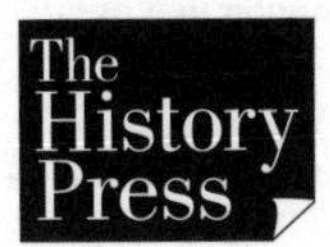

In memory of the women who cared for and consoled the wounded, the sick and the refugees during the First World War.

and for Jeremy; Jonathan, Sarah, Amelia and Alexander; Rupert, Clare, Molly, Jemima and Harriet; Lucinda, Andrew, Edward, Eleanor and Harry

with my love always

First published 2009
This edition first published 2013

The History Press
The Mill, Brimscombe Port
Stroud, Gloucestershire, GL5 2QG
www.thehistorypress.co.uk

British Library Cataloguing in Publication Data.
A catalogue record for this book is available from the British Library.

ISBN 978 0 7524 9360 2

Typesetting and origination by The History Press
Printed in Great Britain

Contents

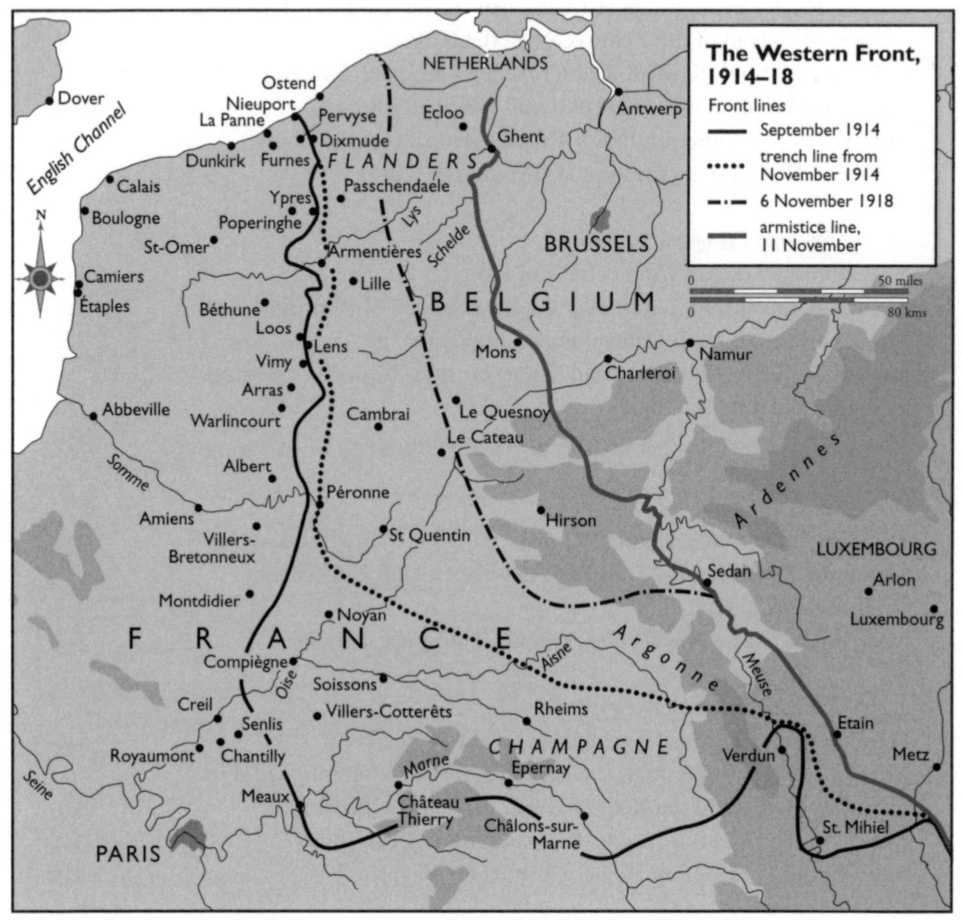
The Western Front, 1914–18
Front lines
September 1914
trench line from November 1914
6 November 1918
armistice line, 11 November
0 50 miles
0 80 kms
NETHERLANDS
BELGIUM
FRANCE
LUXEMBOURG
FLANDERS
CHAMPAGNE
English Channel
Ardennes
Argonne
Dover
Ostend
Nieuport
La Panne
Pervyse
Dixmude
Dunkirk
Furnes
Calais
Boulogne
Ypres
Passchendaele
Poperinghe
St-Omer
Armentières
Camiers
Étaples
Lille
Béthune
Loos
Lens
Vimy
Arras
Abbeville
Warlincourt
Cambrai
Albert
Péronne
Amiens
Villers-Bretonneux
Montdidier
Noyan
Compiègne
Soissons
Creil
Senlis
Villers-Cotterêts
Royaumont
Chantilly
Meaux
Château Thierry
PARIS
Epernay
Châlons-sur-Marne
Rheims
Verdun
St. Mihiel
Etain
Metz
Sedan
Arlon
Luxembourg
Hirson
St Quentin
Le Cateau
Le Quesnoy
Mons
Charleroi
Namur
BRUSSELS
Antwerp
Ghent
Ecloo
Lys
Schelde
Somme
Oise
Aisne
Marne
Seine
Meuse
N

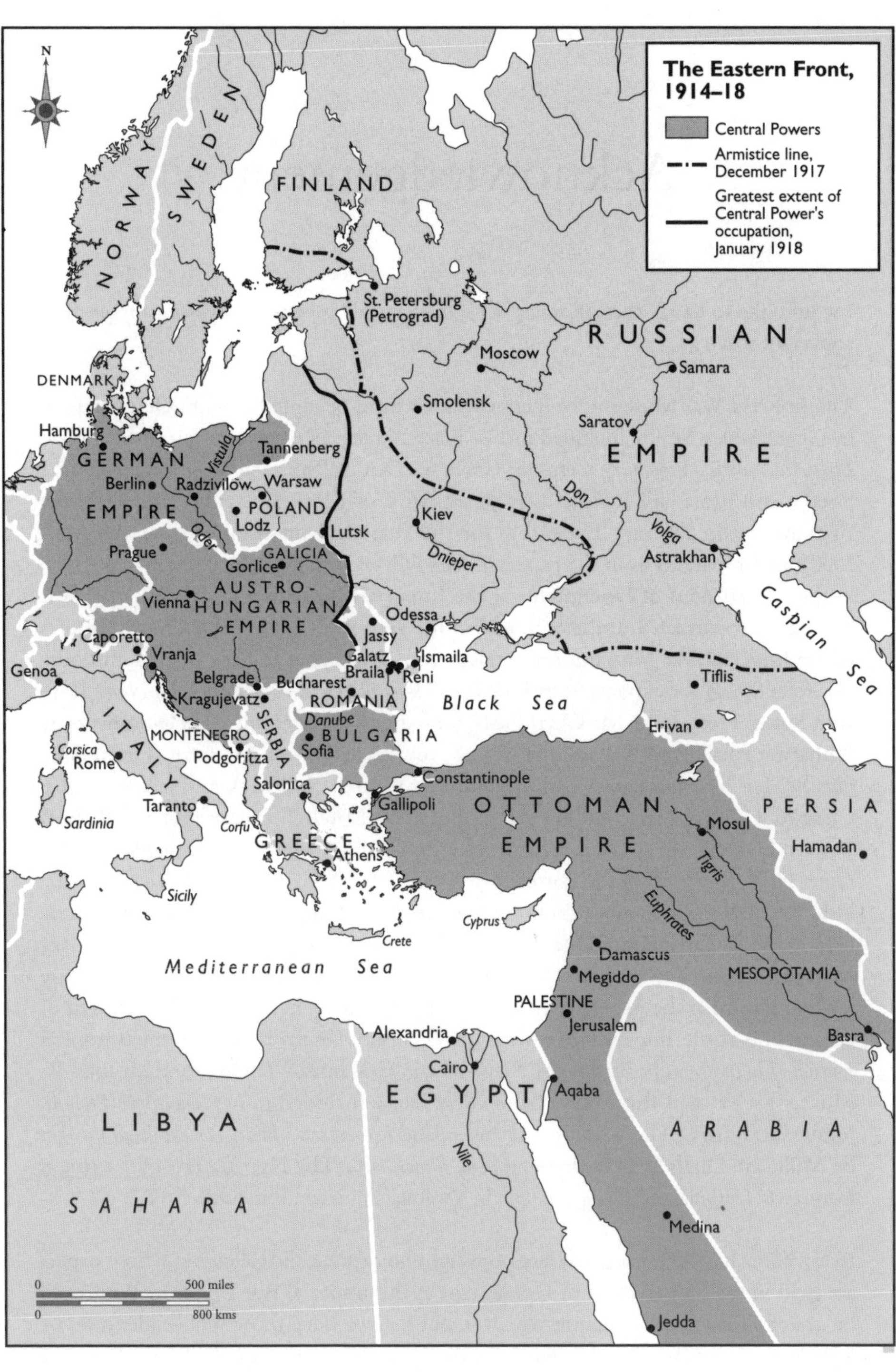

The Eastern Front, 1914–18
Central Powers
Armistice line, December 1917
Greatest extent of Central Power's occupation, January 1918
N
NORWAY
SWEDEN
FINLAND
St. Petersburg (Petrograd)
RUSSIAN
EMPIRE
Moscow
Samara
Smolensk
Saratov
DENMARK
Hamburg
GERMAN
EMPIRE
Berlin
Vistula
Tannenberg
Radzivilow
Warsaw
POLAND
Lodz
Oder
Lutsk
Kiev
Don
Volga
Astrakhan
Dnieper
Caspian Sea
Prague
GALICIA
Gorlice
AUSTRO-HUNGARIAN EMPIRE
Vienna
Odessa
Jassy
Caporetto
Vranja
Galatz
Ismaila
Braila
Reni
Genoa
Belgrade
Bucharest
ROMANIA
Kragujevatz
Black Sea
Tiflis
Erivan
SERBIA
Danube
BULGARIA
ITALY
MONTENEGRO
Corsica
Rome
Podgoritza
Sofia
Constantinople
Salonica
Gallipoli
OTTOMAN
EMPIRE
PERSIA
Taranto
Sardinia
Corfu
GREECE
Mosul
Hamadan
Athens
Tigris
Sicily
Euphrates
Cyprus
Crete
Damascus
Mediterranean Sea
Megiddo
MESOPOTAMIA
PALESTINE
Jerusalem
Alexandria
Basra
Cairo
EGYPT
Aqaba
LIBYA
ARABIA
Nile
SAHARA
Medina
0
500 miles
0
800 kms
Jedda

Acknowledgements

I would like to thank the following who have kindly given permission to reproduce copyright material:

The Imperial War Museum for 'Letter written from occupied Ghent', October 1914, by Grace Ashley Smith, included in *Five years with the Allies (1914–1919): the story of the First Aid Nursing Yeomanry Corps* by Grace McDougall; extracts from Vera Brittain's poetry and prose are included by permission of Mark Bostridge and Timothy Brittain-Catlin Literary Executors for the Vera Brittain Estate, 1970; Mrs Mair McCann for extracts from the papers of Mrs D. McCann (Miss Dorothy Brook), held in the Department of Documents at the Imperial War Museum; the Imperial War Museum for extracts from letters held in the archive of Miss Edith Cavell; trustees of the Imperial War Museum for extracts from the papers of Miss Mairi Chisholm; Mr Peter Spiegl for extracts from *Elsie Fenwick in Flanders: The Diaries of a Nurse 1915–1918*, Spiegl Press, 1980; Mr Chris Furse for extracts from *Hearts and Pomegranates* by Katharine Furse, Peter Davies, 1940; Lady Howard de Walden for extracts from *Pages from my Life* by Margherita Lady Howard de Walden, Sidgwick and Jackson, 1965; Glasgow City Archives and Special Collections, Mitchell Library, for the Report written by Dr Frances Ivens; Eric Dobby Publishing for extracts from *Flanders and Other Fields*, Memoirs of the Baroness de T'Serclaes, M.M., George G. Harrap & Co., Ltd., 1964; Mr Giles Pemberton for extracts from the papers of Miss E.B. Pemberton, held in the Department of Documents at the Imperial War Museum; Mrs Rosemary Marryatt for the letter from Nurse Mildred Rees; Mrs Daphne Loch and family for extracts from the papers of Miss Dorothy Seymour, held in the Department of Documents at the Imperial War Museum; Mrs Nina Theiss Boll for extracts from *A Journal of Impressions in Belgium* by May Sinclair, Hutchinson & Co., 1915; Mr John R. Murray for extracts from Freya Stark's War Diary included in her *Traveller's Prelude*, John Murray, 1950; The Countess of Sutherland for extracts from *Six Weeks at the War* by Millicent, Duchess of Sutherland, *The Times*, 1914; The Hypatia Trust for extracts from *Field Hospital and Flying Column* by Violetta Thurstan, Putnam's, 1915.

Every effort has been made to trace copyright holders for the following whose papers are held in the Department of Documents at the Imperial War Museum. We would be grateful for any information which might help to trace those whose identities or addresses are not currently known: Miss Bickmore; Sister E. Campbell; Miss Florence Farmborough; Miss Margaret Fawcett; Miss K. Hodges; Miss Amelia (Amy) Nevill; Miss F.E. Rendel; Miss Flora Sandes; Mrs M.A.A. Thomas (Miss Swynnerton).

I have been unable to trace a copyright holder for Lady Paget, whose book *With our Serbian Allies: Second Report* is held in the Department of Books at the Imperial War Museum. I thank the Imperial War Museum for permission to quote extracts and would be grateful for any information on Lady Paget.

I have been unable to trace copyright holders for the following whose archives are held in the Liddle Collection, University of Leeds: Sister Burgess; Miss Ida Jefferson (Mrs I. Cliffe); Sister Kathleen Mann.

I acknowledge the following books and periodicals from where extracts were taken. Every effort has been made to trace all copyright holders and we apologise to anyone who inadvertently has not been acknowledged: *A British Nurse in Bolshevik Russia* – The narrative of Margaret H. Barber, April 1916–December 1919, A.C. Fifield, 1920; *Fanny went to War* by Pat Beauchamp, George Routledge & Sons, Ltd., 1940; *Edith Cavell* by Rowland Ryder, Hamish Hamilton, 1975; *War and its Aftermath: Letters from Hilda Clark, M.B., B.S., from France, Austria and the Near East 1914–1924*. Edited by Edith Pye. Privately printed, 1956; *Blackwood's Magazine* articles (1916, 1917, 1918) by V.C.C. Collum; *Letters from a Field Hospital* by Mabel Dearmer, Macmillan and Co. Limited, 1915; *A VAD in France* by Olive Dent, Grant Richards, 1917; *With a Woman's Unit in Serbia, Salonika and Sebastopol* by I. Emslie Hutton, M.D., Williams and Norgate, 1928; *Eighteen Months in the War Zone: The Record of a Woman's Work on the Western Front* by Kate John Finzi, Cassell, 1916; *With the Scottish Nurses in Roumania* by Yvonne Fitzroy, John Murray, 1918; *Dr Elsie Inglis* by Lady Frances Balfour, Hodder and Stoughton, *c.*1920; *A Roumanian Diary 1915, 1916, 1917* by Lady Kennard, Heinemann, 1917; *Diary of a Nursing Sister on the Western Front 1914–1918* by K.E. Luard, William Blackwood and Sons, 1915; *Unknown Warriors: Extracts from the Letters of K.E. Luard, R.R.C., Nursing Sister in France 1914–1918*, Chatto and Windus, 1930; *My War Experiences in Two Continents* by S. Macnaughtan. Edited by her niece, Mrs Lionel Salmon (Betty Keays-Young), John Murray, 1919; *My Experiences on Three Fronts* by Sister Martin-Nicholson, George Allen & Unwin, 1916; *Women as Army Surgeons: Being the History of the Women's Hospital Corps in Paris, Wimereux and Endell Street, September 1914–October 1919* by Dr Flora Murray, CBE., MD., DPH., Hodder and Stoughton, *c.*1920; *Lady Muriel* by Wilfrid Blunt, Methuen, 1962; *The History of the Scottish Women's Hospitals* by Mrs Eva Shaw McLaren, Hodder and Stoughton, 1919; *Four Years out of Life* by Lesley Smith, Philip Allan, 1931; *Miracles and Adventures* by Mabel St Clair Stobart, Rider & Co., 1935; *Red Herrings of 1918* by R.J. Tennent. Privately printed, nd.

Extracts from the letters of Dorothy Higgins held in the Department of Documents at the Imperial War Museum, were first published in an article by Anne Powell in *Hortus: A Gardening Journal* No. 79, Autumn 2006. Edited by David Wheeler.

I would like to thank Sarah Flight and Jaqueline Mitchell at Sutton Publishing who commissioned this book in 2006; and all at The History Press who continued to have faith in the idea and who have helped and advised me over many months. My particular thanks to my editor, Simon Hamlet, and to Jo de Vries, Abigail Wood, Siubhan Macdonald and Robin Harries. I would also like to thank Martin Brown for his work on the maps.

I am very grateful to the following for their help and kindness:
Pauline Allwight, Department of Art, Imperial War Museum; Mark Amory; Judy Bevis, Portsmouth City Council Library Service; Gina Bore and Ginnene Taylor, Authors Licensing Copyright Service (ALCS); Margaret Bowen; Loreen Brown; Jane Conway; Richard Davies, Sam Gibbard, Liddle Collection, Brotherton Library, University of Leeds; Anita Desilva, The Publishers Association; Tabitha Driver, Library of the Religious Society of Friends, London; Caroline Gordon Duff; Ben and Jane Eliot; Melissa Hardie; Jo Howe; Rose Hudson, Society of Authors; Jane Hutchings; Alan Jeffreys; Shirley-Ann Kennedy; Gay Ledger; Gillian Lindsay; Richard Morgan; Lona de Moro; Hew Moseed, The Book Trust; Sybil Oldfield; Philip Oswald; Reading Room staff at the Imperial War Museum; Sara Pons; Paul Preston; Gavin Roynon; Thomas Seymour; Alan Shelley, Bow Windows Bookshop; Jane Smith; Roderick Suddaby, Keeper; Clare Sexton and Sabrina Rowlatt, Department of Documents, Imperial War Museum; David Sutton, Writers and their Copyright Holders (WATCH), University of Reading; Henry Sullivan, Glasgow City Archives and Special Collections, Mitchell Library; Sir Peter Tapsell, M.P.; Canon Michael Tristram; Jean Tsushimo; Wellcome Library staff; Mary Wilkinson, Head of Collections Development, Department of Printed Books, Imperial War Museum; Frances Woodrow, Royal College of Nursing Archives; Jen Young, Curator, Museum and Archives, British Red Cross.

My final thanks are to my beloved family for their love, encouragement and help in so many ways: Jonathan and Sarah for compiling the Glossary; Rupert for tracing biographical details; Lucinda for devoting so much time, yet again, as my 'problem solver' over many computer difficulties and for her ever cheerful guidance and patience; and to Jeremy for his understanding, good humour, practical help and loving care which have sustained me throughout the many stages of preparation for *Women in the War Zone*.

Introduction

Women's involvement in the art of healing stretches back to pre-history. From the Bible we glimpse the well-loved image of Jesus in Bethany a few days before His crucifixion. A woman came to Him carrying an alabaster box which contained ointment made from oil extracted from the aromatic root of the small plant spikenard. The anti-fungal and anti-bacterial properties of spikenard were relaxing and according to the Gospels of Saint Matthew and Saint Mark, the woman poured them on Jesus's head. Saint John wrote that she anointed His feet with the ointment and 'wiped his feet with her hair and the house was filled with the odour of the ointment'.

During the Middle Ages monastries and convents were centres of healing and medical knowledge. Physic plants were grown in the gardens and then gathered, pounded into powder, and mixed with oils, vinegar and wine to produce tinctures and remedies. Diseases and cures were linked to hot, cold, dry and moist elements; and in the sixth century Alexander of Tralles wrote that the duty of a physician was 'to cool what is hot, to warm what is cold, to dry what is moist, and to moisten what is dry.'

Hildegard of Bingen was born in 1098 and at the age of eight she entered the Benedictine monastery at Disibodenberg on the Rhine. By the time Hildegard took her vows when she was fourteen the monastery had extended into a convent. She became Abbess in 1136 and eleven years later she founded her own Abbey at Rupertsberg near Bingen. Already known for her sacred music her fame spread after Pope Eugene III read from her visionary work *Scivas* at the Synod of Trier in the winter of 1147–8. During her early years as a nun Hildegard would have helped in the gardens and the infirmary at Disibodenberg, learning how to tend the plants and the various methods of treating the elderly, infirm, blind, deaf, lame and sick. She became practised in the knowledge of herbal remedies and between 1152 and 1158, when she was abbess at Rupertsberg, she wrote two medicinal works, *Causae et Cyurae,* which examined the causes and cures of diseases, and *Physica* – consisting of nine books on healing. The medical uses and preparations for different remedies are given for plants, trees, fish, animals, reptiles, birds, stones, gems and elements.

In her lifetime Hildegard of Bingen was revered and renowned for her gifts of healing. The physicians of Myddfai, a remote hamlet in the foothills of the Black Mountains in mid-Wales, were active between the thirteenth and nineteenth centuries. They listed over 800 herbal remedies for healing the sick and wounded in body and mind, in a collection of medieval texts. Legend tells that Rhiwallon, the first physician of Myddfai, was the eldest son of a young farmer and the lady of Llyn-y-Fan-Fach. Some years after she returned to the lake the lady appeared to Rhiwallon at Llidiad-y-Meddygon, which is still known as the Physicians' Gate. She told him that he was destined to become a great and skilful physician, who would relieve pain and misery through his gift for healing. She gave him a bag containing herbal remedies and on another appearance took him to Pant-y-Meddygon, the Dingle of the Physicians. She showed him the many plants that grew there and explained their various medical powers. One of these may have been *solidago asteraceae* (golden rod) which originally came from the Middle East, and was later cultivated in Britain for its medicinal properties. It was known as woundwort – a wound-healing plant. A cold compress placed on a fresh wound was believed to be anti-inflammatory. But golden rod is not listed in the Herbal compiled by the first Physicians of Myddfai which gives many remedies for wounds: 'Take wild turnips, pound to a plaster, and apply to the wound: it will open the wound and heal it. Proven'; 'Take the herb called centaury, powder and cast into the wound; by God's help it will cure it.'

The descendants of Rhiwallon and his sons continued to practise medicine in Wales without a break until Dr Rice Williams died in Aberystwyth in 1842, aged eighty-five. He seems to have been the last of the Physicians of Myddfai descended from the legendary Lady of the Lake.

Hildegard of Bingen was known as one of the first women doctors, but over the following eight centuries women struggled continuously in a bitter battle to be accepted by medical schools to train as physicians. In 1865, twenty-three years after the death of the last Physician of Myddfai, Elizabeth Garrett Anderson gained a diploma from the Society of Apothecaries. She then established a dispensary for women in London and seven years later she founded the New Hospital for Women, which was to be staffed only by women. In 1908 women were granted permission to obtain diplomas and fellowships from the Royal College of Physicians and Surgeons. However, they were not accepted into the teaching hospitals in London, Oxford and Cambridge and those who qualified elsewhere were only offered posts not taken up by men – either in the provinces or in some women's hospitals.

Elsie Inglis qualified in medicine in Glasgow in 1892, and became a doctor in Elizabeth Garrett Anderson's New Hospital for Women. By this time the women's suffrage movement in Britain, which had started in 1867, was revitalised by the creation of the National Union of Women's Suffrage Societies (NUWSS). Dr Inglis returned to Edinburgh in 1894 and ran a practice in the city with Dr Jessie MacGregor, an old student friend. She also became honorary secretary of the Edinburgh National Society for Women's Suffrage. In November 1899 she opened her own small hospital in George Square for patients from the poorer areas of the city. After the lease expired she found another suitable property, The Hospice, which opened in January 1904 as a surgical and gynaecological centre with a dispensary and accident department. Five years later, Dr Inglis, by now Edinburgh's most eminent woman doctor, became honorary secretary to the Scottish Federation of Women's Suffrage Societies.

When war broke out on 4 August 1914, the Women's Hospital Corps (WHC) was formed immediately by two women doctors – Louisa Garrett Anderson and Dr Flora Murray. Within weeks, having been rebuffed by the War Office, the WHC was on its way to Paris at the request of the French Red Cross. The seventy-eight-year-old Dr Elizabeth Garrett Anderson, 'a dignified figure, old and rather bent', was on Victoria Station to bid farewell to her daughter and the all-women unit. 'Twenty years younger, I would have taken them myself,' she said.

As there were no vacancies in the WHC for Dr Elsie Inglis she went to Edinburgh Castle and offered her services to the Royal Army Medical Corps. She was rudely rejected with the words: 'My good lady, go home and sit still.' Although angry she remained undaunted and at the Committee meeting of the Scottish Federation of Women's Suffrage Societies on 12 August her proposal was accepted that the Federation should 'give organised help to Red Cross work.' However, the British Red Cross, following the War Office example, refused to allow women doctors to serve with the army overseas. Eight days after the meeting a letter was sent to the Belgian, French, Russian and Serbian embassies offering fully equipped hospitals, staffed entirely by women, to their governments.

An appeal for donations was launched and meetings were held in 'every sort of hall and drawing-room in every part of the United Kingdom'. Money flowed in and by 31 October the first £1,000 had been raised. On the previous day Dr Elsie Inglis formed the Scottish Women's Hospitals (SWH) Committee when it was decided that the uniform should be a grey coat and skirt with Gordon tartan facings. Units were organised; one under Dr Alice Hutchison, and staffed with ten trained nurses, established a hospital in Calais in December 1914 where typhoid patients in the French army were nursed for three months. Also in December 1914 another unit was despatched to France and one was sent to Serbia.

Royaumont, a beautiful, medieval Cistercian abbey, some thirty miles north of Paris, was requisitioned by the French authorities for the SWH. When Elsie Inglis saw the building she wrote that it would be 'one of the finest hospitals in France'. The unit of seven doctors, ten nurses, seven orderlies, two cooks, a clerk, an administrator, two maids and four chauffeurs, arrived at Royaumont at the beginning of December 1914. They found the abbey in a terrible condition with years of dirt and debris in all the huge rooms and realised that an enormous amount of work was needed to convert the Abbey into an efficient hospital. Cecily Hamilton, a forty-two-year-old actress, playwright, writer and suffragist, was Royaumont's clerk and wrote:

> Our only available stove – a mighty erection in the kitchen which had not been lit for a decade – was naturally short-tempered at first, and the supply of hot water was very limited. So, in consequence, was our first washing; at times very limited indeed. Our equipment, after the fashion of baggage in these times of war, was in no great hurry to arrive; until it arrived we did without sheets and blankets, wrapped ourselves in rugs and overcoats at night, and did not do much undressing.

The unit worked through bitterly cold weather, overcoming various setbacks, and on 10 January 1915 Royaumont was recognised as a military hospital. The following day the first six patients were received. The hospital was not closed until March 1919. During these years almost 11,000 patients, mainly from the French and French Colonial armies, were admitted to Royaumont and the additional hospital at Villers-Cotterets.

Over the following four years the Scottish Women's Hospitals cared for wounded soldiers and sick civilians in Serbia, Salonika, Corsica, Russia, Romania and France. They established their hospitals and dressing-stations in disused barracks and schools, in convents, at railway stations, under canvas, on hillsides, in lonely countrysides, in shattered towns and villages, and on occasions found themselves prisoners-of-war.

At home there was an acute shortage of doctors in civilian hospitals when the men joined the Royal Army Medical Corps and women were recruited to take their place. They were also needed in military hospitals and were known as Civil Medical Practitioners (CMPs), but they were granted neither rank nor uniform and their pay was not comparable to that of a male doctor. As the war continued more women were desperately needed in the field of medicine. A circular letter was sent to headmistresses of girls' schools emphasising that there was to be 'a very serious need for women to replace men in Military Hospitals as all eligible men are to be removed from the Home Hospitals for other services'. In July 1915 Dr Mary Scharlieb, an ardent campaigner, spoke at the annual prize-giving ceremony at Manchester High School for Girls, encouraging them to choose a rewarding career as doctors.

By 1916, the War Office was faced with an ever increasing dearth of male doctors, and realising the continued success of the Scottish Women's Hospitals and other voluntary units overseas, reluctantly sent volunteer women doctors to serve with the Royal Army Medical Corps in Salonika, Egypt, India and Malta. They were still refused commissions and had to travel third class while all army nurses and VADs in uniform travelled first class.

In 1917 the Medical Women's Federation (MWF) was formed and continued the struggle to improve the conditions under which women doctors served, but it was not until 1942 that women medical officers' pay was brought into line with their male counterparts. In 1950 they were finally granted commissioned rank.

Before 1660 men joined an army raised to fight a specific war. These soldiers, and the few physicians who accompanied them, returned to civilian life when the war ended. The regular army was established at the Restoration of Charles II and each regiment had a doctor and a primitive mobile hospital staffed by male orderlies. Respectable wives, with their children, and less respectable 'camp followers' accompanied the men overseas and British army wives assisted in military hospitals during the Napoleonic Wars. Until the early nineteenth century the sick civilian population had been treated and nursed in their own homes or in workhouses until voluntary hospitals were set up by various Christian charitable denominations in London and some of the provinces. In 1840 Elizabeth Fry, the Quaker philanthropist, founded the Institution for Nursing Sisters – also known as the Sisters of Charity – and this was followed by other Sisterhoods in various parts of the country where young women were trained to become nurses. In 1877 Mother Mary Potter founded the first Catholic Order of Nursing Sisters in Nottingham. They were called The Little Company of Mary – also known as the Blue Sisters from the blue veils they wore.

By the time the Crimean War started in September 1854, wives still accompanied the regiments, working as cooks, needlewomen, laundresses, and giving some basic nursing. There were no trained military nurses and British soldiers continued to be nursed, for the most part, by male orderlies.

The war correspondent, W.H. Russell, sent dispatches from the Crimea to *The Times* giving vivid accounts of the sufferings of wounded and sick soldiers. There were no preparations for even the most straightforward operations and men were left unattended for many days and often died in agony before they received any medical help. Russell wrote that the medical arrangements made by the French were extremely good and that they 'are greatly our superiors … their surgeons more numerous, and they have also the help of the Sisters of Charity, who have accompanied the expedition in incredible numbers.'

The British public were angry and horrified. *The Times* immediately established a fund to provide more medical aid for those suffering in the Crimea and Florence Nightingale, a thirty-five-year-old woman who had trained with a Nursing Sisterhood in Paris, was asked in October 1854 by Sidney Herbert, the Secretary of State at War, to take a party of thirty-eight women to nurse at the four hospitals at Scutari. Here they found filthy and overcrowded conditions and men suffering more from diseases than wounds. Florence Nightingale supervised the transformation of these hospitals into places of order and cleanliness and ensured that regular supplies of comforts and medical equipment were received. Under her guidance, nourishment and various diets were introduced into hospital food.

Three years after the Crimean war ended, Henry Dunant, a Swiss businessman, was horrified at the suffering the wounded endured in the Battle of Solferino. He suggested the formation of national relief societies, staffed by trained volunteers. The International Committee of the Red Cross was established and the founding charter of the Red Cross was written in 1863. An international agreement, the original Geneva Convention, which recognised the 'status of medical services and of the wounded on the battlefield' was signed in 1864. Six years later the British National Society for Aid to the Sick and Wounded in War was formed.

Many reforms in the army medical services were gradually implemented over the following years. The military hospital at Netley, on Southampton Water had been opened in 1863, followed by more military hospitals throughout the country, and there was an ever-increasing demand for nurses who received their initial training in civilian hospitals.

At the outbreak of the South African war in October 1899 the Army Nursing Services had grown in strength and efficiency and during the following three years almost 2,000 trained nurses served in the war. The vast expanse of veldt meant that it was a long and slow journey on wagons drawn by horses or oxen from the fields of battle to the hospital trains where the wounded were received by Army nursing sisters forbidden to travel any closer to the fighting. The trains then took the patients to base hospitals where conditions had greatly improved since Florence Nightingale arrived at Scutari. Boer and British patients were regularly fed with good food, Florence Nightingale's mantra '*Sanitas Sanitatum*', for scrupulous standards of cleanliness, was generally accepted, and anaesthetics were used. As in the Crimea, there were many more sick than wounded men to be nursed. The soldiers were affected by flies, dust, and veldt-sores, and contaminated drinking water caused dysentry and typhoid fever. It is estimated that only one-third of casualties died of wounds.

Although military and medical authorities now realised that there was a need for a larger and more efficient army nursing service, and that 'in a base hospital the actual nursing should always be entrusted to women', as the twentieth century dawned, nurses still had no rank or status and they were only able to practice their professional skills in areas far from the battlefields.

When the South African war drew to a close in May 1902 high level talks were taking place and a committee was formed to plan the improvement and expansion of the Army Nursing Service. On 27 March 1902 the Service was renamed Queen Alexandra's Imperial Military Nursing Service (QAIMNS). A Matron-in-Chief was appointed to the War Office. In 1905 the British National Society for Aid to the Sick and Wounded in War was renamed the British Red Cross Society.

The First Aid Nursing Yeomanry Corps (FANYs) was established in 1907. The idea was originally conceived by Sergeant Edward Charles Baker who was wounded in Lord Kitchener's Soudan Campaign and realised 'there was a missing link somewhere in the Ambulance Department, which in spite of the changes in warfare, had not altered very materially since the days of the Crimea'. Members of the Corps were required to qualify in first aid and home nursing and pass a course of 'Horsemanship, Veterinary Work, Signalling, and Camp Cookery'. The women had to be between 17 and 35 years of age and at least 5ft 3in in height. They had to provide their own uniforms and first aid outfit. Grace Ashley-Smith, who later commanded the FANYs, wrote that 'it is not a Corps of shirkers, but of workers'.

In 1907 Mrs Mabel Stobart was asked to form the Women's Sick and Wounded Convoy Corps, an off-shoot of the FANYs, which was to be used for service between Field and Base Hospitals in the event of a war. The Corps trained once a week in London and camped for a fortnight annually on the cliffs at Studland in Dorset where the enthusiastic members learned to pitch and strike tents, dig trenches, sleep on the ground without beds or mattresses and live under frugal conditions.

A Territorial Force Nursing Service was established in 1908 and the following year the Voluntary Aid Organisation was formed as part of the Territorial Army Scheme. Both men and women became members of the Voluntary Aid Detachments (VADs), drawn from the British Red Cross Society, the Ambulance Department of the Order of St John of Jerusalem and the Territorial Force Association, and were trained in first aid and nursing.

In 1912 Bulgaria, Serbia and Greece combined against the Turks in the First Balkan War. Mrs Stobart went to Sir Frederick Treves, Chairman of the British Red Cross Society, and offered to take a unit of her Women's Sick and Wounded Convoy Corps to the desperately understaffed hospitals in Bulgaria. She was told that soldiers in the Balkans would object to being nursed by women and that a woman was incapable of operating in a hospital of war. The Bulgarian authorities greatly needed medical assistance and within a few weeks Mrs Stobart and her unit of sixteen women, which included three doctors, six qualified nurses, orderlies and a cook, were asked to set up a hospital in the town of Kirk-Kilisse, the headquarters of the Bulgarian army. After long train journeys the women trekked in rain and through mud for seven days across the Rhodope mountains and the Thracian plains. They passed through many small villages, most of which had been burnt to the ground and were deserted ruins, although occasionally they found bread and cheese. They were accompanied by two soldiers and two policemen, and travelled with all the equipment in forty uncovered ox-carts drawn by eighty oxen or buffalo driven by forty Bulgarian peasants. The unit took over two empty houses in Kirk-Kilisse and were warned to expect a large convoy of wounded. This was the first time that British women had served as doctors and nurses in a hospital close to a front line. Within forty-eight hours of arriving they had scrubbed and scoured the rooms, prepared a kitchen, wards, and surgeries, and unloaded the huge cases of blankets, bed-garments, linen and stores. Over the next weeks they undertook complicated operations and nursed terrible wounds under appalling conditions. They soon realised that the Turkish and Bulgarian soldiers were not only courteous and chivalrous but heartfelt in their gratitude and appreciation of the care given by the British women. After six weeks an armistice was declared. Mrs Stobart and her unit from the Women's Convoy Corps said farewell to their patients and returned to England.

On 4 August 1914, the day Britain declared war on Germany, Mrs Stobart was one of many distinguished women who spoke at a peace meeting at Kingsway Hall in London. The following day she founded the Women's National Service League 'with the aim of providing a body of women qualified to give useful service at home or abroad'. She was again repulsed by Sir Frederick Treves but received a request from the Belgian Red Cross to establish a hospital for French and Belgian soldiers in Brussels.

After war was declared the British Red Cross Society and St John's Ambulance amalgamated and women responded immediately to the various appeals to join the Society. By then some 46,000 women, mostly from the upper and middle classes, were serving in the Voluntary Aid Detachments and were trained 'in the art of improvisation and in coping with emergencies'. They included suffragists, feminists, married and career women, qualified doctors and nurses, and those who felt that serving their country was a release from the genteel role of a daughter destined to run the household for ageing parents. The latter viewed the future as a VAD, whether in a hospital at home or overseas, as an exciting escape from boredom and drudgery. Untrained women worked as cleaners, drivers, and orderlies but their duties became more wide-ranging as they grew more experienced. They supplied food and medical dressings for makeshift ambulance trains, clearing and stationary hospitals, and provided rest stations at train halts. They were also members of the trained medical staff in large hospitals, and ran small hospitals and convalescent homes. Every woman was filled with a sense of responsibility that they were 'doing their bit'. Olive Dent, a young VAD, felt that 'the New Army of men would need a New Army of nurses. Why not go and learn to be a nurse while the Kitchener men were learning to be soldiers'.

Within the first weeks of the war doctors, nurses, and administrators, were already on their way to give medical aid in France and Belgium. Sister Joan Martin-Nicholson, a Red Cross Sister, arrived in Brussels on 9 August 1914; Dr Flora Murray, and her Women's Hospital Corps, opened a hospital in the newly-built, luxurious Hotel Claridge on the Champs Elysees in Paris. Other parties had set off too. Mrs Mabel Stobart, the colourful and intrepid administrator, became a prisoner-of-war when the Germans reached Brussels. Mrs Katharine Furse, the commandant of the British Red Cross VADs, started a rest station at the Gare Centrale in Boulogne; the Duchess of Sutherland took her private ambulance unit to Namur in Belgium; Flora Sandes, accompanied by her violin, went with a St John's Ambulance Unit to a Serbian military hospital; and every unit included young, keen and excited VADs ready to embark on 'an adventure of a lifetime.' It did not take long for the reality to hit them.

Over the next four years this cross-section of women endured homesickness, terrible hardships, exhaustion, and grim conditions; chaotic train journeys in Serbia and Russia; torpedo attacks at sea; life in primitive makeshift hospitals under canvas through bitter winters and sorrow when treating sick and terrified civilian refugees. But above all they felt compassion, anguish and a sense of helplessness when they nursed the appalling wounds suffered by a never-ending stream of casualties in ill-equipped 'wards like battlefields'. K.E. Luard, an experienced Sister in the QAIMNS wrote from an ambulance train that the shrapnel-shell wounds were 'more ghastly than anything I have ever seen or smelt; the Mauser wounds of the Boer War were pin-pricks compared with them'. However, blood transfusions were used to prevent shock and loss of blood and this newly developed expertise saved countless lives.

Yvonne Fitzroy, a young orderly, remembered that 'the nursing conditions are something of a revelation, but what we haven't got we invent, and what we can't invent we do without'. The staple dressing was sometimes just tincture of iodine; anaesthetics, either in short supply or simply not available, were sometimes replaced with brandy. Gas gangrene, which developed from a septic wound, led to innumerable amputations; in the last two months of 1914 there were over 6,000 cases of frostbite on the Western Front and no one was sure of the right cure – four years later tens of thousands of men suffering from the influenza epidemic died in crowded wards; shell-shock was a complex symptom to diagnose; men went down with dysentry and other diseases; jaundice carried by rats, typhus spread by lice, and typhoid caught from impure drinking water were most prevalent on the Eastern Front. Often the sheer volume of casualties was too much to bear. 'One lived very many times in a torrent of emotion', confessed Olive Dent. On many occasions the wounded were so exhausted that they fell asleep as their wounds were being dressed. As one man died on a bed, or mattress on the floor, or on straw in a makeshift dressing-station, it was filled immediately with the next casualty. Almost daily K.E. Luard, by then the sister in charge of a casualty clearing station during the Battle of Arras, put her thoughts and feelings into her diary: 'One has got so used to their dying. It's all very like a battlefield'. She found she could not keep up with the volume of 'Break-the-News-Letters' she had to write late each evening. 'This war is the crucifixion of the youth of the world', wrote Sarah Macnaughtan. Not long before she died of typhoid in Serbia, Mabel Dearmer recorded in a letter that 'the only way to see war is from a hospital'.

In Russia British nurses served alongside Russian Red Cross nurses. Many of these were members of the Russian royal family and aristocracy who were allowed much nearer the firing line than the British and French nurses. Every Russian Regiment had its own doctor and sanitaires (equivalent to RAMC orderlies).

Some of those who served in Russia wrote of their impressions before and after the Revolution. Margaret Fawcett recognised the change in manner of soldiers to their officers; Dorothy Seymour gave a short but graphic account of the circumstances surrounding Rasputin's murder. Those taking part in the various Retreats – in Russia,

Romania and Serbia – were devastated at having to leave wounded men and homeless refugees in abandoned hospitals or dying and starving on roadsides.

There was humour and fun and good times too. Dorothy Brook recalled: 'we were all young and so very enthusiastic about our work and there was always a new adventure'. Regardless of status, but dependent upon where they were stationed, concert parties, visits to theatres, operas, cinemas, boat trips, picnics, tennis tournaments, walking, excursions in cars, and for one young woman, a visit to a harem, provided recreation from the gruelling routine of hospital work. Dorothy Higgins spent peaceful hours creating a garden at the hospital in Rouen. Parties and dances, deemed 'topping' and 'ripping', were enjoyed, although Josephine Pennell, a young ambulance driver in St Omer, soon discovered that dancing in public was not permitted. The girls were, however, allowed to dance in their own ante-room, and a few men from the main dance in the YMCA joined them for a 'very jolly time'. In the instructions handed out to each VAD they were strictly told to 'avoid all intimacy' with patients and officers, but cautious flirtations developed. Pat Waddell, a young FANY, remembered that the girls she knew 'were extremely innocent about the most ordinary sex matters. A kiss was as far as anyone went.' This stage sometimes ripened into more serious romances, which was daring behaviour, especially for VADs who soon found ways round the stringent rules. Vera Brittain on board a hospital ship on the way to Malta wrote with amusement of the couples who were even forbidden to talk to each other on deck, but 'were found in compromising positions beneath the gangways'. Katharine Furse had trouble too amongst her VADs when her ambulance driver became engaged. She was sent home in disgrace. Katherine Hodges wisely refused a bizarre offer of marriage. The Very Adorable Darlings, as they soon became known, were not always found out. Lesley Smith, her VAD friend, and an army major spent an hilarious off-duty afternoon in Camiers avoiding the matron-in-chief. Elsie Fenwick, although a VAD, was a forty-two-year-old married woman and it was accepted that she spent most of her off-duty time in the company of the senior officers from the British Mission in La Panne in Belgium.

Problems and difficulties had to be endured at all levels. There are occasional references to callous treatment from exhausted and overwhelmed surgeons when performing operations. Dr Elsie Inglis, struggling under appalling conditions, and frustrated with the ill-equipped hospitals in Russia and Serbia, succumbed to the occasional bouts of rage. The qualified nurses often resented the younger, untrained VADs, which inevitably led to criticism and jealousy. For a few weeks the nursing staff on board a hospital ship in the Dardanelles had to contend with an alcoholic Senior Medical Officer. Squabbles inevitably developed between women forced to live closely together for months on end under such extraordinary conditions.

Many years ago I vaguely remember my Great Aunt Madge Oswald reminiscing on her experiences as a First World War VAD when nursing with her pre-war friend the Princess Marie de Cröy. She implied that she was also involved in something else at the time, but I was young and busy with my own life and did not question her or even take more than a passing interest. I now greatly regret such a missed opportunity.

With help from other members of the family I have pieced together what may have happened – that Aunt Madge went specifically to help nurse wounded soldiers with the Princess at her home at the Château de Bellignies, outside Mons in Belgium. Possibly the explanation for her hints is that she was aware of, and perhaps assisted with, the underground movement that linked Bellignies with Nurse Edith Cavell in Brussels. I know that Aunt Madge was in England by the time the Germans suspected the connection between Bellignies and Nurse Cavell. I also know that her friendship with Princess Marie de Cröy continued after the war and that she stayed with the Princess in France shortly before her death in April 1967.

We have no letters or papers which could verify these old memories. Many women, however, kept records of their wartime experiences and over the last seven years I have read through at least 200 books and archives of diaries, memoirs and letters. From these powerful and moving personal testimonies the unique stories written by fifty-one remarkable women are included in *Women in the War Zone*. All these are British except for one New Zealander and one Australian. I am sad that I have not been able to include many more.

With a few exceptions, the First World War is seen and written about from a male perspective and women's part in the suffering has not been fully recognised, although many women understood the horrors of the battlefields as they cared for mutilated bodies and tormented minds.

Of all the many thousands of women who served in hospitals during the First World War, a number died before the war ended. Some became disillusioned and went home early. Post 1918 the journey between the two worlds was not easy as the women had to adapt to a new way of life or re-adapt to the one they had known before. Some married men they met while serving; others spent the remaining years with a woman friend who had shared responsibilities and hardships over the four years; many renewed or embarked on various professions and careers. There were those who returned to care for elderly or infirm parents and who settled down to a lonely life at home to 'buy clothes and do the flowers for mother'. All over the world women, who had always known the anxieties and anguish of war, grieved for sons, husbands, lovers and brothers.

The memories of their experiences remained with them for the rest of their lives. They had often been frightened, exhausted, cold, wet, dishevelled and dirty, but through all their adversities they remained resourceful, cheerful, spirited and courageous. They all deserve to be remembered and honoured for their sacrifice and their humanity.

Relevant Dates

1914

28 June	Assassination of the Hapsburg Archduke Franz Ferdinand, heir apparent to Franz Josef, Emperor of Austria-Hungary. During a state visit to Sarajevo in Serbia the archduke and his wife were shot by Gavrilo Princip, a young Bosnian Serb. This was particularly ill-timed as it was a day of national mourning commemorating the anniversary of the Battle of Kosovo when Serbia was defeated by the Turks in 1349.
28 July	After a month of negotiations and ultimatums, Austria-Hungary declared war on Serbia.
30 July	Tsar Nicholas II ordered the mobilisation of the Russian armed forces.
1 August	Germany declared war on Russia.
2 August	Germany demanded that her troops be allowed to march through Belgium (Belgium's neutrality had been guaranteed by Britain in 1839).
3 August	Germany declared war on France.
4 August	British Government's ultimatum that the German Army would not cross into Belgium expired. Britain declared war on Germany. At 4pm German troops marched into Belgium and by midnight five empires were at war – each believed it would be victorious within a few months. Some six million men were mobilised.
12 August	Austrian troops invaded Serbia. They met with strong resistance and retreated within a few days.
15 August	Russian Army advanced into East Prussia.
16 August	British Expeditionary Force landed in France.
20 August	Brussels occupied by the German army.
22 August	At 7am a squadron from the 4th Royal Irish Dragoon Guards fired the opening British shots of the First World War outside the small town of Mons in Belgium.
23 August	Battle of Mons. The British Expeditionary Force confronted the far superior German army. It inflicted, and suffered, heavy casual-

	ties, lost ground, and was forced to retreat south towards Paris. Austrian troops crossed border into Russian Poland.
24–25 August	BEF retreated south from Mons towards the French frontier.
27–30 August	Battle of Tanneberg, East Prussia. Germans halted Russian advance with 50,000 Russians killed or wounded and 90,000 taken prisoner.
5–9 September	First Battle of the Marne. German advance on Paris halted.
13–18 September	Battle of the Aisne.
4 October	Newly formed Royal Naval Division arrived in Antwerp to strengthen resistance.
10 October	Antwerp surrendered to Germans.
15 October	Germans entered Ostend.
19 October	Start of the First Battle of Ypres, which continued until the end of November.
4 November	Turkey declared war on the Allies.
18 November	German and Russian forces fought each other at Battle of Lodz, which was inconclusive although each side lost some 100,000 men.
1 December	Austrian troops invaded and occupied Belgrade, Serbia. The capital was regained by the Serbian army two weeks later and over 40,000 Austrian prisoners were taken.
24–25 December	On Christmas Eve, after five months of ferocious fighting, British and German soldiers called a truce on sections of the front line of the Western Front. They exchanged gifts, food and cigarettes – and in some areas arranged for bodies lying in no-man's-land to be collected and buried.

1915

26 January	Turkish advance on Egypt.
10–13 March	Battle of Neuve Chapelle.
18 March	Naval attack at Dardanelles against Turkish positions.
8 April	On the Eastern Front the Armenian population are blamed by Turkey for co-operating with Russians. Mass murder of Armenian men and deportation of old men, women and children. By September a million had died.
22 April	Second Battle of Ypres. Germans used chlorine poison gas at Langemarck along a four-mile front.
25 April	Allied troops landed on Gallipoli peninsula. The strong Turkish defences prevented the hoped-for swift victory and enormous casualties build up on the beaches over the next months.
1 May	Combined Austro-German offensive to attack Russians in Galicia. Russians driven out of Gorlitse and Tarnow. Gradually Carpathian

	mountain passes are regained by Austro-German troops.
7 May	Cunard liner *Lusitania* torpedoed and sunk by German U-Boat off southern coast of Ireland; 1,198 of the 2,000 passengers were drowned.
9 May	French troops attacked German positions on Vimy Ridge. British attacked opposite Fromelles and La Bassée in an abortive attempt to capture Aubers Ridge.
15–25 May	Battle of Festubert.
23 May	Italy declared war on Austria-Hungary.
5 August	German troops entered Warsaw.
6 August	British forces landed at Suvla Bay on the Gallipoli Peninsula. Two attacks – one by Australians at Anzac Cove – one by British, Australian, New Zealand, Indian and Gurkha troops at Cape Helles. After a four-day battle for Suvla Bay the British and Anzac troops were beaten back, with 2,000 killed and 1,000 wounded.
13 August	Troop transport ship the *Royal Edward* sunk by German U-boat off the island of Kos in the Aegean. Over 1,000 soldiers drowned.
19 August	Continuing Russian losses on Eastern Front culminated with 90,000 officers and men surrendering at the fort of Novo-Georgievsk in Poland.
25 September	Two Allied offensives started on Western Front – British in the Battle of Loos and the French in the Champagne region.
26 September	British advanced in Mesopotamia and took Kut from the Turks
5 October	Austro/German army invaded Serbia. British and French troops landed in Salonika en route to Serbia's aid.
12 October	Bulgaria attacked Serbia. The Retreat of Serbian army and civilians began. Edith Cavell was executed in Brussels.
5 Decemebr	Turks besieged British troops at Kut. Relief force continued to meet fierce opposition.
19 December	Sir Douglas Haig replaced Sir John French as Commander-in-Chief of the British Army in France.

1916

5 January	First conscription bill in Britain.
8 January	Last British troops left Cape Helles, Gallipoli Peninsula after eleven-day evacuation completed with no casualties. During eight-and-a-half-month campaign some 66,000 Turkish, 28,000 British, over 7,000 Australian, over 2,000 New Zealand and 10,000 French soldiers had been killed. Austrian, Bosnian, Muslim and Italian troops attacked Serbia's ally and neighbour, Montenegro. Montenegro surrendered six days later.

13 January	Battle of Wadi, Mesopotamia.
21 January	Battle of Hanna, Mesopotamia. Heavy casualties in both battles and the men trapped at Kut not rescued.
21 February	On Western Front the Germans attacked the French fortress of Verdun. Battle of Verdun continued with attacks and counter-attacks until mid December with appalling loss of life on both sides.
25 February	Germans captured Fort Douaumont, a main fortress at Verdun.
27 February	On Eastern Front Austrian forces attacked Albania.
22 March	Steamer *Sussex* torpedoed and sunk in English Channel.
24 April (Easter Monday)	Easter Rising in Dublin.
29 April	More than 9,000 British and Indian troops surrendered to the Turks at Kut.
31 May–1 June	Naval battle off Jutland.
4 June	On Eastern Front a massive Russian offensive against Austrian Army.
5 June	Lord Kitchener, Secretary of State for War, drowned in North Sea after HMS *Hampshire* sunk by German U-boat off Scapa Flow. Arab Revolt against Turks began outside city of Medina.
7 June	On Western Front the Germans captured Fort Vaux from the French at Verdun.
13 June	Mecca fell to the Arabs.
16 June	Jeddah taken by Arabs.
1 July	First day of the Battle of the Somme. By evening 60,000 British troops were casualties – one third of which had been killed. Offensive finally halted in mid-November when winter weather had set in and battleground was a sea of mud. British and French armies had advanced six miles in the four months. Combined Allied and German losses over a million – 420,000 were British. On Eastern Front the Russian advance against Austrian army continued over the next few weeks.
28 July	On Eastern Front the East Galician town of Brody taken by Russian troops. Heavy losses on both sides.
7 August	General Brusilov's Russian army captured Stanislau in East Galicia with heavy casualties.
27 August	Romania declared war on Germany and Austria-Hungary.
1 September	Bulgaria declared war on Romania.
3 September	Bulgarian aircraft bombed Bucharest.
12 September	French, British, Russian, Serbian and Italian forces attacked on Salonika Front but were driven back.
24 October	On Western Front the French recaptured Fort Douaumont at Verdun.
3 November	French recaptured Fort Vaux at Verdun.
5 December	On the Eastern Front oil from Romanian oil-fields blown up to prevent use by the Germans.

6 December	German troops occupied Bucharest. David Lloyd George replaced H.H. Asquith as Prime Minister.
30 December	Rasputin murdered in Petrograd.

1917

17 February	Revolutionary unrest in some sections of Russian army.
3 March	Riots in streets of Petrograd.
10 March	Authority of the Duma, Russia's Parliament, challenged.
11 March	British troops entered Baghdad shortly after Turkish soldiers left the city.
12 March	Soldiers and civilians demonstrate against Tsar Nicholas II in Petrograd. Start of Russian Revolution – Russia gradually sinks into political turmoil.
15 March	Tsar abdicated. Russia on brink of anarchy.
6 April	United States of America declared war on Germany.
9 April (Easter Monday)	Western Front. First day of Battle of Arras.
14 April	On Western Front Canadian troops took Vimy Ridge.
16 May	In Petrograd Alexander Kerensky became minister of War. His aim was a new Russian offensive against the Austrian army.
22 May	General Brusilov appointed Commander-in-Chief of Russian Army
26 May	First contingent of American troops arrived in France.
27 May	On Western Front sections of the French army mutinied.
7 June	Battle of Messines on Western Front.
10 June	On Eastern Front Italian army fought the Austrians at Trentino, Mounts Ortigaro and Camigolatti.
1 July	General Brusilov launched second offensive against Austrian army on Eastern Front.
2 July	Greece declared war on Germany.
12 July	On Western Front first mustard gas attack by Germans on British troops near Ypres.
16 July	In Petrograd Leon Trotsky supported demands to end war.
19 July	Severe setback in Russian offensive on Eastern Front. Many Russian prisoners taken and thousands of soldiers deserted from battlefields. Russian army in retreat and Austrian army continued to advance. Alexander Kerensky became Prime Minister of Russia.
28 July	General Brusilov replaced by General Kornilov.
31 July	On Western Front Third Battle of Ypres (Passchendaele) opened. Russian retreat continued on Eastern Front.
15 September	Alexander Kerensky declared Russia a republic.
25 October	German troops entered town of Caporetto in Italy after the Italians were defeated at the twelfth battle on the Isonzo front.

26 October	Final British offensive to take the village of Passchendaele began.
31 October	British captured Beersheba and Gaza in Palestine.
7 November	Thousands of Bolsheviks surrounded the Provisional Government in the Winter Palace, Petrograd.
8 November	Bolsheviks took over Winter Palace. Lenin elected Chairman of the Council of People's Commissars, Trotsky Commissar for Foreign Affairs. Red Guards occupied the Kremlin in Moscow and Kerensky fled from Petrograd.
10 November	Battle for Passchendaele ended after Canadian troops advanced 500 yards against huge German bombardment.
19 November	Bolshevik Government in Petrograd asked for immediate armistice on all fronts.
20 November	On Western Front the Battle of Cambrai started and continued until 9 December when it ended in stalemate with heavy casualties on both sides.
9 December	General Allenby entered Jerusalem after the Turkish army left and the city surrendered.
15 December	Bolshevik, German, Austrian, Bulgarian and Turkish Governments announced ceasefire on Eastern Front.
24 December	On Eastern Front an Italian counter-attack succeeded against Austrians.
30 December	Troopship *Aragon* torpedoed and sunk ten miles from Alexandria harbour. The destroyer HMS *Attack* struck a mine and sank as she rescued survivors from the *Aragon*.

1918

31 January	Lenin established Union of Soviet Socialist Republics (USSR).
17 February	Peace negotiations between Germans and Bolsheviks broke down. War started again on Eastern Front.
3 March	On the Eastern Front the Bolsheviks and Germany signed Peace Treaty at Brest-Litovsk.
12 March	Capital of USSR moved from Petrograd to Moscow.
21 March	First day of the German Spring Offensive on the Western Front which continued with fierce fighting until 5 April.
9 April	Battle of the Lys on the Western Front.
16 April	Belgian town of St Omer bombed by German aircraft.
23 April	British naval force stormed the fortified harbour at Zeebrugge, Belgium and sank block-ships.
7 May	Romanian Government signed Peace of Bucharest with Germany and Austria-Hungary.
26 May	Turkish army defeated Armenians. Two days later Armenia declared

	her independence but within two weeks Armenians were massacred by Tatars south of Tiflis. Over 400,000 Armenian civilians murdered three months later when Turkish troops advanced into the Caucasus.
27 May	On the Western Front the Third Battle of the Aisne started. On the following day an American Brigade was in action at the village of Cantigny which they took and held.
1 June	Start of an influenza pandemic which swept through Europe, Africa and Asia. It affected civilian populations and men in all the opposing armies. It was said that more people died in the world epidemic than died in the entire war.
3 June	On the Western Front the Second Battle of the Marne started. American Marine Brigade in action at Belleau Wood.
29 August	Germans started to withdraw on Western Front as Allies continued fierce and sustained attacks against them.
31 August	In Petrograd British naval attache murdered inside embassy by Bolsheviks.
2 September	Bolsheviks announced the Red Terror and many opponents of their regime were executed.
12 September	Fighting on the Western Front continued with the Battle of St Mihiel.
15 September	Serbian, French and Italian offensive against Bulgarians on the Salonika Front.
25 September	British forces occupied Bulgaria. A few days later Skopje regained by French.
28 September	On Western Front British offensive against Germans in Fourth Battle of Ypres.
30 September	Bulgaria surrendered.
1–4 October	Allies advance on all sectors of the Western Front.
24 October	British, French, Czechoslovakian, American, and Italian divisions attacked Austrian positions round Mount Grappa on Italian Front, but Austrians stood firm.
25 October	Generals Foch, Haig, Petain and Pershing met at Senlis in France to discuss their armistice demands.
26 October	Turkish negotiators arrived on the Aegean island of Mudros for armistice talks.
27 October	Italian and British troops crossed river Piave. Austrian troops retreated two days later and were bombarded by Allied aircraft
30 October	Turkey signed armistice.
7 November	Kaiser Wilheim II of Germany abdicated.
11 November	Armistice signed and the First World War ended.

1914
Belgium

Sister Joan Martin-Nicholson

Hôpital Militaire, Brussels, Belgium

Joan Martin-Nicholson, a Red Cross sister, arrived in Brussels on 9 August 1914. After the Germans occupied Brussels on 20 August she was ordered to work at the Hôpital Militaire, where Professor Haeger was in charge.

The large grounds hold one big main building giving on to a stone-paved courtyard, and lines of one-storied wards connected one with another by matting-covered corridors. Kitchens, laundry, and laboratories are separate, each surrounded by trees or lovely flowers, and within its own walls, secluded and peaceful, lies the convent itself, where the Lady Superior had ruled so gently for over sixty years.

I was seated opposite the courteous white-haired old Professor; my luggage had been taken to a sunny, pleasant bedroom on the ground floor in a building on the other side of the grounds, and there remained only a few details to discuss before I took up my duties amongst the most severely wounded. Everything seemed very quiet and peaceful, when suddenly we heard the tramp of many feet. Neither of us spoke as the sound came nearer, but when the door was flung wide open the old man rose and courteously bade the six German officers enter.

Rapid and decisive are the methods of the enemy, as was proved by the orders rapped out by the Colonel upon entering:

'Herr Professor doubtless knows that Brussels is ours. We need a Lazarette for our men coming in from long marches. We have decided upon this place. The entire Belgian staff will leave by four this afternoon. The Herr Professor will hand over all papers and documents, and kindly remove his belongings by the same time. The less injured of the sick will be transported as prisoners to Germany.' Then, turning a small, steely eye upon me as I was waiting to go, he continued:

'The Gnadige Fraulein is, I understand, an English nurse. Our nurses have not yet arrived; you will therefore remain and look after the seriously wounded Belgians until their arrival.'

'I should prefer to go!' I replied in German.

'Ach! You speak our language; that is good. We shall get on well, I think. But Madame must understand that she is a prisoner. She cannot get out, so let her resign herself, and be not afraid if she finds sentries posted outside her door and window, for is she not the enemy? Though' – here the huge man, with breast covered with ribbons, drew himself up and saluted – 'a very charming one.'

As I passed out of the room the other officers also saluted, passing pleasant remarks. I, the one woman in the whole place, for many days was to live and sleep alone amongst more than a thousand of the enemy.

Outside my door I saw a soldier with fixed bayonet, who put out his hand as I approached. 'Your key, Schwester!'

'No man has the key of my room,' I replied icily.

'But I have orders!'

'Well, bring to me the officer who gave them, and I will explain.'

The soldier looked at me in utter astonishment. He hesitated for a moment, and gave a grunt of satisfaction as the Colonel turned the corner.

But his short-lived satisfaction gave way to astonishment as I, in spotless white and blue uniform, gave orders in my turn, as I heard him explaining outside my window later to an almost unbelieving circle of friends, which the Colonel took uncomplainingly, leaving the key in the possession of this strange Englishwoman.

Days of storm and stress followed, filled in with hard work, tears and smiles, brutality and kindness, risk, danger, and sympathy.

The little nun had been banished. Two prisoners had escaped on the first day, so the convent was suspected of subterranean passages; and the next morning, whilst I was talking to the venerable old lady superior, I watched the entry of German officers and soldiers into this cloistered place. Right through the house they went, into the cells where the nuns, kneeling before the crucifix, took no notice of this untoward intrusion; then into the chapel with their caps fixed firmly on their shaven heads; and here a soldier with his bayonet ripped through the drawn curtains of the confessional.

'You will be out of here by this time tomorrow, the lot of you. Until then you are prisoners under lock and key.'

'Where do we go, monsieur?'

'Go? Where you like!'

And so these gentle women were ruthlessly turned out into the burning countryside of devastated Belgium, and I was left alone to strive as best I could for the welfare of my wounded.

That evening as I sat eating my supper with my men, an orderly came to me and saluted.

'The officers' greetings, and will the Gnadige Schwester honour them with her presence at mess from today on.'

A tense silence reigned in the ward. As I shared their pittance of a bowl of coffee without milk and sugar at 8am, a bowl of soup and a bit of bread at 12, a bowl of coffee at 4pm, and a bowl of indescribably disgusting gruel at 8 in the evening, my patients knew how hungry I must be. They knew, too, how good the fare at mess was; for, watching from the windows, they had seen the mess servants running to and fro with meat, and wine, and every delicacy likely to appease the Teuton appetite, and they had noticed how thin and white I had got to look in these past few days in which I had continually fought for them, defying the doctor, who strictly forbade me to touch the dressings, only to find on his visit on the next day that I had done them regularly every four hours night and day, cleaning, cutting, and bandaging wounds that made even him shudder.

I looked across my bowl.

'My sincere thanks to the officers, but I prefer to eat with my patients.'

The snatches of song and coarse laughter, born of much champagne, that floated across to us told me that I had decided wisely, and how grateful my sick were, showing their appreciation by small offerings of their rapidly diminishing store of chocolate and jam, which, added to the gruel, only made it more indescribably disgusting, although I ate it without a sign.

When I went down at midnight to my room, a thunderous knocking made me open my door.

The Colonel stood without.

'Hasten, Gnadige Schwester, to pack your things and come to another room in another building.'

I protested that I was too utterly tired and would like to know the reason why.

For a minute the officer hesitated, then he replied shamefacedly –

'There have arrived six slightly wounded officers in the room opposite yours; you will, I am sure, understand that they have been at the war for many weeks, away from towns, people, and – and women. I could not trust them even though you were behind steel doors.'

I did not speak. I just looked the man in the eyes, bringing a dark flush to the stern face, and turned silently to pack.

My days were a veritable burden on account of the soldier who followed me with fixed bayonet every time I crossed the grounds, my nights were broken every two hours as the sentry was relieved, and the new one challenged me through the window, demanding the watchword.

And yet, as the following incident shows, one sentry at least felt pity for me, the only woman amongst these men, mad with the lust of battle, after hacking a passage of blood through a stricken country.

As I put my key into my door one night, it was rudely snatched from me by a second lieutenant.

'I have orders to see that you are comfortable!'

I vigorously protested, but without avail, and he passed into my bedroom before me. I had just time to beckon to the sentry, praying that his years and the gold ring on his marriage finger might incline him to help me, when the officer, seizing me by the wrist, pulled me into the room and slammed the door. With my back to the wall I waited.

The officer took one step towards me when the door opened, and the sentry stood there, leaning silently on his rifle and seemingly oblivious of the situation.

'Get out of here!' roared the lieutenant.

'I cannot,' the man replied stolidly, 'the Herr Colonel has given me strict orders to look after the Schwester.'

The officer hesitated for one brief second, then, taking me roughly by the arm, threw me across the room, picked up my crucifix and dashed it on to the ground, and, cursing vehemently, stormed out of the room.

I made up my mind. No matter what the result might be, I would protest against this behaviour.

Outside the door the sentry beamed on me, and when I thanked him he replied with pride –

'Ach, Schwester! I have a wife and three daughters, and ach, how they can cook!'

Across the gardens I went, to be caught in a vortex of German nurses; they had just arrived, weary and dusty, and had already heard of the English Sister, and, full of patriotism, they turned and scowled at me.

Straight into the mess I walked.

'Ach, the Madchen has changed her mind,' jocularly remarked one stout young lieutenant.

'Silence!' I rapped, and turned to the Colonel, who rose to his feet as I spoke.

Assured that no such incident would occur again, I went out, running into a major who was joyfully hastening to the food.

'Here, you there! You look fairly intelligent for one of your country!'

There, a lonely woman in the centre of a crowd of about 300 soldiers, I had to stand and listen to the jibes and jeers which this officer so far forgot himself as to throw at me.

He insulted my country, scoffed at my King, jeered at my countrywomen, reviled my Navy. I got whiter and whiter with rage as I stood under the torrent of abuse. I felt rather than saw that the officers at mess had crowded to the window.

'And your Army, ach liebe Gott!'

He stuttered in his rage, almost screamed in his hate; and one soldier put his fingers to his nose and cried, 'Schwinehunden!'

There was one moment of breathless silence as they waited to see what this Englishwoman would say, and then – I left their Kaiser and their country, their Army and their Navy alone, but like a tigress I fastened on their Kultur, their honour, and their faith. My comments were severe, and they emptied the windows of the mess, and so cowed the major and the soldiers that they silently made way for me and allowed me to pass.

As I entered my building a fat little corporal patted me on the back.

'See Schwester, I have a bottle of wine, and you look so tired! Will you not have some? And see, a bit of cake.'

I smiled my thanks and went to my room. As I did so a veritable babel of women's voices broke the air. Too tired to think, I sat on my bed, wondering how much longer I could stand it, when again a thundering knock brought me to the door.

The Colonel begged me to pack at once as the German nurses had gone on strike, refusing to work if the Englishwoman remained.

Joyfully I flung my things into my small trunk. Then I went out into the courtyard, crowded with soldiers bearing torches – hundreds of them. Some officers stood round a car which held an armed escort. When I protested vigorously that I was not a prisoner and was not going to be taken through the town under an armed escort, it was explained that the escort was not for me but for two Belgian civilians who were to be shot at dawn, and that as the hour was so late, I would have to go on the same car to wherever I wanted.

It was one o'clock at night and everything was shut up, and then I remembered an old couple who had begged me to knock them up at any hour I might want help.

The Colonel came to say goodbye; he would not shake hands as doubtless he thought I might object; the officers stood at the salute with complimentary remarks, and soldiers surged round friendly and willing to help to the last moment … I was free …

Millicent, Duchess of Sutherland

Duchess of Sutherland's Ambulance Unit, Namur, Belgium

A few days after war was declared Millicent, Duchess of Sutherland went to Brussels but immediately discovered she was not needed as there were many other Red Cross workers in the city. Dr Antoine Depage, an eminent Belgian surgeon, suggested on behalf of the Belgian Red Cross that she should equip an ambulance unit and go to Namur, a strategically important border town surrounded by nine forts, some thirty-five miles from Brussels. A week later the unit, consisting of the Duchess, as Commandant, a surgeon, eight trained nurses, and a stretcher-bearer, arrived in Namur. They were given rooms in a convent that had been turned into a hospital to nurse the wounded. One of the nurses was Mildred Rees [qv]. Their necessary equipment – medicines, dressings and disinfectant – followed a little later. As they arrived the Germans were advancing – the townspeople were evacuating – and all communications had already been cut.

The Convent of Namur after last week's hurry seemed extraordinarily quiet. Les Soeurs de Notre Dame are scholastic sisters, and they had arranged the school part of the building, which was new and sanitary, as a hospital. My nurses were given a long dormitory where the scholars usually sleep and I had a small dormitory to myself. The nuns treated us most kindly, and said they would do all the cooking for the wounded. In the Belgian Red Cross ambulances and in the military hospital all the nursing is done by partly trained, but willing nuns and ladies. The dressings are done by the doctors.

It was a strange experience next morning to be sitting in the old Convent garden full of fruit trees and surrounded by high walls, whilst the nuns, the novices, and the postulants flitted about the paths with their rosaries and their little books. It was almost impossible to realise that there were nearly 200 nuns in the Convent so quietly did they move. From an upper window the nurses and I watched a regiment of Belgian artillery roll by. It was coming in from the country. 'A big battle rages near Ramillies,' said one nun. 'All the poor families are coming in in carts.' The Belgian military doctor, Dr Cordier, came to inspect our hospital equipment, which only arrived by the last train that reached Namur … He criticised our carbolic, smiled at the glycerine for the hands, and was immensely impressed by our instruments.

It was almost impossible to find out what was really going on. The noise of the motors, the scout motor cyclists, and the occasional whirr of an aeroplane mingled their sounds with a perpetual clanging of church bells. Our nurses were all busy making splints, cushions, sandbags, etc., and generally getting this scholastic side of the nunnery into one of the finest hospitals in Belgium. The English nuns helped us very much. I shall always remember Sister Marie des Cinq Anges and Sister Bernard.

On 21 August there was almost a panic in Namur. All night long the guns had been firing from the forts, and all the morning there was hurrying and scurrying into groups of weeping hatless women and of little children. The great secrecy as to all events that were passing filled them with untold fear.

It was evidently the beginning of a terrible experience. The Germans had been massing on the left bank of the Meuse and had come as close to Namur as circumstances would permit. They had passed through the country carrying off the cattle, burning the villages, cutting the telegraph and telephone wires, and attacking the railway stations. The closeness of the atmosphere had made Namur almost impossible to breathe in, that day. Tired Belgian soldiers came in. They seemed to have so much to wear and to carry. A regiment of Congolais, a Foreign Legion which had been in service in the Congo, marched through with their guns drawn by dogs.

The place was full of refugees who had been brought in from the country in carts. The Germans had burnt the villages of Ramillies and Petit Rosière. The inhabitants had been driven for shelter to Namur with a few poor bundles. They could not be kept at Namur for fear of shortage of food, so they were sent to Charleroi.

In the morning at 7.30 a bomb had been dropped from an aeroplane a few streets from our Convent. It was intended to fall in the Jesuit College, which was temporarily used as Artillery barracks, but it missed the college and dropped near the Academy of Music, breaking all the windows, ploughing a hole in the ground, and badly wounding four artillerymen.

We went over to the Café des Quatre Fils d'Aymond for our two franc dinner. We heard the explosion of another bomb in the next street. People were rushing hither and thither in a distracted manner, but no one could say who had been killed. At the door of the café we looked up, and I saw the Hornet of Hell, as I call the German 'Taube' which had dropped the bomb, floating slowly away. I thought it better to get my nurses to the shelter of the Convent, as German shells directed upon the station were beginning to fly over the town. We heard the long screaming whistle as they rushed through the air like some stupendous firework, and the distant explosion.

On 22 August I wrote my diary in the cellars of the convent. We had taken refuge there with all the schoolchildren, who were very frightened. We sat among sacks of flour, which the military authorities had put in charge of the nuns. Our nurses cut out red flannel bed-jackets and tried to take photographs! The German shells had been whistling ominously over the Convent for 24 hours. They said they were directed against the fort of Maizeret. Rumour had it that Fort Marchevolette had fallen.

One of the strangest parts of all was the fact that we were nursing in the Convent of Les Soeurs de Notre Dame de Namur. Exactly 100 years ago the Venerable Foundress, Mother Julie Billiart, who called herself Sister Ignatius, wrote her experiences of the Napoleonic War in the same Convent.

During those days of penury and distress no one knew how the Venerable Mother contrived to feed her sisters and children. In the same mysterious way today the Reverend Mother contrived to feed the soldiers and children, her 200 nuns, and novices and postulants, and has promised to feed our wounded.

Never shall I forget the afternoon of 22 August. The shelling of the past hours having suddenly ceased, I went to my dormitory. I had had practically no rest for two nights, and after the emotions of the morning I was falling asleep when Sister Kirby rushed into my room, calling out, 'Sister Millicent! The wounded!'

I rushed down the stone stairs. Six motor cars and as many waggons were at the door, and they were carrying in those unhappy fellows. Some were on stretchers, others were supported by willing Red Cross men. One or two of the stragglers fell up the steps from fatigue and lay there. Many of these men had been for three days without food or sleep in the trenches.

In less than 20 minutes we had 45 wounded on our hands. A number had been wounded by shrapnel, a few by bullet wounds, but luckily some were only wounded by pieces of shell. These inflict awful gashes, but if they are taken in time the wounds rarely prove mortal.

The wounded were all Belgian – Flemish and Walloon – or French. Many were Reservists. Our young surgeon, Mr Morgan, was perfectly cool and so were our nurses. What I thought would be for me an impossible task became absolutely natural: to wash wounds, to drag off rags and clothing soaked in blood, to hold basins equally full of blood, to soothe a soldier's groans, to raise a wounded man while he was receiving extreme unction, hemmed in by nuns and a priest, so near he seemed to death; these actions seemed suddenly to become an insistent duty, perfectly easy to carry out.

All the evening the wounded and the worn out were being rushed in. If they had come in tens one would not have minded, but the pressure of cases to attend to was exhausting. One could not refuse to take them, for they said there were 700 in the military hospital already, while all the smaller Red Cross ambulances were full.

So many of the men were in a state of prostration bordering almost on dementia, that I seemed instantly enveloped in the blight of war. I felt stunned – as if I were passing through an endless nightmare. Cut off as we were from all communication with the outer world, I realised what a blessing our ambulance was to Namur. I do not know what the nuns would have done without our nurses at such a moment. No one, until these awful things happen, can conceive the untold value of fully-trained and disciplined British nurses. The nuns were of great use to us, for they helped in every possible tender way, and provided food for the patients. The men had been lying in the trenches outside the forts. Hundreds of wounded were still waiting to be brought in, and owing to the German cannonading it was impossible to get near them. I kept on thinking and hoping that the allied armies must be coming to rescue Namur.

The guns never cease. The heavy French artillery arrived last night, and have taken up the work of the Marchevolette fort, which is reported to be out of action, but one of our wounded tells us that this artillery came 24 hours too late, and that the French force on the Meuse is not sufficient.

The Belgian Gendarmerie have just been in and collected all arms and ammunition.

I have been seeking for the rosaries the patients carry in their purses. They want to hold them in their hands or have them slung round their necks. On the floor there is a confusion of uniforms, kepis, and underclothing, which the nuns are trying to sort. Our surgeon is busy in the operating theatre, cutting off a man's fingers; he was the first to be brought in and had his right hand shattered.

Sunday 23 August. There is a dreadful bombardment going on. Some of our wounded who can walk wrap themselves in blankets and go to the cellars. Luckily we are in a new fire-proof building, and I must stay with my sick men who cannot move. The shells sing over the convent from the deep booming German guns – a long singing scream and then an explosion which seems only a stone's throw away. The man who received extreme unction the night before is mad with terror. I do not believe that he is after all so badly wounded. He has a bullet in his shoulder, and it is not serious. He has lost all power of speech, but I believe that he is an example of what I have read of and what I had never seen – a man dying of sheer fright.

The nurses and one or two of the nuns are most courageous and refuse to take shelter in the cellars, which are full of novices and schoolchildren. The electric and gas supplies have been cut off. The only lights we have to use are a few hand lanterns and night-lights. Quite late in the afternoon we heard a tremendous explosion. The Belgians had blown up the new railway bridge, but unfortunately there are others by which the Germans can cross, and we hear that they are in the town. There is some rapid fusillading through the streets and two frightened old Belgian officers ran into the Convent to ask for Red Cross bands, throwing down their arms and maps. In a few minutes, however, they regained self control and went out in the streets without the Red Cross bands.

Now the German troops are fairly marching in. I hear them singing as they march. It seems almost cowardly to write this, but for a few minutes there was relief to see them coming and to feel that this awful firing would soon cease. On they march! Fine well-set-up men with grey uniforms. They have stopped shooting now. I see them streaming into the market-place. A lot of stampeding artillery horses gallop by with Belgian guns. On one of the limbers still lay all that was left of a man. It is too terrible. What can these brave little people do against this mighty force? Some of the Germans have fallen out and are talking to the people in the streets. These are so utterly relieved at the cessation of the bombardment that in their fear they are actually welcoming the Germans. I saw some women press forward and wave their handkerchiefs.

Suddenly upon this scene the most fearful shelling begins again. It seemed almost as if the guns were in the garden. Mr Morgan, Mr Winser [the stretcher-bearer], and I were standing there. I had just buried my revolver under an apple tree when the bombardment began once more. The church bells were clanging for vespers. Then Whizz! Bang! come the shells over our heads again. Picric acid and splinters fall at our very feet. We rush back into the convent, and there are fifteen minutes of intense and fearful excitement while the shells are crashing into the market-place. We see

German soldiers running for dear life … Women half fainting, and wounded, old men and boys are struggling in. Their screams are dreadful. They had all gone into the Grande Place to watch the German soldiers marching, and were caught in this sudden firing. A civilian wounded by a shell in the stomach was brought into the Ambulance. He died in 20 minutes. We can only gather incoherent accounts from these people as to what had happened. The Germans sounded the retreat and the shelling seemed to stop. At last it leaks out that the German troops on the other side of the town did not know that their own troops had crossed the Meuse on the opposite side. They were firing on the Citadel, an antiquated fort of no value. The shells fell short, and before the Germans discovered their mistake they had killed many of their own soldiers and Belgian civilians who had rushed up to see the German troops. It seems a horrible story, but absolutely true.

Now it is quiet again, save for the sighs of the suffering. All night long we hear the tramp, tramp, tramp of German infantry in the streets, their words of command, their perpetual deep-throated songs. They are full of swagger, and they are very anxious to make an impression upon the Belgians.

Our wounded are doing well, and one must remember that, if their nerves have gone to pieces, to lie in trenches with this awful artillery fire bursting over them, knowing that even if they lifted their heads a few inches it might be blown off, must be an appalling sensation.

The Doctor and I went up into the tower in the dark. The bombardment had ceased, but everywhere on the horizon, there were blazing fires, villages and country mansions flaring in the darkness. Motor cars dashed past. Instead of Belgian, one sees now only German motors filled with German officers. Where are the English and the big French troops? That is what I am wondering.

24 August. The day was peaceful enough after the previous soul-stirring hours. Early in the afternoon a German Count with a Red Cross on his arm came and inspected our ambulance at the Convent. He was perfectly civil, and one had to be civil in return. He drank the beer which the nuns tremblingly pressed upon him, and took a note of the sacks of flour which the nuns were keeping in the cellars.

'Pour l'autorité militair Belge', they said.

'Allemande,' the young Count replied significantly.

I made a mental note to get possession of that flour, for the German troops were rapidly depleting Namur of all its food, and refugees were streaming into the town. We had not seen butter, milk, or eggs for days. Now the nuns came to me and said there was no yeast for the bread, and they were trying various recipes to make bread without yeast.

The German Count adopted a sort of 'charming woman' manner to me; he seemed thoroughly pleased with himself. He said, 'Now the Germans are in possession of Namur all will be quiet and well arranged. There will be no trouble unless the civilians are treacherous and fire on the soldiers. If they do that we shall set fire to the town.' Having said this he clattered out. The Namuriens had suffered so much and had seemed so utterly broken down, it did not strike me that the civilians would venture to fire on these thousands of troops that were filling their streets, their barracks, and their shops. All I kept on thinking was, 'Where are the English and the French?'

It was a hot, still summer night. We had begun to laugh again. We were so interested in our wounded – and we were so relieved at the cessation of firing save of one distant cannon which would not stop and was evidently attacking the last fort.

It was ten o'clock and I decided to go to bed and was nearly undressed when a few rifle shots rang out in the street near the Convent. A pause, and then came a perfect fusillade of rifle shots. It was dreadful while it lasted. Had the Belgians disregarded the warning of the Town Council, of *L'Ami de l'Ordre* [the Namur newspaper], and of the German 'swankers', and refused to take their defeat lying down? If the civilians were firing, it was mad rashness. My door burst open and Mr Winser rushed in calling out, 'My God, Duchess, they have fired the town.'

The Hôtel de Ville was on fire, the market place was on fire. Then came the message that the town was fired at the four corners. One of the buildings of the Convent was absolutely fire-proof and in this portion the worn-out wounded were very quiet. We had about a hundred in a dormitory in an older building. The flames simply shot up beside this and the sparks were falling about the roof. Fortunately the Convent was all surrounded by a garden and the wind was blowing the flames away from us. The whole sky was illuminated; we came to the conclusion that there was nothing to do but to wait and watch the fire, and leave the patients alone until we saw the flames must reach us. It was a terrible hour. The nurses courageously re-assured the wounded and persuaded most of them to remain in bed.

The Padre came in at last and said that the flames would not reach us. In the afternoon we ventured into the smoky street. It was like walking through a dense fog. All the buildings were smouldering. The whole of the market-place and the Hotel de Ville had been burnt and the dear little café where we went for our meals before the bombardment. All the shutters were up on the shops that had not been burnt and one could hardly walk for the number of German troops massed in the streets, bivouacking with their rifles stacked before them. A German officer told me that the town was burnt because some of the civilian inhabitants had been shooting at the soldiers from dark windows.

The Doctor and I thought we had better visit the Commander, General von Bülow. The Headquarters Staff was established at the Hôtel de Hollande. The General apologised for receiving me in his bedroom, so terribly overflowing were all the other rooms with officers. Field Marshall von der Goltz, who arrived en route to take up his duties in Brussels [as Governor], was kept waiting while the General spoke to me.

General von Bülow said he was sure he had met me at Hamburg, and that he would arrange with one of the diplomats to get a telegram through to Berlin, which he trusted would be copied in the London papers, announcing the safety of our Ambulance.

'Accept my admiration for your work, Duchess,' he said. He spoke perfect English. To accept the favours of my country's foe was a bad moment for me, but the Germans were in possession of Namur and I had to consider my hospital from every point of view. Also those who are of the Red Cross and who care for suffering humanity and for the relief of pain and sickness should strive to remember nothing but the heartache of the world and the pity of it.

General von Bülow 'did me the honour' to call the next morning at our Ambulance. He was accompanied by Baron Kessler, his aide-de-camp, who composed the scenario of *La Legende de Josephe*. He had been much connected with Russian opera in London during the past season. It was exceedingly odd to meet him under such circumstances, after having so often discussed 'art' with him in London.

I was able, with the assistance of Mr Winser, whose sister had married a German, to obtain an order that the flour in the cellars might be kept for the use of our Ambulance.

On 27 August the Germans were in full possession of peaceful Namur. We had now over 100 patients. The Germans were occupying the temporary barracks across the road from the Convent which had lately been full of Belgian soldiers. Some German Infantrymen brought us three wounded comrades – an artillery waggon had upset and passed over them.

The walls were pasted with German proclamations. Owing to the shooting of the civilians an order came out that all soldiers, Belgian or French that might be hidden in the houses, were to be given up as prisoners-of-war before four o'clock in the afternoon in front of the prison. If this order were not obeyed the prisoners would be condemned to perpetual hard labour in Germany. If any arms were hidden in houses and were not given up by four o'clock the inhabitants would be shot. All streets would be occupied by German guards, who would take from each street ten male hostages. These hostages would be shot if any other person whosoever fired upon the German troops. No houses could be locked at night. After eight o'clock at night three windows must be lit in every house. Anyone found out in the streets after eight o'clock would be shot. Proclamations of this sort succeeded one another every day. The German authorities fairly tripped over their own regulations. They allowed the Namuriens to have their own Bourgmestre, but when General von Bülow left the town, as he did in a few days, he was succeeded by another Commander, who proceeded to unsew in regulations all that had been sewn up before.

By 3 September Namur had settled down to a certain amount of calm. German sentries stood outside the military hospital, Germans filled every cafe and German troops were perpetually going backwards and forwards through the town. Fresh regiments came up – others disappeared.

A German officer came into our ambulance and said the German wounded that we had there must be taken to the military hospital. They were not really fit to go and I could see that they were very sorry to leave us. I used to go every day and visit the Commander and Dr Schilling [the head doctor of the garrison] and quote the Convention of Geneva and do all I could to lighten the lot of our wounded. In spite of this the Germans soon came and took away as prisoners 30 of those who had nearly recovered. Dr Schilling had a very rough manner, but I do think he had a good heart and positively hated the job in which he was engaged. He was always working to get even the badly wounded sent on as prisoners, 'to evacuate', he said, 'to make room for other wounded'. I asked him if the Belgian and French prisoners were properly looked after in Germany when they were wounded. 'God in Heaven! Madame,' he answered, 'do you take us for barbarians?'

Yesterday a guard of eight German soldiers was sent into our Convent. This was really more than I could bear so I forwarded a message to the Commander and in half an hour the guard was taken away. I asked for two sentries to be left at the door. These men were changed every two hours and I had long conversations with them. They all seemed anxious to go home again and knew nothing of why they were fighting or where they were going to fight.

We were getting very hungry in Namur. An order had gone out from the Commander to re-victual the town, but it was easier said than done. With the destroying of the surrounding villages and with so many troops in the town, there was hardly anything left to eat, although the nuns always managed to provide coffee and bread for the wounded. There was no milk. I had fortunately brought down some biscuits and jam from Brussels, and the nuns fed us with all they could let us have and gave us lots of fruit.

Mr Winser was at last able to go to Brussels in a Red Cross motor. He brought back a ham, a cheese, and some marmalade … He fetched from the American Legation a *Weekly Dispatch* of 30 August and in this I learnt of the French reverses near Charleroi and of the English difficulties at Mons and St Quentin.

My whole mind was now bent upon getting to Mons. Comtesse Jacqueline de Pourtales had come back with Mr Winser from Brussels. She said the city was full of German wounded, but no English. She told me that Miss Angela Manners and Miss Nellie Hozier [the sister-in-law of Winston Churchill] had gone down with a small ambulance of London Hospital nurses to Mons, having got the permit from the German authorities through freely using Mr Winston Churchill's name.

We heard bad news of the burning of Louvain. Some of our patients were Louvain University students and they were miserable at the burning of the University and their wonderful and world-renowned library. Some say the Germans saved the books and took them to Germany.

I wished to see the English wounded and on 5 September I obtained a permit from the Commander to visit Mons in a motor car with a German soldier as guard. I asked for the guard, as I knew by this means our car would be able to pass everywhere in safety.

All the way to Charleroi from Namur along the banks of the unhappy Sambre the country was desolate. I shall never forget the burnt houses, the charred rubbish, the helpless-looking people. There had been fearful fighting in the suburbs of Charleroi. The fields were full of German graves. The persistence of the glorious weather made the contrast more tragic.

Mons is an attractive town with large avenues of trees. At the very first Red Cross Ambulance I found five British privates – two Royal Scots, two of the Irish Rifles, and one of the Middlesex Regiment.

The Belgian Red Cross ladies were more than kind to them but the trouble was that they could not speak English and the soldiers could not speak French. I understood from Miss Manners and Miss Hozier that there were about 200 British wounded in the town, and that a whole ward of the civil hospital was full of British wounded. They were well looked after by Belgian doctors and were clean and comfortable. I gathered from every man I asked that they had been surprised by the Germans on 22 or 23 August. They had killed a great number but they had got separated from the remainder of the British force, and knew nothing of the sequel of the fight.

I had to leave Mons without seeing all the English wounded. I wanted to get as near to the frontier as possible on my way back to Namur, in case of coming across any out-lying wounded. The big siege cannon were still firing at Maubeuge, evidently the forts had not yet fallen.

Presently we came to a country house embedded in trees with a Red Cross flag flying. I drove up and found the place belonging to Count Maxine de Bousies at Harvengt. He was nursing here 20 English wounded of the Irish Rifles, Irish Guards, Coldstream Guards, and others. Nuns were in charge, and the men assured me they were splendidly taken care of.

When I got back to Namur I found the Germans had been busy; taking advantage of my absence they had announced their decision to close all private ambulances in Namur. They said they would group the wounded in two big 'Lazarets' or German military hospitals. Our wounded would have to be taken to the College of the Jesuits under German control before they entrained for Germany as prisoners.

I felt furious at this news, but it was too late to do anything that night as the fatal hour of 9 was passed, when all who ventured into the streets were shot.

In the morning I went to Dr Schilling. He said that we could have a room at the Jesuit College in which to put all our wounded, and he gave me a note to the head German doctor at the College to this effect, but he would make no exception for our ambulance to keep it open …

Miss Sarah Macnaughtan

Mrs Stobart's Hospital Unit, Antwerp, Belgium
Dr Hector Munro's Flying Ambulance Corps, Furnes, Belgium

On 20 September 1914 Sarah Macnaughtan, a well-known author, musician and painter, and member of the British Red Cross Corps, arrived in Antwerp to serve as a senior orderly with Mrs St Clair Stobart's Unit – which was made up of women doctors, nurses and orderlies. They brought a large store of medical equipment and immediately started to scrub floors and set up operating theatres, receiving rooms, kitchens, bathrooms and wards in a large, empty philharmonic hall that the Belgian authorities had commandeered for a hospital for Belgian and French casualties. Beds were ranged in rows, each with clean sheets and a bright counterpane and on 24 September the first fifty wounded men were received. Some of the staff lived in rooms over the philharmonic hall and others in a nearby convent.

28 September

Last night I and two orderlies slept over at the hospital as more wounded were expected. At 11pm word came that 'les blessés' were at the gate. Men were on duty with stretchers, and we went out to the tram-way cars in which the wounded are brought from the station, twelve patients in each. The transit is as little painful as possible, and the stretchers are placed in iron brackets, and are simply unhooked when the men arrive. Each stretcher was brought in and laid on a bed in the ward, and the nurses and doctors undressed the men. We orderlies took their names, their 'matricule' or regimental number, and the number on their bed. Then we gathered up their clothes and put corresponding numbers on labels attached to them – first turning out the pockets, which are filled with all manner of things, from tins of sardines to loaded revolvers.

We arranged everything and then got Oxo for the men, many of whom had had nothing to eat for two days. Their absolute exhaustion is the most pathetic thing about them. They fall asleep even when their wounds are being dressed. When all was made straight and comfortable for them, the nurses turned the lights low again, and stepped softly about the ward with their little torches.

A hundred beds all filled with men in pain give one plenty to think about. I was struck by the contrast between the pillared concert-hall where they lie, with its platform of white paint and decorations, and the tragedy of suffering which now fills it.

At 2am more soldiers were brought in from the battlefield, all caked with dirt, and we began to work again.

At five o'clock I went to bed and slept till eight. Mrs Stobart never rests. I think she must be made of some substance that the rest of us have not discovered. At 5am I discovered her curled up on a bench in her office, the doors wide open and the dawn breaking.

2 October

At 7am the men's bread had not arrived for their six o'clock breakfast, so I went into the town to get it. The difficulty was to convey home twenty-eight large loaves, so I went to the barracks and begged a motor car from the Belgian office and came back triumphant. The military cars simply rip through the streets, blowing their horns all the time. Antwerp was thronged with these cars and each one contained soldiers. Sometimes one saw wounded in them lying on sacks stuffed with straw.

After breakfast I cleaned the two houses, as I do every morning. When my rooms were done I went over to the hospital to help prepare the men's dinner, my task today being to open bottles and pour out beer for 120 men. Afterwards I went across to the hospital again and arranged a few things with Mrs Stobart. I began to correct the men's diagnosis sheets, but was called off to help with wounded arriving, and to label and sort their clothes.

The men's supper is at six o'clock, and we began cutting up their bread-and-butter and cheese and filling their bowls of beer. When that was over and visitors were going, an order came for thirty patients to proceed to Ostend and make room for worse cases.

The Germans have destroyed the reservoir and the water-supply has been cut off, so we have to go and fetch all the water in buckets from a well. After supper we go with our pails and carry it home.

The shortage for washing, cleaning, etc., is rather inconvenient, and adds to the danger in a large hospital, and to the risk of typhoid.

4 October

Winston Churchill is here with Marines. They say Colonel Kitchener is at the forts.

The firing sounds very near. Dr Hector Munro and Miss St Clair [May Sinclair qv] and Lady Dorothie Feilding came over today from Ghent, where all is quiet. They wanted me to return with them to take a rest, which was absurd, of course.

Some fearful cases were brought in to us today. My God, the horror of it! One has heard of men whom their mothers would not recognise. Some of the wounded today were amongst these. All the morning we did what we could for them. One man was riddled with bullets, and died very soon.

It is awful work. The great bell rings, and we say, 'More wounded', and the men get stretchers. We go down the long, cold covered way to the gate and number the men for their different beds. The stretchers are stiff with blood, and the clothes have to be cut off the men. They cry out terribly, and their horror is so painful to witness. They are so young, and they have seen right into hell. The first dressings are removed by the doctors – sometimes there is only a lump of cotton-wool to fill up a hole – and the men lie there with their tragic eyes fixed upon one.

The lights are all off at eight o'clock now, and we do our work in the dark, while the orderlies hold little torches to enable the doctors to dress the wounds. There are not half enough nurses or doctors out here. In one hospital there are 400 beds and only two trained nurses.

5–6 October

I think the last two days have been the most ghastly I ever remember. Every day seems to bring news of defeat. It is awful, and the Germans are quite close now. As I write the house shakes with the firing. Our troops are falling back, and the forts have fallen. Last night we took provisions and water to the cellars, and made plans to get the wounded taken there.

All these last two days bleeding men have been brought in. Today three of them died, and I suppose none of them was more than 23.

The guns boom by day as well as by night, and as each one is heard one thinks of more bleeding, shattered men. It is calm, nice autumn weather; the trees are yellow in the garden and the sky is blue, yet all the time one listens to the cries of men in pain. Tonight I meant to go out for a little, but a nurse stopped me and asked me to sit by a dying man. Poor fellow, he was twenty-one, and looked like some brigand chief, and he smiled as he was dying.

7 October

It is a glorious morning: they will see well to kill each other today.

At lunch-time today firing ceased, and I heard it was because the German guns were coming up. We got orders to send away all the wounded who could possibly go, and we prepared beds in the cellars for those who cannot be moved. The military authorities beg us to remain as so many hospitals have been evacuated.

The wounded continue to come in. All the orderlies are on duty in the hospital now. We can spare no one for rougher work. We can all bandage and wash patients. There are wounded everywhere, even on straw beds on the platform of the hall.

At 7 last night the guns were much louder than before, with a sort of strange double sound, and we were told that these were our 'Long Toms', so we hope that our Naval Brigade has come up.

We know very little of what is going on except when we run out and ask some returning English soldiers for news. Yesterday it was always the same reply: 'Very bad'. One of the Marines told me that Winston Churchill was 'up and down the road amongst the shells', and that he had given orders that Antwerp was not to be taken until the last man in it was dead.

The Marines are getting horribly knocked about. Yesterday Mrs O'Gormon went out in her own motor car and picked wounded out of the trenches. She said that no one knew why they were in the trenches or where they were to fire – they just lay there and were shot and then left.

On Wednesday night, 7 October, we heard that one more ship was going to England, and a last chance was given to us all to leave. Only two did so; the rest stayed on. Mrs Stobart went out to see what was to be done.

At midnight the first shell came over us with a shriek, and I went down and woke the orderlies and nurses and doctors. We dressed and went over to help move the wounded at the hospital. The shells began to scream overhead; it was a bright moonlight night, and we walked without haste – a small body of women – across the road to the hospital.

Nearly all the moving to the cellars had already been done – only three stretchers remained to be moved. One wounded English sergeant helped us. Otherwise everything was done by women. We laid the men on mattresses which we fetched from the hospital overhead, and then Mrs Stobart's mild, quiet voice said, 'Everything is to go on as usual. The night nurses and orderlies will take their places. Breakfast will be at the usual hour.' She and the other ladies whose night it was to sleep at the convent then returned to sleep in the basement with a Sister.

We came in for some most severe shelling at first, either because we flew the Red Cross flag or because we were in the line of fire with a powder magazine which the Germans wished to destroy.

We sat in the cellars with one night-light burning in each, and with seventy wounded men to take care of. Two of them were dying. There was only one line of bricks between us and the shells. One shell fell into the garden, making a hole six feet deep; the next crashed through a house on the opposite side of the road and set it on fire. As long as we stayed with the wounded they minded nothing. We sat there all night. We just waited for daybreak. When it came the firing grew worse. Two hundred guns were turned on Antwerp, and the shells came over at the rate of four a minute. They have a horrid screaming sound as they come. We heard each one coming and wondered if it would hit us, and then we heard the crashing somewhere else and knew another shell was coming.

The worst cases among the wounded lay on the floor, and these wanted constant attention. The others were in their great-coats, and stood about the cellar leaning on crutches and sticks. We wrapped blankets round the rheumatism cases and sat through the long night. All spoke cheerfully, and there was some laughter in the further cellar.

At six o'clock the convent party came over and began to prepare breakfast. The least wounded of the men began to steal away. Mrs Stobart was walking about for three hours trying to find anything on wheels to remove us and the wounded. At last we got a motor ambulance, and packed in twenty men – that was all it would hold. We told them to go as far as the bridge and send it back for us. It never came.

We got dinner for the men, and then the strain began to be much worse. I told Mrs Stobart we must leave the wounded at the convent in charge of the Sisters, and this we did, telling them where to take them in the morning.

About five o'clock the shelling became more violent, and three shells came with only an instant between each. Presently we heard Mrs Stobart say, 'Come at once', and we went out and found three English buses with English drivers at the door. They were carrying ammunition, and were the last vehicles to leave Antwerp. We got into them and lay on the top of the ammunition, and the girls began to light cigarettes! The noise of the buses prevented our hearing for a time the infernal sound of shells and our cannons' answering roar.

As we drove to the bridge many houses and sometimes a whole street was burning. No one seemed to care. No one was there to try and save anything. We drove through the empty streets and saw the burning houses, and great holes where shells had fallen, and then we got to the bridge and out of the line of fire.

We set out to walk towards Holland, but a Belgian officer got us some Red Cross ambulances, and into these we got, and were taken to a convent at St Gilles, where we slept on the floor till 3am. At 3 a message was brought, 'Get up at once – things are worse.' Everyone seemed to be leaving, and we got into the Red Cross ambulances and went to the station.

9 October
We have been all day in the train in very hard third-class carriages with the RMLI. The journey of 50 miles took from five o'clock in the morning, when we got away, till twelve o'clock at night, when we reached Ostend. The train hardly crawled. It was the longest I have ever seen. All Ostend was in darkness when we arrived – a German airship having been seen overhead. We always seem to be tumbling about in the dark. We went from one hotel to another trying to get accommodation, and at last (at the St James's) they allowed us to lie on the floor of the restauarant. The only food they had for us was ten eggs for twenty-five hungry people and some brown bread, but they had champagne and I ordered it for everybody, and we made little speeches and tried to end on a good note.

10 October
Mrs Stobart took the unit back to England today.

12 October
Everyone has gone back to England except Sister Bailey and me. She is waiting to hand over the wounded to the proper department, and I am waiting to see if I can get on anywhere. It does seem so hard that when men are most in need of us we should all run home and leave them.

The noises and racket in Ostend are deafening, and there is panic everywhere. The boats go to England packed every time. Some ships lie close to us on the grey misty water, and the troops are passing along all day.

Later. We heard tonight that the Germans are coming into Ostend tomorrow, so once more we fly like dust before a broom. It is horrible having to clear out for them.

This evening Dr Hector Munro came in from Ghent with his oddly-dressed ladies, and at first one was inclined to call them masqueraders in their knickerbockers and puttees and caps, but I believe they have done excellent work. It is a queer side of war to see young, pretty English girls in khaki and thick boots, coming in from the trenches, where they have been picking up wounded men within 100 yards of the enemy's lines, and carrying them away on stretchers.

Dr Munro asked me to come on to his convoy, and I gladly did so: he sent home a lady whose nerves were gone [Miss May Sinclair] and I was put in her place.

13 October
We had an early muddly breakfast. Afterwards we all got into our motor ambulances en route for Dunkirk. The road was filled with flying inhabitants, and down at the dock wounded and well struggled to get on to the steamer. People were begging us for a seat in our ambulance, and well-dressed women were setting out to walk 20 miles to Dunkirk.

I began to make out of whom our party consists. There is Lady Dorothie Feilding – probably 22, but capable of taking command of a ship, and speaking French like a native; Mrs Decker, an Australian, plucky and efficient; Miss Chisholm [qv], a blue-eyed Scottish girl, with a thick coat strapped around her waist and a haversack slung from her shoulder; a tall American, whose name I do not yet know, whose husband is a journalist; three young surgeons, and Dr Munro. It is all so quaint. The girls rule the company, carry maps and find roads, see about provisions and carry wounded.

We could not get rooms at Dunkirk and so came on to St Malo les Bains, a small bathing-place which had been shut up for the winter. The owner of an hotel there opened up some rooms for us and got us some ham and eggs, and the evening ended very cheerily. Our party seems, to me, amazingly young and unprotected.

St Malo les Bains. 14 October
Lady Dorothie Feilding is our real commander, and everyone knows it. She goes to all the heads of departments, is the only good speaker of French, and has the only reliable information about anything. All the men acknowledge her position.

16 October
Today I have been reading of the 'splendid retreat' of the Marines from Antwerp and their 'unprecedented reception' at Deal. Everyone appears to have been in a state of wild enthusiasm about them, and it seems almost like Mafeking over again.

What struck me most about these men was the way in which they blew their own trumpets in full retreat and while flying from the enemy. We travelled all day in the train with them and had long conversations with them all. I find the conceit of it most trying. Belgium is in the hands of the enemy, and we flee before him singing our own praises loudly as we do so. The Marines lost their kit, spent one night in Antwerp, and went back to England, where they had an amazing reception amid scenes of unprecedented enthusiasm!

I could not help thinking, when I read the papers today, of our tired little body of nurses and doctors and orderlies going back quietly and unproclaimed to England to rest at Folkestone for three days and then to come out here again. They had been for eighteen hours under heavy shell fire without so much as a rifle to protect them, and with the immediate chance of a burning building falling about them. The nurses sat in the cellars tending wounded men, whom they refused to leave, and then hopped on to the outside of an ammunition bus.

21 October
Firing has begun again. This afternoon we came out in motors and ambulances to establish ourselves at Furnes in an empty Ecclesiastical College. Nothing was ready, and everything was in confusion. Night was falling as we came back to Dunkirk to sleep (for no beds were ready at Furnes).

Today I see tired dusty men, very hungry looking and unshaved, slogging along, silent and tired, and ready to lie down whenever chance offers.

23 October
The guns are nearer today or more distant, the battle sways backwards and forwards, and there is no such thing as a real 'base' for a hospital. We must just stay as long as we can and fly when we must.

About 10am the ambulances that have been out all night begin to come in, the wounded on their pitiful shelves.

All day the stretchers are brought in and the work goes on. It is about five o'clock that the weird tired hour begins when the dim lamps are lighted, and people fall over things, and nearly everything is mislaid, and the wounded cry out, and one steps over forms on the floor. From then till one goes to bed it is difficult to be just what one ought to be, the tragedy of it is too pitiful.

Blood-stained mattresses and pillows are carried out into the courtyard. Two ladies help to move the corpses. There is always a pile of bandages and rags being burnt, and a youth stirs the horrible pile with a stick. A queer smell permeates everything, and the guns never cease. The wounded are coming in at the rate of 100 a day.

The Queen of the Belgians called to see the hospital today. Poor little Queen, coming to see the remnants of an army and the remnants of a kingdom! She was kind to each wounded man, and we were glad of her visit, if for no other reason than that some sort of cleaning and tidying was done in her honour. Tonight Mr Nevinson [the war artist] arrived, and we went round the wards together after supper. The beds were all full – so was the floor. The doctors said, 'These men are not wounded, they are mashed.'

The surgeons are working in shifts and can't get the work done. One can only be thankful for a hospital like this in the thick of things, for we are saving the lives of men who perhaps have lain three days in a trench or a turnip-field undiscovered and forgotten.

As soon as a wounded man has been attended to and is able to be put on a stretcher again he is sent to Calais. We have to keep emptying the wards for other patients to come in, and besides, if the fighting comes this way, we shall have to fall back a little further.

26 October. My birthday
We started early in the ambulance today, and went to pick up the wounded.

The churches are nearly all filled with straw, the chairs piled anywhere, and the sacrament removed from the altar. In cottages and little inns it is the same thing – a litter of straw, and men lying on it in the chilly weather. Here and there through some little window one sees surgeons in their white coats dressing wounds. Half the world seems to be wounded. We filled our ambulance, and stood about in curious groups of English men and women who looked as if they were on some shooting-party. When our load was complete we drove home.

21 November. Furnes Railway Station
I am up to my eyes in soup! I have started a soup-kitchen at the station, and it gives me a lot to do.

Our kitchen at the railway-station is a little bit of a passage, which measures eight feet by eight feet. In it are two small stoves. One is a little round iron thing which burns, and the other is a sort of little 'kitchener' which doesn't. With this equipment, and various huge 'marmites', we make coffee and soup for hundreds of men every day. The first convoy gets into the station about 9.30am, all the men frozen, the black troops nearly dead with cold. As soon as the train arrives I carry out one of my boiling 'marmites' to the middle of the stone entrance and ladle out the soup, while a Belgian Sister takes round coffee and bread.

These Belgians (three of them) deserve much of the credit for the soup-kitchen, as they started with coffee before I came, and did wonders on nothing. Now that I have bought my pots and pans and stoves we are able to do soup, and much more. The Sisters do the coffee on one side of eight feet by eight, while I and my vegetables and the stove which goes out are on the other.

After the first convoy of wounded has been served, other wounded men come in from time to time, then about four o'clock there is another train-load. At 10pm the largest convoy arrives. The men seem too stiff to move, and many are carried in on soldiers' backs. The stretchers are laid on the floor, those who can sit on benches, and every man produces a 'quart' or tin cup. One and all they come out of the darkness and never look about them, but rouse themselves to get fed, and stretch out poor grimy hands for bread and steaming drinks. There is very little light – only one oil-lamp, which hangs from the roof, and burns dimly. Under this we place the 'marmites', and all that I can see is one brown or black or wounded hand stretched out into the dim ring of light under the lamp, with a little tin mug held out for soup. Wet and ragged, and covered with sticky mud, the wounded lie in the salle of the station, and, except under the lamp, it is all quite dark … and then the train loads up, the wounded depart, and a heavy smell and an empty pot are all that remain. We clean up the kitchen, and go home about 1am. I do the night work alone. I have a little electric lamp, which is a great comfort to me, as I have to walk home alone. The villa is a mile from the station.

1 December
Mrs Knocker [qv] and Miss Chisholm [qv] and Lady Dorothie went out to Pervyse a few days ago to make soup etc. for Belgians in the trenches. They live in the cellar

of a house which has been blown inside out by guns, and take out buckets of soup to men on outpost duty. Not a glimpse of fire is allowed on outpost duty. Fortunately the weather has been milder lately, but soaking wet. Our three ladies walk about the trenches at night.

The piteous list of casualties is not so long as it has been. A wounded German was brought in today. Both his legs were broken and his feet frost-bitten. He had been for four days in water with nothing to eat, and his legs unset. He is doing well.

8 December

Unexpected people continue to arrive at Furnes. Mme Curie and her daughter are in charge of the X-ray apparatus at the hospital.

Today I was giving out my soup on the train and three shells came in in quick succession. One came just over my head and lodged in a haystall on the other side of the platform. The wall of the store has an enormous hole in it, but the thickly packed hay prevented the shrapnel scattering. The station-master was hit, and his watch saved him, but it was crumpled up like a rag. Two men were wounded, and one of them died. A whole crowd of refugees came in from Coxide, which is being heavily shelled. There was not a scrap of food for them, so I made soup in great quantities, and distributed it to them in a crowded room whose atmosphere was thick. Ladling out soup is great fun.

25 December

My Christmas Day began at midnight, when I walked home through the moonlit empty streets of Furnes. At 2am the guns began to roar, and roared all night. They say the Allies are making an attack.

I got up early and went to church in the untidy school-room at the hospital, which is called the nurses' sitting-room. Mr Streatfield had arranged a little altar, and had set some chairs in an orderly row, and white artificial flowers in the vases, and there were candles and a cross. We were quite a small congregation. Inside we prayed for peace, and outside the guns went on firing. Prince Alexander of Teck came to our service – a big soldierly figure in the bare room.

After breakfast I went to the soup-kitchen at the station, as usual, then home – i.e. to the hospital to lunch. At 3.15 came a sort of evensong with hymns, and then we went to the civil hospital, where there was a Christmas tree for all the Belgian refugee children.

Every man, woman and child got a treat or a present or a good dinner. The wounded had turkey, and all they could eat, and the children got toys and sweets off the tree. I suppose these children are not much accustomed to presents, for their delight was almost too much for them … Without homes or money, and with their relations often lost. The bigger children had rather good voices, and all sang our National Anthem in English. 'God save our nobbler King' – the accent was quaint, but the children sang lustily.

We had finished, and were waiting for our own Christmas dinner when shells began to fly. One came whizzing past Mr Streatfield's store room as I stood there with him. The next minute a little child in floods of tears came in, grasping her mother's bag, to say 'Maman' had had her arm blown off. The child herself was covered with dust and dirt, and in the streets people were sheltering in doorways, and taking little runs for safety as soon as a shell had finished bursting. The bombardment lasted about an hour, and we all waited in the kitchen and listened to it.

About 8.15 the bombardment ceased, and we went in to a cheery dinner – soup, turkey, and plum-pudding, with crackers and speeches.

At 9.30 I went to the station. It was very melancholy. No one was there but myself. The fires were out, or smoking badly. I got things in order as soon as I could and the wounded in the train got their hot soup and coffee as usual, which was a satisfaction. Then I came home alone at midnight – keeping as near the houses as I could because of possible shells – and so to bed, very cold, and rather too inclined to think about home …

Miss May Sinclair

Dr Hector Munro's Ambulance Unit, Ghent, Belgium

May Sinclair, aged 51 and an established novelist, became the 'Secretary and Reporter' to the thirteen strong ambulance unit raised by Dr Hector Munro when war was declared. Her role was to keep the accounts, write Dr Munro's reports, and articles for the daily newspapers. After initial doubts the British Red Cross agreed to buy the ambulances and the unit arrived in Ostend towards the end of September 1914. The members included Mairi Chisholm [qv], Elsie Knocker [qv] and Lady Dorothie Feilding. The Unit's first Headquarters were in Ghent at the magnificent Flandria Palace Hôtel where some were given bedrooms and private sitting-rooms, although all the fine furniture and draperies had been removed to make an auxiliary hospital. The billiard-room was an operating theatre, the dining-room, reception rooms and some bedrooms became wards. There were only about 100 wounded when they arrived but they were told to be ready to drive out to collect casualties. May Sinclair had a room at the Hôtel Cecil.

Sunday, 11 October 1914
8am
Antwerp has fallen. Taube over Ghent in the night.
We expect that we may have to clear out of Ghent before tomorrow.

4.45pm
Went over to the Convent de Saint Pierre, where Miss Ashley-Smith [qv] is with her British wounded. I had to warn her that the Germans may come in tonight. I had told the Commandant [Dr Munro] about her yesterday, and arranged with him that we should take her and her British away in our Ambulance if we have to go.

The Convent is a little way beyond the Place on the boulevard. I knew it by the Red Cross hanging from the upper windows. Everything is as happy and peaceful here as if Ghent were not on the eve of an invasion. The nuns took me to Miss Ashley-Smith in her ward. Absolutely unperturbed by the news, she went on superintending the disposal of a table of surgical instruments. She would not consent to come with us at first. But the nuns persuaded her that she would do no good by remaining.

I am to come again and tell her what time to be ready with her wounded, when we know whether we are going and when.

The night goes on. I sit with Mr —— for a little while. It is appalling to me that the time should seem long. For it is really such a little while, and when it is over there will be nothing more that I shall ever do for him … He holds out his hands to be sponged, 'if I don't mind'. I sponge them over and over again with iced water and eau de Cologne, gently and very slowly. I am afraid lest he should be aware that there is any hurry. The time goes on.

It is time that I should go round to the Convent to tell Miss Ashley-Smith to be ready with her British before two o'clock …

It is nearly two o'clock. Downstairs, in the great silent hall two British wounded are waiting for some ambulance to take them to the Station. They are sitting bolt upright on chairs near the doorway, their heads nodding with drowsiness. One or two Belgian Red Cross men wait beside them. Opposite them, on three other chairs, the three doctors sit waiting for our own ambulance to take them. They have been up all night and are utterly exhausted. They sit, fast asleep, with their heads bowed on their breasts.

Outside, the darkness has mist and a raw cold sting in it.

A wretched ambulance wagon drawn by two horses is driven up to the door. It had a hood once, but the hood has disappeared and only the naked hoops remain. The British wounded from two other hospitals are packed in it in two rows. They sit bolt upright under the hoops, exposed to mist and to the raw cold sting of the night; some of them wear their blankets like shawls over their shoulders as they were taken from their beds. The shawls and the head bandages give these British a strange, foreign look, infinitely helpless, infinitely pitiful.

Nobody seems to be out there but Mrs Torrence [Mrs Knocker] and one or two Belgian Red Cross men. She and I help to get our two men taken gently out of the hall and stowed away in the ambulance wagon. There are not enough blankets. We try to find some.

At the last minute two bearers come forward, carrying a third. He is tall and thin; he is wrapped in a coat flung loosely over his sleeping-jacket; he wears a turban of bandages; his long bare feet stick out as he is carried along. It is Cameron, my poor Highlander, who was shot through the brain.

They lift him, very gently, into the wagon.

Then, very gently, they lift him out again.

This attempt to save him is desperate. He is dying.

Presently they carry him back into the Hospital.

They can't find any blankets. I run over to the Hôtel Cecil for my thick, warm travelling-rug to wrap round the knees of the wounded, shivering in the wagon.

It is all I can do for them.

And presently the wagon is turned round, slowly, almost solemnly, and driven off into the darkness and the cold mist, with its load of weird and piteous figures, wrapped in blankets like shawls. Their bandages show blurred white spots in the mist, and they are gone.

It is horrible.

I go over and pack and dress for the journey. I leave behind what I don't need and it takes seven minutes.

Now it is time to go and fetch Miss Ashley-Smith and her three wounded men from the Convent.

They are all there, ready and waiting. And the Mother Superior and two of her nuns are in the corridor. They bring out glasses of hot milk for everybody. They are so gentle and so kind that I recall with agony my impatience when I rang at their gate. Even familiar French words desert me in this crisis, and I implore Miss Ashley-Smith to convey my regrets for my rudeness. Their only answer is to smile and press hot milk on me. I am glad of it, for I have been so absorbed in the drama of preparation that I have entirely forgotten to eat anything since lunch.

The wounded are brought along the passage. We help them into the ambulance. Two are only slightly wounded; they can sit up all the way. But the third is wounded in the head. Sometimes he is delirious and must be looked after. A fourth man is dying and must be left behind.

Then we say goodbye to the nuns

The other ambulance cars are drawn up in the Place before the 'Flandria' waiting.

We arrange for the final disposal of the wounded in one of the Daimlers, where they can all lie down.

It is quarter to three.

They are all ready now. The Commandant is there giving the final orders and stowing away the nine wounded he had brought from Melle. The hall of the Hospital is utterly deserted. So is the Place outside it. And in the stillness and desolation our going has an air of intolerable secrecy, of furtive avoidance of fate. This Field Ambulance of ours abhors retreat.

It is dark with the black darkness before dawn.

And the Belgian Red Cross guides have all gone. There is nobody to show us the roads.

At the last minute we find a Belgian soldier who will take us as far as Ecloo.

The Commandant has arranged to stay at Ecloo for a few hours. Some friends there have offered him their house. The wounded are to be put up at the Convent there. Ecloo is about half-way between Ghent and Bruges.

We are not going so very fast, not faster than the three cars behind us, and the slowest of the three (the Fiat with the hard tyres, carrying the baggage) sets the pace. We must keep within their sight or they may lose their way. But though we are not really going fast, the speed seems intolerable.

Somewhere on this road the Belgian Army has gone before us. We have got to go with it. We have had our orders. The Belgian Army is retreating, and we are retreating with it.

If it had occurred to me to stay behind for the sake of one man who couldn't be moved and who had the best surgeon in the Hospital and the pick of the nursing-staff to look after him, I think I should have disposed of the idea as sheer sentimentalism.

When I was with him tonight I could think of nothing but the wounded in the Convent of Saint Pierre. And afterwards there had been so much to do.

And now that there was nothing more to do, I couldn't think of anything but that one man.

The night before came back to me in a vision, or rather an obsession, infinitely more present, more visible and palpable than this night that we were living in. The light with the red shade hung just over my head on my right hand; the blond walls were round me; they shut me in alone with the wounded man who lay stretched before me on the bed. And the moments were measured by the rhythm of his breathing, and by the closing and opening of his eyes.

I thought, he will open his eyes tonight and look for me and I shall not be there. He will know that he has been left to the Belgians, who cannot understand him, whom he cannot understand. And he will think that I have betrayed him.

I felt as if I had betrayed him.

I am sitting between Mr Riley [a stretcher-bearer] and Miss Ashley-Smith. Mr Riley is ill; he has got blood-poisoning through a cut in his hand. Every now and then I remember him, and draw the rug over his knees as it slips. Miss Ashley-Smith, tired with her night watching, has gone to sleep with her head on my shoulder, where it must be horribly jolted and shaken by my cough, which of course chooses this moment to break out again. I try to get into a position that will rest her better; and between her and Mr Riley I forget for a second.

Then the obsession begins again, and I am shut in between the blond walls with the wounded man.

I feel his hand and arm lying heavily on my shoulder in the attempt to support me as I kneel by his bed with my arms stretched out together under the hollow of his back, as we wait for the pillow that never comes.

It is quite certain that I have betrayed him.

It seems to me then that nothing that could happen to me in Ghent could be more infernal than leaving it. And I think that when the ambulance stops to put down the Belgian soldier I will get out and walk back with him to Ghent.

We have got to Ecloo before we seem to have put 3 miles between us and Ghent.

Still, though I'm dead tired when we get there, I can walk 3 miles easily. I do not feel at all insane with my obsession. On the contrary, these moments are moments of exceptional lucidity. While the Commandant goes to look for the Convent I get out and look for the Belgian soldier. I tell him I want to go back to Ghent. I ask him how far it is to walk, and if he will take me. And he says it is 20 kilometres. I am just sane enough to know that I can't walk as far as that if I'm to be any good when I get there.

We wait in the village while they find the Convent and take the wounded men there; we wait while the Commandant goes off in the dark to find his friend's house.

The house stands in a garden somewhere beyond the railway station, up a rough village street and a stretch of country road. It is about four in the morning when we get there …

Our kind Dutch host and our kind English hostess have got up out of their beds to receive us. This hospitality of theirs is not a little thing when you think that their house is to be invaded by Germans, perhaps today.

They have only one spare bedroom, which they offer; but they have filled their drawing-room with blankets; piles and piles of white fleecy blankets on chairs and sofas and on the floor. And they have built up a roaring fire. It is as if they were succouring fifteen survivors of shipwreck or of earthquake. To be sure, we are flying from Ghent, but we have only flown 20 kilometres as yet.

I don't know how I got through the next three hours, for my obsession came back on me again and again, and as soon as I shut my eyes I saw the face and eyes of the wounded man.

I remember finding myself in the garden, at sunrise.

The next thing I remember is the Chaplain coming to me and our going together, into the dining-room, and Miss Ashley-Smith joining us there. My malady was contagious and she had caught it, but with no damage to her self-control.

She says very simply and quietly that she is going back to Ghent. And the infection spreads to the Chaplain. He says that neither of us is going back to Ghent, but that he is going. With difficulty we convince him that it would be useless for any man to go. He would be taken prisoner the minute he showed his nose in the 'Flandria' and set to dig trenches till the end of the War.

Then he says, if only he had his cassock with him. They would respect that (which is open to doubt).

We are a long time discussing which of us is going back to Ghent. Miss Ashley-Smith is fertile and ingenious in argument. She is a nurse and I and the Chaplain are not.

And while we are still arguing, we go out on the road that leads to the village, to find the ambulances and see if any of the chauffeurs will take us back to Ghent. I am not very hopeful about the means of transport. I do not think that Tom or any of the chauffeurs will move, this time, without orders from the Commandant. I do not think that the Commandant will let any of us go except himself.

And Miss Ashley-Smith says, if only she had a horse.

If she had a horse she would be in Ghent in no time. Perhaps, if none of the chauffeurs will take her back, she can find a horse in the village.

She keeps on saying very quietly and simply that she is going and explaining the reasons why she should go rather than anybody else. And I bring forward every reason I can think of why she should do nothing of the sort.

I abhor the possibility of her going back instead of me.

And in the end, with an extreme quietness and simplicity, she went.

We had not yet found the ambulance cars, and it seemed pretty certain that Miss Ashley-Smith would not get her horse any more than the Chaplain could get his cassock.

And then, just when we thought the difficulties of transport were insuperable, we came straight on the railway lines and the station, where a train had pulled up on its way to Ghent. Miss Ashley-Smith got on to the train. I got on too, to go with her, and the Chaplain, who is abominably strong, put his arms round my waist and pulled me off.

I have never ceased to wish that I had hung on to that train.

On our way back to the house we met the Commandant and told him what had happened. I said I thought it was the worst thing that had happened yet. It wasn't the smallest consolation when he said it was the most sensible solution.

And when Mrs Torrence for fifteen consecutive seconds took the view that I had decoyed Miss Ashley-Smith out on to that accursed road in order to send her to Ghent, and deliberately persuaded her to go back to the 'Flandria' instead of me, for fifteen consecutive seconds I believed that this diobolical thing was what I had actually done.

And on circumstantial evidence the case was black against me. When last seen, Miss Ashley-Smith was entirely willing to be saved. She goes out for a walk with me along a quiet country road, and the next thing you hear is that she has gone back to Ghent. And since, actually and really, it was my obsession that had passed into her, I felt that if I had taken Miss Ashley-Smith down that road and murdered her in a dyke my responsibility wouldn't have been a bit worse, if as bad.

And it seemed to me that all the people scattered among the blankets in that strange room, those that still lay snuggling down amiably in the warmth, and those that had started to their feet in dismay, and those that sat on chairs upright and apart, were hostile with a just and righteous hostility, that they had an intimate knowledge of my crime, and had risen up in abhorrence of the thing I was.

And somewhere, as if they were far off in some blessed place on the other side of this nightmare, I was aware of the merciful and pitiful faces of Mrs Lambert and Janet McNeil [Mairi Chisholm].

Then, close beside me, there was a sudden heaving of the Chaplain's broad shoulders as he faced the room.

And I heard him saying, in the same voice in which he had declared that he was going to hold Matins, that it wasn't my fault at all – that it was he who had persuaded Miss Ashley-Smith to go back to Ghent.

Then Mrs Torrence says that she is going back to protect Miss Ashley-Smith and Ursula Dearmer [Lady Dorothie Feilding] says that she is going back to protect Mrs Torrence.

And there can be no doubt that three motor ambulances, with possibly the entire Corps inside them, certainly with the five women and the Chaplain and the Commandant, would presently have been seen tearing along the road to Ghent, one in violent pursuit of the other, if we had not telephoned and received news of Miss Ashley-Smith's safe arrival at the 'Flandria' and orders that no more women were to return to Ghent …

Miss Grace Ashley-Smith

First Aid Nursing Yeomanry Corps, Antwerp and Ghent, Belgium

In 1910 Grace Ashley-Smith became one of the organisers of the First Aid Nursing Yeomanry Corps (FANYs). She was at sea on the way to South Africa when war was declared and sent a wireless message to Cape Town to book her a return passage as soon as possible after arrival.

By mid-September she was in a Belgian ambulance rescuing casualties from the battlefields round Antwerp and working in a 300-bed hospital in the city. After the retreat from Antwerp on 10 October 1914 she was based at Ghent.

My adventures have come thick and fast within the last ten days. I date the most thrilling from Monday a fortnight ago, on the 19th, my first day actually under fire. The English and Belgians were fighting in the trenches round Lierre, and I went out with a Belgian motor ambulance to look for wounded. I was accompanied by a Belgian gentleman who works for the Red Cross and a Belgian driver. We were bound for Buckerout, where a sort of collecting hospital was being run, about 7 kilometres from Lierre. On our way two cyclists stopped us – Belgian soldiers (one came on the car to show us the way), and told us of wounded at an outpost 3 kilometres from Lierre. They asked if I was afraid, and, of course, I said we must go. It was a quick run out along a lonely road, and we stopped the ambulance under cover of a brick building, stables or something. The trenches were 200 yards away, and my Belgian friend and the chauffeur, with our soldier guide ran off at once. I pelted after them, and suddenly realised that the noise all round was shells and shrapnel flying. For a moment terror seized me. I had a silver medal hanging from a button on my uniform, and I stopped to hide the glitter of it in my pocket. A mechanical action, naturally … Then I ran on hard, and whilst the men picked the worse wounded up I helped a man whose right leg was torn fearfully. He leant on my shoulder and hopped on the other leg. Suddenly there was a deafening crash, and for a few seconds I stood blinking my eyes, wondering where my man with the bad leg had vanished to. Looking round I saw him lying flat in a big ditch by the side of the field; and the other men all there too. Then it struck me a shell had burst close to us, and I ran and sat down in the ditch also. However, by this time they were crawling out, and with three soldiers I made a dash down the road and across to a thin tree. The three Belgians hung on to the tree, and I stood in front of them, and looking at their white faces and wild eyes I realised from the tension round my heart that I must be as white and scared looking and suddenly I laughed, for the absurdity of the little thin tree affording protection to four big people reminded me of a cinematograph film. Well, we made other dashes after that, and got to our motor ambulance and returned in triumph. This time we struck Buckerout and English marines and doctors, and filled up with more wounded. I rode into Antwerp standing on the step, as every seat was taken for wounded.

Next day we returned to Buckerout, and found a big rush of wounded to be patched up and sent to Antwerp.

I commandeered a big GS waggon full of bread, turned out the bread, got mattresses and pillows and blankets from an empty house, and filled it up with wounded. Two motor 'buses full of wounded went off also. The motor ambulance I was with went too, and still more arrived. Poor men, some were too far gone to be saved. All of them, English and Belgian, showed wonderful courage. They were brought in on waggons and motors etc. Then came a lull in the day's work, and later a message came there were two wounded about 2 kilometres farther on. So off I went with my motor ambulance, and we met a motor car returning with one man on a stretcher. We got to a little house by itself, and found there a few Belgian soldiers and an Englishman who is attached to the Belgian Army. We took cover under a stone wall whilst a Priest and a soldier went to bring in the wounded. From where we stood we saw a shell explode quite close and tear up the road. The Englishman had a big shrapnel that had come down without bursting and was guarding it as a trophy! All round us in the air we saw the little clouds of smoke that denote the presence of shrapnel. The sound grew so familiar I miss it here in Ghent. The sharp, hissing shizz-zz-zz-boom and the moment's suspense – the involuntary holding of one's breath until the shrapnel has fallen.

The English doctors were splendid – so brave – and one I heard had worked all night long in the trenches in the most dangerous places. The others had had little or no sleep, and no time for food. The St John's men were there too; brave and ready for any emergency. It was nice to work amongst our own men. The Belgians are splendid and cannot do enough for one, but one's heart warms to the khaki and blue and our own men. One St John's man insisted on my accepting a bar of chocolate from him and a sailor made me a present of two pears, and a soldier in khaki came to me with a shy smile and a bunch of mignonette. I think they, too, were glad to see my khaki uniform, and know I was their own countrywoman.

All the way into Antwerp we ran through lines of blue jackets just arrived, and how they cheered their little sister in khaki.

Next day (Wednesday) I ran out in my motor ambulance in the same direction, but alas, what a change. Troops coming into Antwerp retiring, and one lot of men coming back at the double. At Vieux Dieu what a contrast! Yesterday all had been activity – khaki everywhere – the English headquarters full of life and bustle. Today, empty streets, the whiz-zz-zz boom of shrapnel overhead; the English headquarters deserted. I met a car full of English staff officers coming towards Antwerp, and stopped to ask them if they knew where the collecting station was, or where there were wounded. One of them said abruptly, 'There are no wounded, and it is not safe for an ambulance, the firing line is 200 yards further on.' We went on a little further, and some Belgians told us there were wounded 8 kilometres farther on, so we ran on through Buckerout. But, what a desert! No hospital, no troops, no ambulances; a few stray dogs, and a few dead horses. We came on little groups of soldiers. One poured out his tale at once. Retreat. God knows I have seen dreadful things: the horrors and suffering of War, dead and dying. I have held my breath at the approach of shrapnel, but never till that moment had tears come to my eyes. My Belgian orderly and my Belgian chauffeur tried to check the narrator. They silently tried to show their sympathy with me. Then we got in the two wounded, and went off. We overtook a party of English marines (Red Cross mostly), wheeling a wounded Belgian on a barrow, and carrying their stretchers.

The run back was as thrilling as the run out, and right glad I was to get inside the barricades and see our sailors working on the trenches. We made a few excursions in all directions to find wounded but were happily disappointed.

That afternoon I spent at the forts – the ambulance being useful in fetching dressings and medical stores for the English doctors; and also I got some loaves of white bread, cheese and butter brought out, and very thankfully they were received after days of biscuits and bully beef. The poor Red Cross Company had no rations with them, as they had lost their own company – they were the men we had overtaken in the morning.

On our way back to Antwerp we overtook an English naval officer on his way to headquarters with a despatch, and we gave him a lift. We were stopped in the town of Vieux Dieu to deal with a Belgian thief who had looted a house where there were only two women. That little affair settled and the thief arrested and left with Belgian soldiers, we got to the English headquarters. There a jolly Jack Tar found me a cup of delicious coffee, and was quite sad because I wouldn't have chicken broth prepared too. A trusting ADC, Vere Harmsworth, confided his sword to my charge, and we set off again with our despatch bearer – got him safely into a car to take him to his fort, and returned to Antwerp. We were late, and my Belgian hosts had fled, so I gratefully accepted a bed in the cellar of the house next to the hospital for the night. That was Wednesday. On Tuesday I had a suite of rooms – on Wednesday a cellar.

I was late and had hardly finished my journal when twelve o'clock struck, and whiz-zz-boom came the first shrapnel over Antwerp! I leapt up and turned on my light and had no time to don a dressing gown before father, mother, five sons, daughters, grandmother, servants, and another nurse from the hospital came tumbling into the cellar! I seized my clothes and bolted upstairs to dress. Then the other nurse and I went to the hospital and helped to carry down all the wounded to the cellars and kitchen passages. What a night it was! About 2.30 we had some coffee, and then scattered ourselves to try and rest. I went to the courtyard and lay on a wooden bench, and cringed at each whizz of shrapnel overhead. Later I went in and lay on the stone floor behind the front door near one of the doctors and sister. At 5.30 two cars left and took three wounded with them. The bombardment continued; at 10.30 three English soldiers came in wounded and said there were lots of wounded in the trenches, so I walked down to the Place de Meir (Red Cross Headquarters) to try and get my motor ambulance, which should have called for me at nine o'clock. It was a weird experience to walk along the almost empty streets and hear the shrapnel overhead and all round; see, too, houses falling, and poor people fleeing wildly away with a few belongings tied up roughly. At the Red Cross Headquarters all was confusion – nobody knew where anybody else was to be found. As I turned to leave two English doctors, Dr Soutter and Dr Beavis, came in, and almost at the same moment, a shell burst outside with a deafening crash, killing two people. I was more than grateful when they called to me they would take me back in their car. That ended the Red Cross for the moment; we three English were left alone, as everyone made a hurried exit.

The rest of that day we spent in loading wounded into motor 'buses – an unhappy proceeding, for instead of allowing the worst cases to be left with one or two people to take care of them, all were bundled in, and a sad procession left Antwerp. The roads were rough – the way was long, doubly so, for a wide detour was necessary to avoid Germans – the cold was intense – over that night it is better to draw a veil of silence. For we who were strong it was hard, for the wounded, God help them. Hell and the tortures of the damned used to be expressions conveying nothing to my mind – but now I can realise what hell means.

We arrived at Ghent at 5.30 on Friday morning, and panic seemed to prevail. Everyone declared the Germans would arrive in three hours. Wounded were left here and there – exhausted, tired out – after that night of horror, and the motor 'buses and the staff went on to Ostend.

In Ghent our troops and the French came in on Friday, and on Saturday everywhere the Belgians gave them of their best – coffee, tea, fruit, chocolates and cigarettes. Loud cheers greeted every British regiment. On Sunday it seemed likely the wounded might be moved. On Sunday afternoon the English Consul got a telephone message from Ostend to leave. On Sunday, at midnight, I was offered places for myself and the English wounded I was looking after in some English ambulances. Miss May Sinclair [qv] the novelist, kindly remembered me in that trying hour – she was with Dr Hector Munro's Ambulance Fleet. At 2.30am Monday, they called for me [at the Convent de Saint Pierre], and at 5.30 we stopped at Ecloo, 25 kilometres away. There was a hard frost, the cold was intense. We were taken into an English house with a big fire blazing, and blankets and pillows were handed round. Then it appeared that the ambulance party had come away [from the auxiliary hospital in the Flandria Palace Hôtel] leaving behind an English officer [Lieutenant Richard Foote] who was too ill to be moved. There were seven women and about ten men in their personnel – and one lady, Miss Sinclair, wanted to return but knew nothing about nursing. A young clergyman also spoke of returning. They had been kind to think of me, a stranger, and I was grateful to them for their thought – but there was only one thing to do. I walked out and down the road – this lady and the clergyman with me – got to Ecloo Station, and luckily found a train just starting for Ghent, so I jumped in. I was frightened. I admit my heart was in my boots – I was cold and hungry and very tired – and I felt forlorn indeed. Two Flemish peasants came from a third class car and looked at my khaki uniform and my Red Cross and tried to be nice to me. I got out at Ghent, and all the people stared. I got to the Flandria; and the relief of the young Englishman when I entered repaid me tenfold for the terrors I had undergone. All was in disorder and confusion. I had to go and get water, and look for everything I wanted. There were a few Belgian ladies left. About eleven o'clock we carried my Englishman on a stretcher to a nursing home near, and there, to my intense relief, I found a Scotswoman, Miss Maud Fletcher of Guy's Hospital. The reaction was almost too great. I suddenly realised I had had no breakfast; that I was no longer a forlorn Scotchwoman awaiting with horror the arrival of wicked enemies. I had found friends where I had looked for nothing but hard treatment.

The Germans came; but the wounded officer was in good hands, and I slept off all the night's fatigue. Next night I sat up with him; and seven Germans were quartered in the house. Each time a footstep passed, I wondered, 'Is this the end?' But dawn came, and we had not been molested. What was more, he still lived, though the doctor had thought he would not see another day. Next night I watched again – but alas! Though the night passed, the morning brought death in its train. I wanted to go and ask the German General for a Military funeral. I wanted a Union Jack … and I was so strongly urged against both courses, I left it. I went out disguised in mufti to make the necessary arrangements. I asked the American Consul to come to the funeral, but he said he couldn't. So next day a gallant officer was buried by three women – a Scotch nurse in Guy's Hospital uniform, a Belgian nurse (also trained at Guy's) in the same, and I, in my khaki First Aid Nursing Yeomanry uniform. We followed his hearse – we passed through lines of German soldiers, who eyed my khaki with amazement, but did not molest us – and there in a foreign cemetery we came to a plot of ground set aside for soldiers. There were ten graves already, and into one we lowered our countryman's body, and I, a woman in my khaki British uniform, supported by two Guy's nurses, read the burial service over him. It was a sad, and a strange scene, on a dismal autumn day, a group of poor Flemish people standing near in reverent silence, and German soldiers in their drab uniform all round. So we left him at rest; and my heart was very sad thinking how different this ending was to his dream of war when he left England ten days before. Two other Englishmen lie near him – one an 'unknown' ambulance man, the other a sailor.

After that my work was done, so I drove to the Spanish Consul, whom the American Consul said was entrusted with English interests, but there I was told the Spanish Consul had nothing to do with English interests; so I drove to the German Staff Headquarters, walked through the sentries in my khaki uniform, and asked to see the General. I was conducted to a group of officers, most of whom spoke perfect English. They opened their eyes wide at my khaki, and saluted me. I told them I had been here to nurse English wounded, and now I wanted to go back to England, and asked for a passport. They were very polite, and almost sympathetic, but said no one was allowed Eastwards. I must go to Brussels, and perhaps get papers there to permit me to go to Germany, and from thence to England. I assured them I had no wish to go to Brussels, and still less to go to Germany, and suggested that they should let me go to Holland. However, they assured me that was impossible. One young officer asked how I would go to Brussels – it was very far to walk. I politely assured him that I did not want to go to Brussels, and if they wanted me to go there they would have to send me. They assured me that they were grieved I could not go to England, but – it was war! We parted with salutes, and I swanked out through rows of Germans as if the earth was indeed mine, for being the only possessor of khaki in Ghent I felt I must live up to it.

Today I went out openly in my khaki. The Germans all looked wildly amazed when they caught sight of me; one man jumped violently. I think he thought me a British soldierman; only two have scowled on me. For the most part they seem to be 'en bon camarade'. One Sergeant drew up his men to attention and saluted! And several of the soldiers saluted me in the streets. It is rather humorous to see me marching along in khaki, typically English, and hundreds of German soldiers swarming round me. The Belgians think me quite mad I expect; they come and ask me if I am not afraid: they cannot do enough for me; and to see me and German officers making purchases side by side or travelling on the same tramcars is decidedly funny. I am more than surprised they permit it; but I must say their behaviour is admirable. They open doors for women, they make way for women to pass. The soldiers quartered here actually go on tiptoes in the corridors because we have invalids who have just had operations.

At the German Headquarters yesterday, there was a jolly old General with twinkling eyes, who seemed hugely to enjoy the whole situation, and I am certain he would have let me go back to England if he could. I suppose really it was rather unique – a Scotch girl in khaki walking calmly into the enemy's stronghold and demanding a pass to England!

Mrs Elsie Knocker

Advanced Dressing Station, Pervyse, Belgium

Mrs Elsie Knocker, divorced from her husband, was a trained nurse and midwife, and an expert driver and mechanic by the time war was declared in August 1914. She had been one of the first women to take up motorcycling seriously and owned a Chater Lea motorcycle. She joined Dr Hector Munro's Ambulance Corps which had already been rejected by the War Office, British, French and American Red Cross. When the Belgian Red Cross accepted their services the British Red Cross gave its blessings and paid for some ambulances to go to Belgium.

Helen Gleason, Lady Dorothie Feilding, May Sinclair [qv], and Mairi Chisholm [qv], an eighteen-year-old Scots girl, were also members of the corps. Miss Chisholm was a good driver and mechanic and before the unit set off for Belgium, she and Mrs Knocker, who were already friends, drove as despatch riders in London as part of the newly-formed Women's Emergency Corps.

On the evening of 11 October, at the auxiliary hospital in the Flandria Palace Hôtel, Mrs Knocker was nursing a young British subaltern who had been riddled with machine-gun bullets. She was told that the Germans were expected in Ghent in five hours and that every British soldier in the hospital who could be moved was to be evacuated in the ambulances. However, the subaltern was too badly wounded to be moved, and although several members of the unit offered to stay with him, the Belgian doctors assured them he would be cared for by themselves and the Germans and that it would be too complicated and dangerous for the unit to stay. [See Grace Ashley-Smith's and May Sinclair's account of this incident].

The convoy of retreating ambulances also took Grace Ashley-Smith [qv] and the wounded British patients she was nursing in the Convent de Saint Pierre. They reached Ostend just before the Germans arrived, and managed to send the wounded off in a small ship sailing to England.

The ambulance unit was then based at a Hospital in Furnes which was housed in a Convent and a school and was 'pitifully inadequate'.

The remnants of the Belgian army and a few French troops held the eastern end of the front line which stretched from Nieuport to Dixmude and on to Ypres, and the drivers of the Munro Ambulance Corps were immediately sent into action, driving the ambulances, day and night, in bitterly cold weather to gather casualties from the Dixmude sector. As soon as they set down the wounded Belgian and French soldiers and German prisoners at the hospital, they returned again to the battlefields.

Mrs Knocker drove a heavy Napier ambulance and 'other strange vehicles at a moment's notice – including Daimlers, Wolseleys, Mercedes, Pipes, Sunbeams, and Fiats'. She became increasingly appalled by the casualty rate, the lack of medical facilities, and the chaotic conditions in the hospital.

I wanted to set up a first-aid station (or Advanced Dressing Station, as it was called) where the wounded could rest and recuperate before being jolted over the roads to the operating table. I had noticed how many of them died of superficial hurts, a broken arm, perhaps, or a gash. They died on the way to hospital, or on the pavements or the floors, and I knew why this happened. They were the victims of shock – the greatest killer of them all.

At first it seemed that I would never get even a cellar to work in. I went to Dunkirk to badger Sir Bertrand Dawson, medical chief of the BEF, and talked to Prince Alexander of Teck. Both were sympathetic, and gave me all the support in their power then and later, but they were so busy with a multitude of things. Admiral Ronarch [commander of the French Fusilier Marin garrisoned at Dixmude] who happened to be present when I was pleading with Sir Bertrand, scoffed openly, and became very angry when I persisted. He had never heard anything quite so absurd. Surely I knew that women were not allowed in the trenches? They had to be at least 3 miles behind the lines. If I chose to disobey orders I could expect no assistance, and that meant no rations and no medical supplies.

I firmly believed in my mission – for such it had become to me after much thought – I would go, with or without assistance.

I made my preparations, undeterred by the fact of Dr Munro's disapproval.

The next thing was to find a suitable place to start a post. I was fortunate to meet a Belgian Army doctor, Dr Van der Ghinst, who fully agreed with my plan. He had spent weeks in Dixmude and knew that I was not talking out of the back of my head. He suggested that a village called Pervyse might be the spot, and we drove out there to have a look. There was not a house which one could even pig it in – it was just one huge fallen mass, heaped-up bricks and stones. The dead horses, cows, and sheep looked so pathetic.

Yet behind the intervening floods the Belgians had set about fortifying the place. The crude earthworks thrown up in the heat and hurry of battle were being linked and converted into a system of trenches and dug-outs. Two houses, both with deep, damp but safe cellars, remained fairly intact. In one of them some Belgian officers had their quarters. The other one was offered to me, and with it went the good wishes and a promise of co-operation from the officers and men to whom Dr Van der Ghinst introduced me and explained my idea.

'Our house' – for it was soon settled that Mairi Chisholm, who had proved herself brave and steady as well as being an excellent driver, should accompany me – was a woeful sight. There was not a pane of glass left whole, the roof had fallen in, the walls were ominously cracked, and everything that was any good had been taken or looted. It was right at the edge of the village, nearest the tottering church and the trenches, and the stream of shells which the Germans lobbed across the water meant that we should have to sleep, cook, and nurse in the cellar.

The cellar was about ten feet by twelve, dimly lit by gratings set into the pavement above. Two soldiers, Alphonse and Désiré, who had been sleeping there on some straw, rustled up a table and a few chairs for us, and some boards to surround our sleeping straw, which they renewed as often as possible. The stove sometimes smoked badly, but in that icy winter of 1914 we were able to overlook such trifles. We slept in our clothes, and cut our hair short so that it would tuck inside our caps. Dressing meant simply putting on our boots. Most nights Tom Woffington, our Cockney driver, and Alexandre, the 18-year-old cook who was assigned to us, slept in the cellar too.

Ablutions were infrequent and difficult. Alexandre sometimes managed to heat some ditch water, and we would try to wash down in a huge old copper while he kept watch at the top of the steps and prevented any new patients from coming down before we were decent. Now and again we would get to Furnes or Dunkirk for a good soak, but there were times when we had to scrape the lice off with the blunt edge of a knife, and our underclothes stuck to us.

There was no sanitation, and for some time we had to go down a convenient shell-hole to relieve nature while Alphonse or Desire kept guard. Later, this devoted couple brought us a magnificent commode which they had somehow managed to find, complete with a screen which they had made out of some old sheets.

Disposing of soiled bandages was a problem, but after a while in Pervyse one forgot the niceties. The village had been taken and retaken several times in the Battle of the Yser, and the graveyard was choked with corpses of several nationalities, exposed by the heavy rains. Our only available water-supply ran through the middle of the courtyard, and even when it had been boiled it had a horrible taste.

We soon contrived to make the house cheery, by hanging on the walls the flags of Belgium, France, and Scotland and a fine defiant Union Jack. Spoons, forks, and crockery were discovered in a derelict farmhouse, and Alphonse and Desire scraped up some vegetables from the abandoned gardens. Alexandre boiled up a great soup stew in his copper in a lean-to outhouse at the back. Every night more horses were killed bringing up food and ammunition, and they provided the meat on the menu. Now that he had been appointed cook, Alexandre took on a new dignity. He was no longer a private – he was a chef, a man of importance.

The trenches were only five yards away, and in those first days we took jug after jug of soup or hot chocolate to the men on watch. When they were relieved the men would come over to the Cellar House, as it became known, and queue up with their mugs. At night we took hot drinks to the sentries in the outposts at the end of the causeways which ran out into the floods. An officer accompanied us through the icy and often misty darkness, giving the password as we were challenged. The machine-gunners had scooped a dug-out of sorts: a hand would emerge, grasp the jug, and draw it in. In a few seconds it would be returned empty. All was done in silence, and when the odd star shell curved down towards us inquisitively we would have to stand stock still.

The soup and the chocolate made us known and welcome, but they were only a sideline.

The fearful winter of 1914 brought us more casualties than German bullets or shells. The men's clothes were hopelessly inadequate for the intense cold. Frostbite, pneumonia, and bronchitis followed nights of exposure, and I spent many a spare moment writing to friends and acquaintances at home begging for warm clothes. Men came in with festering sores after scratching themselves on barbed wire, or in agony with swollen, inflamed feet. Sometimes a soldier would have no obvious symptoms, except that he was 'quite done-up' and incapable of any exertion. We put such cases of trench fatigue on clean straw in the corner, covered them with blankets, arranged a good supply of hot-water bottles, and let them sleep round the clock. More often than not they were new men when they got up.

There were curious accidents. One man fell down a deep crater in the dark, and gashed his head badly on a jagged piece of shell. Another came in with his hand in an appalling state: he had been wearing gloves at the time of the explosion, and bits of glove were mixed up with shredded flesh, and had to be picked out. Stray shrapnel and a moment of carelessness brought some horrible casualties. A piece of shell had penetrated one young fellow's head and blinded him …

Mme Curie, who, with her daughter, was running an X-ray unit in Furnes, was most interested in the work, and did me the honour of visiting the Cellar House. She was only five feet tall, soft-spoken and gentle in manner. We had a long and most interesting technical talk about methods of treatment, and she agreed with me that the three great priorities of nursing were quiet, rest, and warmth.

The shelling got so bad that we were forced to move to the other house farther back in the village, while keeping our first cellar as a forward dressing-station. The Daimler ambulance was riddled with shrapnel, and we got quite sentimental over it, for it was like seeing an old friend wounded …

Our daily work taxed us to the limit of our physical strength. Mairi and I often went out to help bring in the wounded, and between us lifted a man in full field kit with rifle and tin-hat. There was the first wrenching jerk from off the ground to waist-level, and then the stumbling over mud and slush and cratered roads.

Many people, especially British officers, thoroughly disapproved of our being at Pervyse. It just did not fit in with their conventions, and they would start off by wasting a great deal of breath in arguments which simply ran like water off a duck's back. I let them get on with it, and then asked them to contribute something to keep the work going, instead of grumbling about it. Most of them responded very well with gifts of food and drink – much needed in the first months when we had to depend on scrounging for our own food: Alphonse once spent a whole day shooting twelve sparrows which he brought to us for supper.

Naturally I was more concerned about getting official approval for our mission. Sir Bertrand Dawson visited us several times and told me that he had noticed that wounded who had been nursed at Pervyse arrived at hospital in far better condition. He had put in a favourable report but it was now up to the Allied Council in Paris to decide whether or not to let us continue.

Weeks later Sir Bernard called. I was particularly busy bandaging a nasty chest-wound, and could not get away. I knew what his mission was, and he gave me such a wonderful warm smile that I guessed it was all right – and so it was. My work had been recognised, and in the most flattering terms. Mairi and I were to be allowed to stay where we were – the only exceptions on the whole of the Western Front. I was to have rations and any help I needed with medical supplies, and to be taken on the strength of whichever unit took over that part of the line.

Straight away I wrote to the British Red Cross Society, and from then on I had their full support, and could add the Red Cross flag to our array. They sent me a fine lot of equipment, even including a complete set of dental instruments. To my surprise I found them very easy to use. If you have a strong wrist, the right weapon, and a decisive mind the tooth comes out. My fame as a dentist spread far and wide, and I pulled out many teeth which were causing a lot of discomfort and even suffering. We had no anaesthetic, but for particularly nervous cases or tough pullings we would, if we had any, give the patient a swig of brandy or whisky.

Ours was an ever-open door. It was nothing unusual to be woken up in the early hours of the morning and to hear a voice saying, 'Wake up, Sister; I'm wounded! …'

1914
France

Dr Flora Murray

Hospital in the Hôtel Claridge, Paris, France

Dr Flora Murray, a physician, and Dr Louisa Garrett Anderson, a surgeon (daughter of Dr Elizabeth Garrett Anderson), were militant suffragettes in the years preceding the outbreak of the First World War and understood the prejudices and stereotyped outlook held by men in government departments. When war was declared they realised their offer to serve as doctors in hospitals for the wounded would only be rebuffed, so they approached the French Red Cross who asked them to organise a unit to go to Paris. The Women's Hospital Corps was then hastily but efficiently assembled. Within two weeks £2,000 had been subscribed to buy all the necessary equipment, the staff was engaged and a uniform carefully chosen. The uniform consisted of a short skirt and loose-buttoned tunic in a light, durable green-grey material. The medical officers had red shoulder straps with 'W.H.C.' stitched in white, and the orderlies had white collars and shoulder straps with red letters. Small cloth hats with veils and overcoats to match completed the outfit.

The unit arrived in Paris on 14 September. The newly-built, luxurious Hôtel Claridge, on the Champs Élysées, had been commandeered as a hospital for Allied soldiers. The floors were still covered with debris and men were working on electric installations.

The second morning in Paris found the Corps busily engaged at the Hôtel Claridge. There was a great deal of cleaning to do and many arrangements to make before the place would be habitable. In the centre of the building was a handsome paved hall with a many-coloured marble table and enormous glass chandeliers. Out of this four good-sized salons opened, and it was in these that wards were first arranged.

The salons were only divided from one another by plate glass; and some degree of privacy is necessary for a ward. Doctors and nurses alike put on aprons and rolled up their sleeves, and while some cleaned the whitening off the glass, the others pasted the lower part over with white paper. With help from the Belgian refugees, who were lodged on the seventh story, the floors were cleaned and polished, beds were put up and order began to be evolved.

The ladies' cloakroom, with its pavement, its hot-water supply and basins, was converted into the operating theatre. A gas steriliser and a powerful electric light were fixed in. Though small, it proved serviceable and well equipped.

The cleaning was sufficiently advanced to allow the Corps to move into its quarters on the first floor next day, and they spent the morning carrying bedding and furniture down to the wards. These at once began to have a professional look, and by concentrating on two wards they were successful in getting fifty beds prepared for patients by the evening.

The work of preparation was at its height when a doctor from the American hospital walked in. Upon the outbreak of the war, the American colony in Paris had organised their fine hospital in the Lycée at Neuilly and had established a fleet of ambulances. Their ambulances enabled them to carry hundreds of men from the fighting line in to Paris. Both French and British wounded were in terrible straits; for there was no organised motor transport service, and the Armies depended on the railways for the removal of the sick and injured. The long delays and the conditions under which the men lay whilst waiting for removal were fatal, and the American service was the means of saving numbers of lives.

When trains were available the wounded were packed into them and despatched to distant places in the interior. As they passed Paris, those who were so severely wounded that they were unlikely to survive a long journey were left at the stations on the Circle Railway round the city. There they would lie on straw or sacks, waiting for friendly ambulances to come out and bring them in.

In those first weeks there was no system of communication between the hospitals and the stations; the French ambulances were small and bad, and the British had none available for Paris. The matter depended largely upon individual effort, and the ambulances of the American and other voluntary hospitals played a devoted and humanitarian part.

The doctor from Neuilly was in charge of the ambulance service. The American hospital was already very full of French and British, but, in response to a message which he had received, he was sending out his cars that day, and he hoped that there might be beds ready for some of the cases at 'Claridge's'.

As those first stretchers with their weary burdens were carried in, a thrill of pity and dismay ran through the women who saw them. The mud-stained khaki and the unshaven faces spoke to them no less than the wounded limbs and shattered nerves. Here, for the first time, they touched the wastage and the desolation of war. In every wounded man they saw some other woman's husband or son, and the thought of those other women made a double claim on their energy and sympathy. The battered, inarticulate, suffering men who lay there needed service, and they braced themselves for the work before them.

Organisation developed automatically: nurses for night duty were sent to rest; the theatre sister began to sterilise; chloroform, instruments, drugs and dressings were produced and distributed.

Late in the afternoon a message from the Chief Surgeon was brought from the wards: 'Dr Anderson wishes to know if the theatre is ready and if she can operate tonight.'

'It is ready now,' was the answer.

And the surgeons operated till a late hour that night.

The hospital was a smooth-running concern by the end of the week. Nurses and patients had settled down in the wards; work in the operating theatre was going well;

and though it was far from perfect in all its details, the comfort of the officers and men was assured.

The uniform of the Women's Hospital Corps soon became known, and secured a cordial reception for its members in the bureaux and offices which they had to visit, as well as on the boulevards. Strangers would offer them gifts of socks and mittens. Shopkeepers asked about 'les blessés' and sent presents of sweets and biscuits. The greengrocer added an extra cauliflower to the purchase. Flower-women ran after them and pressed bunches of roses into their hands.

At the entrance of the Hôtel when ambulances were unloading, elderly men in silk hats and black kid gloves would crowd round and offer to carry the stretchers, or would follow the bearers inside, with the kit – often a very dirty kit – in their arms. The sight of the suffering moved them so that they turned aside and wept. They brought violets and roses and cigarettes for the men. They stood outside the doors to listen to them singing, and they wrung the hands of the doctors silently and went.

To all of them, officers and men alike, hospital was a haven of peace and security. It was heavenly to lie in clean beds, to be cared for by Englishwomen, to be rid of regimental discipline and for the moment of responsibility too. The severity of their wounds, the operations, the pain were minor matters; for the time being they had found comfort and rest. Probably none of them had been in contact with women doctors before; but that did not make any difference. They trusted the women as they would have trusted men – passing the bullets which had been extracted from their persons from bed to bed and pronouncing the surgeon to be 'wonderfully clever'.

The condition of the men was, if possible, worse than that of the officers. They had laid in queer wayside stations, waiting for trains, or on straw in stables and churches, hoping for transport. At Villeneuve, on the Paris railway circle, there was a goods shed with straw on the ground, in which officers lay at one end and men at the other. An RAMC doctor and a few men did what they could for them, and when the ambulances came out from Paris, the worst were picked out; but, for the rest, the weary waiting for a train continued. At Creil, 40 miles from Paris, the accommodation was an open shed filled with straw. French and British lay huddled in groups, some covered by blankets, others by dirty sacks. A doctor of the French Army, very dapper in his red and blue plush cap, sorted them into trains, when any trains came. Several French soldiers stirred a mess of potage with a dirty stick. But of dressings or nursing there was no sign. Patiently and uncomplainingly these sufferers waited, often fifteen, twenty-four or more hours, while the rain poured down on the roof of their shed, and the wind swept drearily through the station.

At last, septic and wasted by fever, they were jolted by the ambulances over the ill-paved roads to Paris and hospital. Lieutenant Lowe, whose only chance lay in getting into hospital without further delay, was brought down from Compiègne on a stretcher laid across an ordinary motor car and held in position by an American doctor and a man with one hand. His thigh was badly fractured and very imperfectly supported; but with the help of morphia he endured the journey. From the first there was little hope of his recovery, but he lingered for some weeks, during which his sister was able to be with him, lavishing care and tenderness upon him to their mutual comfort.

The men were dirty and half-fed; many had not had a change of clothes or socks since they left England; but they were absolutely uncomplaining and began at once to appreciate their hospital surroundings.

Women doctors were a novelty which served to enhance the importance and the grandeur of the gilded and marbled halls in which they found themselves. 'The doctors is ladies', they wrote in their letters home.

They found comfort in the presence of women and repose in the care lavished upon them, and with the philosophy of the soldier they let it rest there.

Towards the end of September, the War Office sent over a representative to examine into existing conditions, and to inspect and report on the auxiliary hospitals, of which Claridge's Hôtel was one.

The 'Milord' selected for this mission made a handsome, martial figure as he strode through the streets of Paris. He was resplendent in khaki and brass hat, and a beautiful order hung round his neck. Rumour said he was the Duke of Connaught or Lord French or Sir Frederick Treves or Mr Bottomley! But whoever he was, his appearance commanded great respect. He was saluted on all sides, and men stepped from the pavement to let him take his noble way.

The first hospital which he visited was Claridge's. He was an imposing figure as he entered the central hall. His spurs rang on the pavement and his steps re-echoed in its vastness. He fixed a suspicious blue eye on the senior medical officers who went to meet him, and interrogated them sternly:

'Who is in charge of this place?'

'What are you doing here?'

'What have you got behind there?' pointing at the glass partition rendered opaque by white paper.

'A French hospital! How can it be a French hospital? You're British.'

'All women! No proper surgeons?'

'Have you British soldiers here? Any officers?'

'What are you doing with them?'

'Where do they go when they leave you?'

'Versailles! Who told you to send them to Versailles?'

'Colonel Smith! How do you know about Colonel Smith?'

Curt, sharp questions that met with curt, sharp answers.

At this moment Madame Perouse [President of the French Red Cross], who had been notified of his visit, arrived. He greeted her with the most delightful courtesy, and withdrawing with her to a little distance, asked if these women were really practical surgeons and if it were possible that the soldiers tolerated such an arrangement.

The poor old lady was rather flustered, but she declared that this was her 'meilleure installation' and that the organisation was 'parfaite'. He was only half-convinced by the assurances which she gave him, but his manner became more ordinary, and turning to Dr Flora Murray and Dr Garrett Anderson, he announced his intention of going through the wards. He was accompanied by a doctor, a civilian, whom he introduced as being 'unconverted to women doctors'. These pleasing preliminaries being concluded, he was conducted into the hospital.

It was the rest hour, when many patients were asleep, and an air of peace and comfort was over everything. Sisters moved softly whilst tending the more seriously ill, and those who were awake lay quietly reading and smoking. The handsome wards with their flowers and coloured blankets looked charming: for they were in perfect order, and there were no visitors so early in the day. The men when questioned spoke of their 'good home' with grateful appreciation. The officers expressed their satisfaction in cordial terms; and as 'Milord' went from ward to ward, he became silent and thoughtful. He finished his inspection without relaxing the severity of his aspect and took a graceful farewell of Madame Perouse, leaving her much mystified as to the reason of his visit and his apparent displeasure.

Two days later the 'unconverted doctor' called again, bland and eager for conversation. He explained that he and his companion had been sent over by the War Office, and he talked of the intentions of 'K' [Kitchener] with regard to the hospitals. He said they wanted to know whether the Women's Hospital Corps could increase its beds, and whether it could move its hospital forward if needed. The astonished organisers were given to understand that if any auxiliary hospitals were moved forward, Claridge's would be the first to be invited to move, and that the British Army would not hesitate to make use of it, supposing that the matter could be arranged with the French Red Cross.

The 'unconverted one' still seemed, however, to be tormented with uncertainty as to the attitude of men when called upon to accept treatment from women doctors. In order to reassure him, he was pressed to visit the officers' ward by himself. He went, and, to the amusement of all concerned, returned an agreeable and equable convert …

Mrs Katharine Furse

No. 1 British Red Cross VAD Unit based at Gare Centrale, Boulogne, France

Katharine Furse, Commandant of the British Red Cross VADs, arrived in Boulogne in October 1914. She and her party of VADs started a Rest Station at the Gare Centrale in 'three trucks and two second-class coaches on a siding'. The Unit consisted of twenty-five nurses, eight orderlies, one cook, two Quarter-Masters and Commandant Furse. Colonel Wake, the Red Cross Commissioner, kept a boat in reserve to evacuate the Unit if the Germans marched into Boulogne.

Those three trucks on the siding to the south of Boulogne Town station were the beginning of something which spread rapidly and usefully along the British Lines of Communication, and to the work of that small unit of VAD pioneers must be due, I believe, the credit for paving the way to the more extensive use of our organisation. We certainly were pioneers because we were the first VAD members to be sent abroad officially and very few among the Army authorities knew anything about the basis on which we were formed.

Our trucks never moved from Boulogne. We divided them into kitchen, dispensary and staff room, combined with stores, and we furnished them as best we could with what we thought would be necessary for the supply of comforts to limited numbers of wounded, including such surgical attention as could be rendered by our trained nurses, who worked in the dispensary which was our chief pride.

The kitchen van with Stephenson and Lyne in charge depended entirely on two or three Primus stoves for cooking and lotions. Water was already laid on to the platform, and we used the sanitary arrangements of the station, being allowed a key to one cubicle; we slept and ate at our hotel.

Our two second-class coaches were not much use to us but for a time the Director of Medical Services, Lines of Communication, slept in one and orderlies in the other, and then all sorts of stranded people took refuge in them and they became verminous.

We received our first wounded on 27 October and from that date we were fully occupied. As ambulance trains came in at any hour day or night, we divided our unit into two shifts and were on duty all the time in case we might be needed. To make our presence better known, we hoisted the Union Jack and Red Cross flags side by side by day, and two lanterns at night, as we had been taught to do. The lanterns were a great difficulty to us, as they would go out when the wind blew, but I insisted on them being kept going until we learned by experience that such details are best omitted when energy is scarce owing to the staff being overworked.

Our brand-new Union Jack was much coveted by a Naval gun crew, who had their armoured train on a siding near us, and we finally agreed to exchange our new flag for their smoke-black tattered one which had seen active service up the line.

Being in charge of the Rest Station, I used to go to it at any hour, day or night, and often wonder at the friendly welcome given to me as, when inspecting, I used at first to expect parade-ground manners and was very upset if everyone did not stand at attention and show respect for their Commandant. So much of it was play-acting and very unnecessary but, pompous and boring as it was, I believe that it started us on the right lines; it could not outlive the real pressure of work when we got busy. As a start off, it gave us the right tone and we soon settled down to a more simple way of life in which the leaders took their share of the drudgery together with all the other members, which I believe to be one of the most important factors in leadership.

Early on 2 November, when I went to the Rest Station, there were only two or three cooks on duty in the trucks, the rest of the unit, both day and night shifts, being at the other side of the station giving hot drinks to a great crowd of supposedly walking wounded who had arrived unexpectedly from the battle of Ypres, and who were travelling further to the base hospitals at Rouen. I went across and found our VADs in the midst of hundreds of men for whom they were ladling out tea and cocoa, which was gratefully accepted, these wounded having come directly from field dressing-stations and many being in a terrible condition with only their first field dressings on what were often very severe wounds. The medical officers who had brought them down were dog-tired and wanted to get a wash and breakfast, and I do not remember seeing any orderlies with them. The men had just been put in an empty stores train, and were glad enough to have got away however uncomfortably.

When I told the Senior MO that we had two trained nurses at the Rest Station who could see to dressings, he was very relieved, and told the men to go to our trucks, which they did, those who could walk helping those who couldn't, and they lined up in a queue along our platform, waiting for their turn for attention. It was a most amazing day, as two or three more similar trains drifted in, and we were kept indescribably busy. The nurses worked magnificently, and all the VADs helped. In some cases the men's wounds showed signs of gangrene, and we got them accepted by the Military Hospital, but though I went repeatedly to the DAMS. office, I could get no help, because the officers were busy elsewhere and the NCOs could not take action. Our greatest difficulties were to provide enough boiling water for lotions and for drinks, as well as to get rid of soiled and soaked dressings. For the former we had only our Primus stoves, and for the latter we built a fire in the station yard, having two railway lines as foundation and getting faggots from a baker, and coal from a kindly French engine-driver.

Cocoa ran out, and we had to send our ambulance driver to buy up every quarter-pound packet that she could find at all the small grocers. At one moment, about midday, I felt so heavily responsible that I insisted on seeing Colonel Wake and shifting the responsibility on to him. I remember the feeling of standing in his office, my hands stiff with carbolic and the weight of the world on my back. He promised me two surgeons and three trained nurses who were arriving by the afternoon boat. When they came, all dressed up, I almost regretted that we had practically finished our job and that there were no wounded left for them to attend to, when another train steamed in unexpectedly. Late into the night the surgeons were operating on the platform under the arc lamps, and we all looked and felt very unreal. That one day we fed 2,300 men and did over 200 dressings, and the news of our work having at last spread officially, by the evening the DMS appeared and with him Miss McCarthy, Principal Matron in France, Red Cross Officials and others.

The poor men who could not walk and had to be put back on straw in cattle-trucks had suffered so terribly from lack of orderlies' routine attention, and the numbers were so large, that we could do nothing but feed them and see to their dressings, and we wished we had orderlies to do all else which was necessary for their comfort. It is a nightmare to look back on that day, and the only consolation is knowing that our training had prepared us a little to cope with what came to us, for I am convinced that had Cantlie not taught us the importance of improvisation we should not have been able to face the situation efficiently, for we were but ill-prepared with the usual forms of equipment in sufficient quantities. [Sir James Cantlie was the pioneer of First Aid in England].

By the time the last train of that lot had steamed out of the station on its long way to Rouen, we had time to look round, and found ourselves to be the heroes of the hour. Everyone congratulated us on what we had done, but what was much more to the point, they also offered us anything we needed to make our work easier in the future; we then and there asked for more trucks, stoves, medical stores, cocoa, condensed milk and whatever else we could think of in what seemed to us to be vast quantities. We were allowed two more trucks then and three more later, making eight in all. These were on two sidings with the platform between them.

We also got a squad of boys as orderlies who slept in hammocks in two of the new trucks, who proved to be more trouble than they were worth and we soon distributed them, keeping four men for definite duties with a SM [Sergeant Major], Mr Edgar Woolcombe, the brother of one of our cooks, to look after them and to help us generally.

We now had one whole truck for reserve stores, and filled it so full with our cocoa and condensed milk that it sat right down on its springs; I was amused to find how soon this stores truck took on the smell and the atmosphere of a village shop. What we dreaded was that the French railway officials might object to their wagon risking its springs being ruined. One truck was a Staffroom with camp beds, etc., another QM's daily store and one a workshop where we made all sorts of furniture out of packing cases, the two Miss Barbers being our very competent carpenters.

We fitted stoves into our kitchen truck and also the staffroom and dispensary, cutting holes in the roofs for the chimneys to go through …

[Extract from a letter to her son]
I have been given two cars and have Preston and a man chauffeur ready to drive them. Preston has been using an ambulance lately and has driven numbers of stray cases to hospital, as well as all our stores.

I have collected such a lovely lot and mean to keep it all locked up, for no one has any conscience. We all loot. The other night two of our stretchers were not returned, so we picked the best two stretchers we could find in a pile. The same with the blankets. Only the wounded man gains. He gets the best of everything.

Talking of looting. Hitherto all the coal we burn has appeared somehow. We bought none till yesterday when we wanted to fill the dog boxes in our vans as a reserve.

Grateful stray patients such as a sailor, (English, who appears most days to have a poisoned finger dressed), bring lumps of coal picked up somewhere for us. Slabs of bacon arrive. Four sacks of potatoes left by some men who were leaving. Masses of stuff comes like this.

And we go and wander round the huge BRCS store and ask for what we fancy and I must say they give us all they can.

Tomlin and I searched about 20 shops and bought all there was. Also carbolic. But we want everything. Nothing comes amiss. I now indent for everything in doz., gross and cwt. The Society is very generous and we get all we want, but with delay sometimes. We need pillows. Even stuffed with paper. They do for stretcher cases. Everything gets so soiled and there is no means of disinfecting so one has to destroy. We do spray a great deal.

Today they have started painting the inside of the dispensary all white. It is really a mail van and has endless little shelves and pigeon holes for sorting letters. These when painted are perfect for keeping packets of dressing in. Rachel [Rachel Crowdy who later became Commandant] loves her dispensary of course and she makes up all the lotions, etc. …

The difficulty of Rest Station work, like so much emergency work, was that it was so uneven. Sometimes we had great rushes, and then long pauses with only routine work.

As Boulogne settled down to a long period of war the Military Base Hospitals settled in and our work was mainly confined to giving hot drinks to walking cases passing through, so then we took to odd jobbing to be of more use. First of all we tried to make the Rest Station itself attractive, in which we succeeded so well that it became one of the sights of the town. The men loved it, and used any excuse to come for a chat with the 'sisters', as they called us all.

The 'souveniring' habit came out with regard to the Red Cross mugs we used, as the men coming from the front having lost all their belongings would pocket them; so we thought of our 'tinkering' and decided to convert empty condensed milk tins into mugs, turning over the edges to prevent their cutting and devoting one tin to handles, which were soldered on to the others, so that a perfectly serviceable though rather rough small mug was produced for practically nothing. The work helped to fill the empty hours at night, and presently our members were producing mugs by the hundred and thousand, and we no longer minded how many were souvenired.

From the beginning we determined to fill every gap which could be filled by the amateur and our oasis gradually became a centre for all who needed help. When the regular hospital trains were running, we acted as an exchange for the nurses' laundry, taking their bundles when they came into Boulogne, getting it washed by French women and keeping it ready for when their train came in again. We also served as a lost luggage office and a cloakroom, taking care of every possible bit of luggage, umbrellas, etc. The French civilians began to use us, bringing us their cuts and hurts, and asking us to visit them in their homes, to do dressings, etc., and even to set the leg of an old lady lying in a bed some 4 feet high. They brought their donkeys and their cats and their dogs to us, and no help was refused, because we wanted to prove our readiness to do anything which could be done under the Geneva Convention.

Our great dread was that if we were too idle we should get into mischief. So we forbade smoking, and forbade association with men, with the result that our nickname was 'the Starched Brigade'. Poor Preston, our very fine ambulance driver, was a great anxiety to us, because she could not adapt herself to the rigid rules. I was faced with a love affair at the very beginning. Preston got engaged and I imagined that our reputation might be ruined and that we might all be sent home in disgrace, so I sent Preston home. She was furious and several other people thought me ridiculous, but I had to make an example of a VAD who so far forgot herself as to get engaged while on active service.

However, Sir Alfred Keogh [Director General of Medical Services at the War Office], as he showed in the following note, thought us too severe:

> How dreadful! What an irreparable disgrace to the Red Cruisers! It is your fault, you take out a charming Eve and she meets Adam. I don't mind tackling fashionable London, but I can't take Cupid on. I give it up. But is it not cruel to send her home, poor girl? She couldn't help it.

Preston married Dr Graham Jones later and had a family and forgave me. It was not narrow prudishness which made me so severe. I knew enough about men and women and their relationships to be tolerant of perfectly natural behaviour and I did not read immorality into every love affair or mutual attraction. But I was sure that for uniformed women sent out to pioneer in new work it was essential, if they were to be successful and pave the way to an extension of their employment, that they should establish a reputation for almost exaggerated seriousness, and that this was safer than too great leniency at first.

For Christmas, 1914, we thought we must do something special for the ambulance trains which came through on Christmas Eve, so Edith Crowdy [Rachel Crowdy's sister] collected a small fund at home and sent out candles and crackers, as well as a great many cheap presents, and we put fir trees on our trek carts, of which we had two in the Station; as the trains came in we pushed the carts along, as usual, ladling out cocoa, and then we gave each man a cracker and a present. Mouth organs were the favourite. Their joy was pathetic to see; they were just as much children as we felt ourselves to be this strange Christmas Eve …

Miss Eleonora B. Pemberton

No. 1 British Red Cross VAD Unit based at Gare Centrale, Boulogne, France

No. 7 Stationary Hospital, Boulogne

Eleonora Pemberton, a member of Katharine Furses's VAD unit, arrived in Boulogne in October 1914. For the first few months the unit ran a canteen on the railway station providing food for the sick and wounded on ambulance and passenger trains that passed through the station, and helped to dress wounds at the dispensary on one of the platforms. They also distributed newspapers and magazines to the various trains and hospitals in the town itself and in the neighbourhood of Boulogne. During this time Eleonora Pemberton wrote long letters home.

23 October 1914
The trains draw up right on the quay – regular hospital trains with Army Sisters in charge and the stretchers are taken straight from the train on to the hospital ships alongside and they go to Southampton, which is said to be a more central starting place for England in general than Folkestone.

Altogether life is very varied and all very interesting. This place swarms with men in khaki, a certain number of French soldiers, English soldiers, and packs of motor ambulances. Our hotel immediately faces the quay and the ambulances pass up and down, up and down, almost continuously taking bad cases from the trains to the hospitals and then the ones who are better from the hospitals to the hospital ships. There are four of the latter. There is always one in and she usually starts about 9pm for

Southampton. It takes 10 hours there and 10 hours back and they stop 6 hours, so she is away 26 altogether and is then ready for another load.

Hospital trains come in at all hours of the day and night; some have kitchens on board and then they are all right. Others have not and it is then that our work comes in. Of course the trains are fearfully uncertain. One was expected at 9pm the night before last and only came in at 6am the next morning, so our cooks find it somewhat difficult to manage the hot drinks. We have tea, cocoa and soup going as a rule and lots of bread.

We have been given three luggage vans and a good many ordinary railway carriages. The former are used as store room, kitchen and dispensary respectively, and there is always a trained nurse, head cook and quartermaster in charge, and about 4 lesser lights who do as they are told. The shifts are from 8.30–8.30 day and night, and the night people mostly sleep in the carriages until notice comes from the RTO (Railway Transport Officer) that a train of so many hundred is expected. From today onwards the day people are, if possible (i.e. if there is not too great a rush) to have two hours off each and four of us are doing relief, 2 from 10–2 and the other two from 2–6 and this ought to work quite well. It will not be able to last very long however I expect, as we have been asked to form a second Rest Station and then every available member will be wanted to complete day and night shifts.

Yesterday was my first day there since last Monday when I had been in charge of the spring cleaning gang who wrestled with the pristine grubbiness. They have worked simply wonders since then and it is a regular Swiss Family Robinson encampment now. We have four men Red X orderlies attached to us under Mr Woolcombe, two at a time and they have to keep a large fire going outside with great 'Dixies' boiling on it. In addition to this we have two stoves and any number of methylated ones in the kitchen and they are all wanted when the rush comes. The trains do not of course draw up conveniently at one platform! Not a bit of it, they are sometimes about a quarter of a mile away. The one I was summoned to yesterday morning was quite that distance but we were luckily able to wheel most of the stuff down on a trolley and only carry the additional supplies that were wanted. It is just lovely to see how the men appreciate the hot drinks, and it is awfully interesting talking to them and hearing all their different experiences and opinions.

The London Scottish went up on Tuesday and we have had some back again wounded on Friday, so you see we are not far from the fighting. There were a lot of H.A.C. men here at the beginning of the week.

On Monday a message came down from the senior medical officer (Major Miles) to Colonel Wake, our chief, asking whether some of us could possibly go and help at No. 7 Stationary Hospital as Matron was so short staffed. Accordingly six of us were summoned amidst great jubilations and trotted off, to be told when we got there that we were to go on night duty. This, to me, was better news still as it meant an absolutely and entirely new experience, and nine o'clock saw me almost chattering with excitement.

We were allotted to different floors and I went to the 3rd where the staff consisted of a nice kind Sister, a staff nurse, two orderlies and myself. In military hospitals the orderlies are supposed to do all the cleaning and a good deal of the other work which in an ordinary civilian hospital falls to the share of the probationers.

We had not been there more than long enough for me to fly round finding out where a few things were kept when the stretchers began to arrive. The lift here was too small to take them so each one had to be carried up. In this hospital also the wards consisted of a perfect rabbit warren of small rooms leading out of one another which makes it much more difficult both to get the stretchers in and out and also to keep an eye on everybody and hear when they call.

That night we took in 26 new cases which filled up our 40 beds and they all had to be undressed and washed ready for the doctors. It took us till about 2.30 as it is not a quick job when you have to be so careful about moving them and also when you have to change the water about 4 times for each case on account of the grime.

Most of the men had not washed for weeks, many had their socks sticking to their feet, all the clothes were filthy, clotted with blood and very odiferous and it was just a joy to get them off and make the poor fellows a bit clean and fairly comfortable, but it brought war home to one in a way that nothing else, short of the actual battlefield could. When you turn down the blanket to wash an arm and find no arm only a soaking bandage that was once white, or you go to feed 'No. 14' and find that he has only half a face and cannot swallow but tries to speak and you strain to understand. It fills you with a fury against the devillish ingenuity which conceived the perfection of the weapons which have caused this devastation and a loathing of the man who set loose these fiends of hell.

One and all, nurses, doctors, orderlies – many who were all through the S. African War – say that there never, never have been wounds like this, and I cannot think that there ever could be worse.

I am thankful to say that it has not affected my nerve in the very least, and the sights, and what is much worse, the smells, leave me untouched from a nursing point of view and I have been able to handle anything and see anything without flinching – but the smells stick in one's nostrils (it is the sloughing and the gangrene) and I have found Formamint very essential in keeping off the 'hospital sore throat' which so many of the nurses have been getting.

The second night I was there the staff nurse was crocked up so it only left the Sister and myself who knew the cases a bit and two more of our detachment were sent up to help. It was a wonderful chance for me, as Sister was busy at one part of the landing and told me to attend to the doctors who were coming to perform two operations in a ward the other end. It was an experience that I might have waited years for in an ordinary hospital. One case was a fractured femur and that has been put up with an actual rifle as a splint. One has always heard of rifle splints but except in war time one would hardly ever have the chance of seeing one. The man was given chloroform and then the rifle was taken off. I helped to pad a long splint (having to find everything that was wanted myself) and then held the leg and helped to bandage. Of course there was a nasty wound on the outside as well but it was not as septic as many.

When that was finished the man in the next bed was also given chloroform and had his arm dressed – a very bad wound near the elbow which is giving him a terrible lot of pain and he may have to lose it. It is his left arm, and his right leg has also a bad wound so he can only lie on his back, which is of course very tiring and makes him ache all over, poor man. We had to improvise an angle splint for the elbow and while this was done the Dr told me to clean up the wound.

All the time the others kept popping in to ask where things were kept and how they were done and who might have what. It was a case of the blind leading the blind, but Sister was too busy always to attend to details and I was the only other one who had been there the night before.

Another interruption during the whole 5 nights was in connection with two wounded Germans whom we had. No one either on night or day duty could understand much less talk to them. The orderlies were awfully good to them and tried hard to find out what they wanted, but they often had to come for assistance and the Germans were so glad to find someone who could understand, but when it comes to exhaustive enquiries as to symptoms it is not too simple! and I wished I had studied up some bedside German as well as French.

So far we have had no French at all and I believe they are all being sent to Calais and Bercque and down south.

3 Nov. c/o BRCS, Hôtel de Paris, Boulogne
We had a busy time yesterday. I went on duty at the station at two o'clock and found the whole place simply swarming with wounded. The dispensary was hard at work doing dressings and the cooks were labouring with might and main to feed them all. We got back here at 9.40 having fed 2,300 with soup, cocoa and tea and bread and dressed the wounds of perhaps 150. It was an extraordinary sight, particularly when it got dark and the station lights were lit. Everywhere there were men, sitting on trucks and barrows and the few chairs we could offer them, standing about with heads, arms, shoulders tied up, limping about and even lying on the platforms just as they were. One man I saw lying flat with his head pillowed on a loaf of bread. They had come straight down from Ypres where they say a terrific battle, worse even than Mons and Le Cateau is raging, and they were being taken on to Havre. Altogether 3 train loads came in and some of our people were working there from 8.30am till we all left. They could not even spare anyone to come back during the morning to fetch those of us who were off duty.

One poor man died in the station, one or two were off their heads, all had more or less severe wounds though the majority could get about with assistance. The hospitals here are so full that they could only take in the very worst cases and the rest had to go on. Of course we could not possibly change all or anything like all the dressings, although three nurses and two doctors were fetched during the pm. It was however working under awful difficulties; first the swarms of people through whom you had to push your way; then the shortage of hot water in sufficient quantity (such masses were required for the feeding as well as the dressings, the water here is so bad that we are not allowed to use it unless boiled for dressings or even for cleaning our teeth!); then the almost complete absence of instruments – very few of us had thought of bringing anything down as this had never happened before; then the fact that every lot of dirty water or lotion or blood or anything had to be carried down to a drain and emptied.

It was really wonderful the way our store of wool gauze and antiseptics held out, but it taxed them very severely and we have got to lay in heaps more. I made and applied a jaw bandage out of another one and the nurse was quite surprised to find that I knew how!

Miss Crowdy [who later took over from Katharine Furse as Commandant of the VAD in France and Belgium] was simply splendid over the dressings. She is a born nurse.

As it got late and another train load came in the doctors said some of the nurses had better just do dressings for the very worst out on the platform, so we carted some of the things up to the part under the lamps, trolleys served both as seats and tables, and the work went on, only it was a little more difficult as it doubled the distance for emptying things and fetching supplies. However the men were so good and so grateful and patient that nothing seemed too much to do, and it really did ease them a lot. I only wish we could have done many, many more. While our own two nurses, the three fetched ones and the two doctors assisted by some of us, were just racing through dressings, the rest of the party were going down the train feeding the hungry and they managed to get through the whole lot – which does them immense credit – before the train went off.

Miss Kate Finzi

No. 13 Stationary Hospital, Boulogne, France

Kate Finzi, a British Red Cross nurse, arrived in Boulogne in October 1914. She wrote that she was part of 'the tattered remnants of a once-flourishing Red Cross detachment whose energies and equipment alike had been left behind at the enforced evacuation of Ostend.'

As the fight for Calais raged, thousands of wounded men were brought down to Boulogne by trains. Many were left helpless on their stretchers on the quayside waiting to be taken off on hospital ships. The hotels, taken over as makeshift hospitals, were overcrowded 'with wounded who lay so close together in the corridors that it was necessary to climb over one stretcher to reach the next patient, and often stand astride the pallets to dress the wounds'. The casino was opened as a hospital but soon became as overcrowded as the hotels. Then a disused sugar shed was requisitioned as a clearing station.

29 October

Let me tell the tale of No. 13 Stationary Hospital. It should go down to posterity as a memorial of what British resourcefulness may achieve, even if its existence was the outcome of the proverbial British state of unpreparedness. For what in the annals of History has equalled the holocaust and chaos of modern warfare, of which there was no precedent, of which everything has had to be learned by the bitterest experience?

A vast wooded barn whose cracked cement floor is piled high with dust, whose smashed glass roofing is besmirched with dirt, is hardly an ideal site for a hospital, but it is the best thing to hand, and the Major commandeered it, and here, before the lumber had been cleared, before the glass had been repaired or the walls whitewashed, the wounded began to tumble in. It wasn't much of a place, but it was out of the torrential rain which had set in and bade fair to continue, and it was less cold than the open air.

By day and night the orderlies worked, alternately preparing the place and attending to the wounded. A solitary English girl who happened to be on the spot had volunteered her services, and was doing her best single-handed in the wards. One day the Major, walking on the quay, saw some Red Cross nurses. On hearing they were waiting for their orders, and that they were all qualified women, he commandeered them, even as he had commandeered his barn. Back they came to Headquarters to fetch more assistance.

'Why don't you come too? It's a case of all hands aboard!' said one. It was thus I came to work at the first clearing station at the base. Such was the stationary hospital when, laden with all the loaves we could carry to supplement the ration biscuits, we set to work in the 'casualty ward' this afternoon.

For the thousand wounded likely to come through daily there are six fully-trained nurses and myself, besides the male staff of RAMC doctors and orderlies, and two or three Red Cross surgeons and lady doctors.

Ten beds and a number of sacks of straw form the main equipment. Planks, supported by two packing-cases, are the dressing-table. At one end men are engaged in putting in three extemporary baths, others whitewashing the walls.

A boatload had just left for England as I came in, and we proceeded to get a meal for those who remained. But it was a struggle to get sufficient tea out of the orderlies, who had been working all night and were dead beat. The men's delight at the bread and old newspapers we had brought in was incredible.

Those who were able to clustered round the solitary stove in the centre. Great, rough, bearded fellows, covered with mud from the trenches in which they have lived for weeks, how different they look from those who set out! The worst cases lay on their stretchers as they had arrived. One said simply as I took him his tea, 'This is heaven, Sister.'

A tall, dark man entered – the CO, someone said. 'Take those two Germans down to the boat,' I heard him order. Then, turning to us, 'You'd better come to our mess-room and get some tea yourselves,' he said. 'Four train-loads are expected in shortly.'

We trooped into the small sanctum dignified by the name of 'mess-room', where the Major's orderly was busy preparing tea on a Primus stove. There was no milk, but the bitter black beverage out of the large tin mugs was welcome none the less. Someone had secured a cake that we cut with a sword as the cleanest thing present.

Next to the mess-room are the officers' quarters (into which we were privileged to take one glance) – small whitewashed cubicles furnished with a camp bed, a shaving-glass about three inches by six inches in size, and an old sugar-box converted into a washstand.

Tea finished, we set to work to get 'beds' ready for the next batch, the first of the four train-loads expected. Ten bedsteads for a thousand men! It sounds almost incredible, but it is nevertheless true; and although we are told that more are expected at any moment, we have only wooden pallets at present and a limited supply of blankets. One to lie on, two for cover, a coat for a pillow was the order of the day until a pile of mattresses came in.

30 October

We worked till midnight and were on duty again by 7.30 this morning. From our billets to the hospital is nearly half an hour's walk, which, over the rough cobblestones in the blinding rain, is hardly attractive. At any rate, it has the advantage of clearing the haunting smell of the gas-gangrene out of our nostrils.

The worst part of the wounds is the fearful sepsis and the impossibility of getting them anything like clean.

'First time I've had my boots off for seven weeks!' is the kind of exclamation that recurs all day, as we literally cut them off. Hardly any of the boots have been off for three weeks, with the result that they seem glued on, whilst the feet are like iron, the nails like claws.

Some of the men have not had their wounds dressed since the first field dressing was applied, for the simple reason that the rush on the hospital trains makes it impossible to attend to any but the worst cases, many of whom, as it is, are dying of haemorrhage, accelerated by the jolting on the journey.

There is no time to do anything but the dressings, and if we did want to wash the patients there is nothing but the red handkerchiefs we hang round the lights for shades by night, for towels by day.

Water, especially boiling water, is at a premium, as it all has to be fetched from outside where the veteran cook stokes hard all day in the driving rain, ladling us out a modicum into each bowl from his cauldrons.

'I never thought to see such sights,' exclaimed a nurse of thirty years' experience as a new trainload came in. But we have no time to think of our own sensations.

Fingerless hands, lungs pierced, arms and legs pretty well gangrenous, others already threatening tetanus (against which they are now beginning to inoculate patients), mouths swollen beyond all recognition with bullet shots, fractured femurs, shattered jaws, sightless eyes, ugly scalp wounds; yet never a murmur, never a groan except in sleep. As the men come in they fall on their pallets and doze until roused for food.

Quite a number of prisoners who had been taken near Lille were brought into the clearing station this morning. Being the only linguist present, I was installed as interpreter.

31 October

Who could believe, had they not seen for themselves, the manifold horrors of war? The vermin [lice], against which there is no copy, vermin that in ordinary times one never saw. The men are alive with them, so are we, a fact which necessitates a tremendous 'search' at every available opportunity. Even amputated limbs are found to be crawling.

The girl who was working single-handed in this barn until we arrived was walking along the quay yesterday when a feeble voice called her from a stretcher. It was her brother. He died in the night, but she is on duty all the same.

All day long the rush continues. The question 'Shrapnel or bullet?' rings incessantly in our ears as each man comes up to get his dressing done.

One boy of nineteen had no fewer than six bullet wounds in one arm and two in each leg. It took two of us an hour to dress his wounds.

Towards sunset I was called to the side of a youthful Saxon already rigid with tetanus.

Through his clenched teeth he could still groan to the orderly's command to lie still: 'Ich kann nicht still liegen' ('I can't lie still').

At seven o'clock (after nearly twelve hours' work) we went home to dinner, and, it being our turn to take night shift, were back again at our posts, with clean aprons and a satisfied inner man, two hours later. The orderly officer called for any who had not yet had their second anti-typhoid injection, and I, being one of them, was injected on the spot.

During the long night, as we hurried from patient to patient in the darkened cry-haunted ward, covering the restless sleeping figures, moving them into more comfortable positions, with a prayer for each one's mother, I could screw up no feeling of resentment towards the dying Saxon boy.

By midnight things were quiet enough to allow us to cut up dressings as best we might. By this time, owing to there not being a chair in the place, I confess my legs were almost giving way. Moreover, the injection took speedy effect, and a stiffening arm and rising temperature do not facilitate work of this kind. Frankly, I do not think any of us will ever be as busy again, and our one prayer was for strength to 'carry on'. Many of the men were tormented by coughs that kept the others awake. All we had to give them was lukewarm water and the rinsings of a condensed milk tin. (For euphony we called it 'milk'.)

Those who could not sleep for vermin lit cigarette after cigarette until their supply ran out. At 2am we retired to the nurses' 'bunk' – a whitewashed, rat-ridden, ill-smelling partitioned compartment, whose sole furniture consisted of two shelves – until someone was inspired to fetch the 'dressing-table' (two empty boxes – oh, joy of joys! upon which we took it in turns to sit) – and a coke fire, on which we boiled eggs for our midnight meal. Half-way through my egg the orderly called me: 'The prisoner can't last much longer. Will you come and speak to him, Sister?' It seemed as if the ward were one huge battlefield, for cries greeted me on all sides. 'Get at 'em, lads!' shouted the burly Scot in the corner as he urged forward his comrades in his sleep. 'Christ help us', groaned an armless dragoon, coming round from the anaesthetic.

I soothed the dying German as best I could when the awful spasms came, and through his clenched teeth he signified the pain in the 'kreuz' (small of the back). What could I say but 'Guter Junge – bleib still' ('It will not last long now!'). With his remaining hand he pressed mine as I wiped the pouring sweat from his brow. After all, suffering is a great leveller.

The orderly, an old South African campaigner, looked at the light that began to flood the sky.

'They usually go West at this hour,' he remarked grimly, with a shudder. I shuddered too; the place was alive with spirits.

For a moment we seemed to hear the sigh of the departing, feel the rushing of many wings as they brushed past. Then a gaunt, muffled figure appeared at the door bearing a lantern, for all the world like a hoary figure of 'Time', and we awoke to reality.

'I've brought down a trainload,' he said. 'A round dozen of them are urgent cases and must have beds.'

Perforce we had to shift the sleeping forms on to the concrete floor, all bruised and torn and bleeding though they were, cutting shorter their all too short rest.

An officer was brought in wounded in the abdomen, but cheerfully talking of getting home. He, too, passed away before eight o'clock.

From the nursing point of view the work is most unsatisfactory, as disinfectants, to say nothing of dressings, are continually at low ebb. Today the iodine ran out. One of the surgeons came round and signified his intention to dress a bad femur case. I had got together what things I could when he called for iodine. There being none to be had, he sighed resignedly, and saying, 'Then we will leave the dressings for the present', walked off, only to return an hour later with a quantity he had found in the town.

Of course there can be no attempt at asepsis in a place so ill ventilated, or, rather, not ventilated at all, for there are no side windows, and, although the skylight is sufficient for lighting purposes, the ventilation is effected by means of the excessively draughty entrances.

It is distinctly unhealthy, and the odours in the place are indescribable and never to be forgotten. There is no lavatory accommodation – although latrines are situated along the quay, whither the blind are led by the armless, the lame carried on orderlies' backs.

Refuse of all sorts that cannot be burned in the incinerator is disposed of in the sea, and it is good to note that the sacks of straw are being gradually replaced by real beds and the supply of blankets is greatly augmented.

Unsatisfactory, too, from the nursing point of view, is the fact that the men pass through the clearing station so rapidly that we seldom do the same dressing twice; and though there are days when, owing to rough seas or overladen boats, we are able to watch the progress of the patients, for the most part it is only the immovable cases that remain, and the rest are hurried through, leaving one wondering how they will get on.

Did I say hurried through? There is no need to hurry the men who are to go home, for no sooner is a boat announced than a general scramble ensues, and they will leave their breakfast, clothing, even their treasured trophies behind, in order not to be late.

There follows the inspection of labels (for each man is labelled for his destination: blue for England, yellow for Havre, white for a convalescent depot), and sad indeed are the faces of those to whom the medical officer has not vouchsafed the coveted blue ticket.

Just as day dawned, with a last spasm, more awful than the others, the little Saxon prisoner died.

I asked for his corpse number, but it was not to be found. In my heart I wished the boy's mother could have known he died well cared for. It is all very primitive; we have no screens to hide what once was mortal from the others.

We came off duty at 10am, just as another batch of 1,100 men began to arrive and on our way home caught a glimpse of K of K [Kitchener of Khartoum], who is paying an incognito visit, as he stepped from a destroyer.

1 November

It is impossible to keep note of the daily occurrences. Things move too quickly out here – besides, if the spirit is willing the flesh is very exhausted. Nevertheless, not for a moment do our spirits flag; on the contrary, the worse things grow the more cheerful do we become, the more determined to make the best of things. It is strange that all the years we worked hard to amuse ourselves at home not one brought an eighth of the satisfaction of this.

There is a wonderful dearth of utensils, though the store grows larger daily. It is no infrequent occurrence to have to sally out to the nearest chemist to buy air cushions, eye baths, etc., as they are required.

Night, and the wards are full. Another train disgorges its burden. The stretcher cases have to remain on stretchers. The walking cases are huddled round the stove, extended on the concrete, their blood-stained, bug-ridden greatcoats for coverings.

Without, for a moment, the rain has ceased, and in the clear night the moon smiles peacefully over the silver, gleaming sea.

What a contrast to the scene within! The restless figures of the wounded – the busy nurses.

Everyone is exhausted, for it is an almost superhuman task for seven women to tackle by day and night; but they say the Army Nursing Service will be here in sufficient numbers soon. The lady doctors have been invaluable, their zeal unflagging. They are splendid operators, and in the midst of the worst rushes never careless. Besides their work here they spend much time at the 'Women's Hospital' at a château some 3 miles out of Boulogne, where everything is run by volunteer women workers, who act as doctors, nurses, orderlies and quarter-masters.

The theatre looks quite smart, with the large sterilisers that have been installed and the operating table. What tales those whitewashed walls could tell!

Will those who are knitting away at home ever realise the value of their own handiwork, I wonder?

If they could but see the eager faces of the men as the meagre stores are issued, and they receive those ill-fitting coats, and socks, and card-board-footed shoes; could they for a single moment glance at the contented expression of the 'movable cases' as they wriggle out of their creeping shirts, so torn, so stiff with congealed blood and stained with Flanders mud, into garments that are both soft and warm, all those hours of patient knitting would be well rewarded; they would know they are not labouring in vain.

2 November
Someone has been asked to volunteer to run the military baths. I, being the one whose work in hospital must be of least value, naturally did so, and was accepted.

7 November
I am now installed as 'Lady Superintendent of Military Baths', an entirely new post!

The scene of my activities is the public baths in the Rue des Vieillards, that have been rented from the old proprietress. With six orderlies to do the rough work – the washing of towels, the cleaning of the twenty baths, and my own spacious office in which to do the men's dressings – things are cheerful enough.

About 100 men come through each day – the convalescents in the morning, so that the whole forenoon is taken up with dressings.

The difficulties at first were many, a fact which considerably enhanced the joy of the work.

1. To get the place clean was a veritable chef-d'oeuvre.
2. Drawing things from the Ordnance is no easy matter. One must not buy what may be drawn; and as I have no notion of what can be drawn there is often considerable delay.
3. Persuading the orderlies that water for dressings must be boiled, and not lukewarm, is likewise far from easy.

The days are no longer so strenuous. I arrive at eight to see that the men are getting on with their work, cut up dressings, leave out and mark towels until ten o'clock, when the convalescents begin to arrive.

By 3.30 I am able to go down to the clearing station to write letters for the helpless …

8 November. On the Ramparts of Boulogne
After the hush of the unornamental cathedral the soft autumn breezes out here are refreshing. Even in the well-ventilated baths the pungent smell of segregated humanity permeates.

What a strange place is Boulogne now, the city of hospitals, every hotel a hospital, every road thronged with troops and nurses!

23 November
The baths closed most suddenly and unexpectedly last night. The owners' exhorbitant demands for money – damages for towels which we have not even used, walls, ceilings, windows etc., that are in the same good repair as when we came – have made it imperative to commandeer the place or, to avoid friction and expense, erect new ones.

After the Major and his interpreter driver (a dentist who volunteered his services) had spent nearly two hours haranguing Madame and her hommes d'affaires, we cleared the place out.

Snow fell for the first time during the night, and it is freezing so hard this morning that the hot water thrown over the stones outside for cleansing purposes becomes ice at once …

Miss Bickmore

Ambulance Trains, France

Miss Bickmore served as a Nursing Sister on an ambulance train in France between 1914 and 1917. In January 1918 she wrote:

The experience is much sought after and the majority find their anticipation realised. There are a few to whom the life is too confined and limited and upon whose nerves the constant noise and movement of life on railway lines has a disturbing effect. These, however, are in the minority. To others there is a strange, inexplicable fascination in it, which quite supersedes the discomforts and limitations …

It is a life of uncertainty. A Sister receives orders she is to join a certain train – where is the train? No one knows. Where, when and how can she join it? No one knows. Who arranges where and when an individual ambulance train shall run? (I say individual advisedly – for the train on which one lives becomes as much an individual companion or friend as one's horse or motor car).

The OC of an ambulance train is not allowed to send telegrams stating where his train is likely to be on a certain date: therefore any member of the staff wishing to join it must patiently wait at some Base Station until Fortune sends it that way, or pursue it like a will o' the wisp in a maddening and exhausting circle. Five days, a week, a fortnight is often thus spent by fresh or returning members of the staff.

To the waiting Sister the longed for intelligence comes at last, and an order to be at such and such a place at a certain time. Probably the time is night, or early on a dark and cold morning. Personal belongings are reduced to a minimum; a car or an ambulance drops the seeker at the nearest point to the garage, and in darkness a perilous foot journey intervenes, among and across railway lines, moving trains, shunting trucks, points and signal wires, clutching suitcase and hold-all, before the train is boarded.

A first class coach then becomes home and a very comfortable and happy one it can be.

The Staff Coach is usually in the middle of the train and is occupied by the Medical Officers and Nursing Sisters. It has a corridor and the compartments are transformed into bed-sitting rooms and mess rooms.

Away from this centre, at either end, runs the long, long train – a shining, vibrant, living creature of sinuous grace. It is a very patient and long-suffering creature, for it has many and various drivers – some French, some English, some who understand its brakes and ways, some who do not, and like a well or badly driven horse, so it responds. But it has no vice and when bumped and jerked and broken, it still holds its load safely. Thus it winds its way, up hill and down, through woods and vales and towns; along single lines or threading, bumping, grating its mysterious track among labyrinths of metals, into great junctions. Dashing at high speed 'Empty' to a far advanced Casualty Clearing Station (CCS) to gather a 'Crisis Load'; or returning at 10 miles an hour, bearing within it the shattered remnants of those who so proudly and bravely sallied forth against the foe on the battlefields a few short hours before. Sometimes under shell fire, sometimes under raiding or fighting aeroplanes it serenely 'carries on'.

On arriving at the 'Rail Head' where the Casualty Clearing Stations lie, the work for the staff begins.

The patients are brought to the train in ambulances or on little trolleys run on light rails. They lie on stretchers and are passed into the coaches or 'wards' of the train and are then transferred to the beds. The Sisters receive them and examine their medical cards, decide what diet they should have and arrange their shattered limbs, by means of bandages, pillows, sand bags etc., to travel with as little suffering as possible.

Mud, blood and sweat clothe them still, and the tormenting parasites accompany them unless they have been detained for a period at the CCS until fit to undertake the journey, in which case they have been cleansed and clothed afresh.

No tongue can tell what these patients have been through, and none who have not at least seen them in their battle-field array can form any conception of it.

The Medical Officers see each case personally and order the treatment, which the Sisters carry out, while the orderlies attend to food, drink and general wants.

The space is very confined. 'Stretcher cases' fill up the floors of the wards, in addition to the occupied beds which are arranged in tiers like the bunks in a ship's cabin. Water is heavy and difficult to carry; it therefore must be used economically – sterilising or boiling of water for fomentations, tea or bovril, has to be done on a Primus stove, in the midst of the crush and in spite of the swaying, jerking train, helpless patients to be fed in almost inaccessible positions, carrel tubes charged, splints adjusted, dressings attended to by Sisters in acrobatic and perilous positions. But whatever is done is so necessary and so joyously and gratefully received, that the handicaps, limitations and crass imperfections of the nursing, per se, are compensated.

But it is these great and unavoidable imperfections that distress the nurse, and the consciousness of how very little she can do compared to what requires to be done. On the other hand the ambulance train is the easiest and best attended phase of the period of transportation, from the spot on which the wound is received, to the Hospital, which being beyond the Fighting Area, can have and do all that science and skilled attendance demand.

It usually takes about two hours to load and two to unload an ambulance train and the journeys (loaded) last anything between six and thirty-six hours. The average length of time is probably twelve hours for a journey loaded.

The ambulance train comes fourth in the Traffic Schedule, and is often held back for troops, ammunition and supply trains which have precedence. A loaded ambulance train has a speed limit also. But long though such journeys are for sick and wounded, the patients are so much more comfortable than they have been for many long weary days and nights on active service, that they sleep and rest, thankful to have done their bit, and to be getting away from the horror of it all for a while.

The return runs empty; from the Base to the CCS takes, generally, eight or ten hours.

On reaching its destination the loaded train becomes again like a beehive in swarm. In the early morning hours, dark and cold and wet, the unloading usually takes place.

Ambulances, stretchers and stretcher-bearers appear like a waiting shadow crowd, as the train glides into her berth, but soon, under a few dim lights, the shadows spring to life. Ambulances hum, bearers shout and moving lights and vague forms thread a maze-like dance, which to the uninitiated, must look weird and dangerous in the extreme. The engine is taken off and the train seems dead, though every door is flung wide open and a constant stream of stretcher-borne, blanket-wrapped figures pass out from the hands of the train orderlies to those of the platform stretcher-bearers.

Meantime, the Sisters keep watch over the moving and arranging of the patients, until they are safely in the Ambulance, while the Medical Officers patrol the platform, keeping all under observation.

Once in the ambulance, the train staff has no more jurisdiction over the patients. Slowly and carefully they are driven away; the train staff knows not whither. The order as to which Hospital each loaded ambulance is bound for are given by an officer at the station exit.

The train is now 'empty', except for its permanent dwellers. These return to their various quarters and labours.

Pending the arrival of an engine, the wards are swept and the blankets shaken by the orderlies, while official and domestic matters are taken in hand by the various departments, after which breakfast and a much needed wash (no baths and not much hot water!) lead to bed and a rest, when possible. At times the ambulance train is taken into garage and awaits orders from the mysterious Headquarters which deals with ambulance trains; at times a return journey is ordered at once to take up another load. During these intervening periods in garage, cleaning and preparation for the next 'load' proceeds. Occasionally the train loads again within a couple of hours at the Base, to which it has just discharged its sick and wounded from the Front. Now the load consists of patients leaving the Base Hospital for 'Blighty'. These, indeed, are happy loads and the travellers can be recognised from afar, not only because they look so clean and have so many labels attached to them – Oh no! – not those reasons – but by the 'Blighty Smile' which diffuses their whole person.

The engine driver, French or English, is the best authority as to the destination of an ambulance train and even he is not to be relied upon, as he may only drive to a certain point and then hand over to another authority and driver, French or English.

Also the hour at which an ambulance train starts is as uncertain as the weather. Information may be given to the Officer Commanding that the engine will not come on for a couple of hours at least.

The OC, thereupon, having due regard for the health and necessities of his Staff, allows certain members, Sisters and others, to go out; but it is quite possible that, during their absence, long before the stated hour, those left on the train will feel the familiar little thud and vibration, which means 'Engine on – we're off!' and regardless of the feelings or inconveniences of anyone, 'off' we are, and 'on' the absentees are not.

These are exciting moments. By means, however, of telephones, cars and messengers, the missing members are usually retrieved before the train has crawled, bumped, laboured and shrieked its long length over points, paused at signal boxes and got up speed.

Two hours only is the regulation leave of absence from the train and often it is impracticable to take that. Sisters are not allowed 'out' singly except at the Base towns and one Sister must always remain on the train.

The rules regulating the social life of the Sisters are very severe and social intercourse with the Medical Officers is prohibited. It is, therefore, especially essential that the Sisters should have resources in themselves and be on friendly terms.

The constantly varying scenes and changing surroundings form an endless interest. Flourishing towns and fair rich country in the peace areas give place to desolation, chaos and ruin as the track of the Armies is followed up. Traces of German occupation and ruination give way to British occupation and re-construction, followed by re-possession by French. Shattered villages with ruins, barely marking out former streets, in seas of mud, thronged with khaki clad troops, living in cellars or roofless, almost wall-less rooms;

among them the few French women and old men, who braved all, rather than leave their wrecked homes, with their tiny displays of goods to tempt the Tommy: the forlorn and homeless cats, the booming of big guns, the rattle of machine guns, the hum of aeroplanes, the cram and crush and crowd of the high roads; troops marching or riding in old London buses, cavalry, motor lorries and cars, bicycles, German prisoners. As the Army presses on, a forlorn and haunted emptiness, till safety being assured, the inhabitants begin to creep back again; the awful aspect of shell-destroyed land under winter snow and mud, retreats before the miracle of Spring when nature throws a veil of beauty over the hideous desolation and ruin, making the remembrance of what was seem impossible before what is. And in addition the short visits to villages while the train lies in garage, in some lonely country spot and acquaintances with the charming independent French peasantry. All constitute a kaleidoscopic interest that never fails.

This account of ambulance train work would be incomplete without a reference to the special difficulties attached to the work on 'French' trains that have been adapted to this use, as against khaki or 'English' trains, built for the purpose.

The khaki trains have a corridor passing down their whole length and many special arrangements facilitating the work.

The adapted French train is merely an ordinary non-corridor passenger train. Thus each ward or coach becomes self-contained and isolated from others. Two orderlies are in charge of each coach and the MOs and Sisters visit their appointed number in turn. This necessitates constant jumping up and down when the train is standing, in rain, wind or snow, unspeakable mud, daylight or pitch black night, or 'foot boarding' from coach to coach.

The lights of the train are closely veiled. If an air-raid takes place over and around it, all lights are extinguished and like a long dark snake it squats on the lines, waiting till the danger is passed.

Thus the difficulties, fatigue and danger of the work on a 'French' train are considerably added to by its construction – so also are the interest and the 'thrill'.

Sister K.E. Luard

No. 5 Ambulance Train, France and Belgium

Sister Luard, an experienced nursing Sister in the QAIMNS, served during the South African war. She arrived in Le Havre on 20 August 1914 and at the beginning of September was sent to St Nazaire where she became increasingly frustrated with the situation. There seemed to be no work for her until 13 September, when she received orders to go by train to Le Mans where she arrived two days later.

Tuesday, 15 September

The train managed to reach Le Mans at 1am this morning. At 7am a motor ambulance took us up to the Hospital, which is a rather grimy Bishop's Palace, pretty full and busy.

Wednesday, 16 September
We explored the Cathedral, which is absolutely beautiful, perched high up over an open space – now crowded with transport and motor ambulances.

I have just been to High Mass (Choral).

There is any amount of work here at the Bishop's Palace; more than they can get through on night duty with bad cases, and another Jesuit College has been opened as a Stationary Hospital.

Sunday, 20 September
Began with an early service at the Jesuit School Hospital at 6.30, and the rest of the day one will never forget. The fighting for these concrete entrenched positions of the Germans behind Rheims has been so terrific since last Sunday that the number of casualties has been enormous. Three trains full of wounded, numbering altogether 1,175 cases, have been dressed at the station today; we were sent down at 11 this morning. The train I was put to had 510 cases. You boarded a cattle-truck, armed with a tray of dressings and a pail; the men were lying on straw; had been in trains for several days; most had only been dressed once, and many were gangrenous. If you found one urgently needed amputation or operation, or was likely to die, you called an MO to have him taken off the train for Hospital. No one grumbled or made any fuss. Then you joined the throng in the dressing-station, and for hours doctors of all ranks, Sisters and orderlies, grappled with the stream of stretchers, and limping, staggering, bearded, dirty, fagged men, and ticketed them off for the motor ambulances to the Hospitals, or back to the train, after dressing them. The platform was soon packed with stretchers with all the bad cases waiting patiently to be taken to Hospital. We cut off the silk vest of a dirty, brigandish-looking officer, nearly finished with a wound through his lung. The Black Watch and Camerons were almost unrecognisable in their rags. The staple dressing is tincture of iodine; you don't attempt anything but swabbing with lysol, and then gauze dipped in iodine. They were nearly all shrapnel shell wounds – more ghastly than anything I have ever seen or smelt; the Mauser wounds of the Boer War were pin-pricks compared with them. There was also a huge train of French wounded being dressed on the other side of the station, including lots of weird, gaily-bedecked Zouaves.

There was no real confusion about the whole day, owing to the good organising of the Clearing Hospital people who run it. Every man was fed, dressed and sorted. They'll have a heavy time at the two hospitals tonight with the cases sent up from the trains.

M. and I are now – 9pm – in charge of a train of 141 (with an MO, and two orderlies) for St Nazaire; we jump out at the station and see to them, and the orderlies and the people on the stations feed them; we have the worst cases next to us.

Tuesday, 22 September
Got back to Le Mans at 2am. We have been two days and two nights in our clothes; food where, when, and what one could get; one wash only on a station platform at a

tap. One cleaning of teeth in the dark on the line between trucks. They have no water on trains or at stations, except on the engine, which makes tea in cans for you for the men when it stops.

We are to rest today, to be ready for another train tonight if necessary. The line from the front to Rouen – where there are two General Hospitals – is cut; hence this appalling over-crowding at our base. When we got back this morning, nine of those we took off the trains on Sunday afternoon had died here, and one before he reached the hospital – three of tetanus. Some of the amputations die of septic absorption and shock. I went to the nine o'clock Choral High Mass this morning at that glorious Cathedral. It was very fine and comforting.

Thursday, 24 September, 3pm

Taking 480 sick and wounded down to St Nazaire, with a junior staff nurse, one MO, and two orderlies. Just been feeding them all at Angers; it is a stupendous business. The train is miles long – not corridor or ambulance; they have straw to lie on the floors and stretchers. The MO has been two nights in the train already on his way down from the front (4 miles from the guns), and we joined on to him with a lot of hospital cases sent down to the base. I've been collecting the worst ones into carriages near ours all the way down when we stop; but of course you miss a good many. Got my haversack lined with jaconet and filled with cut-dressings, very convenient, as you have both hands free. We continually stop at little stations, so you can get to a good many of them, and we get quite expert at clawing along the footboards; some of the men, with their eyes, noses, or jaws shattered, are so extraordinarily good and uncomplaining. Got hold of a spout-feeder and some tubing at Angers for a boy in the Grenadier Guards, with a gaping hole through his mouth to his chin, who can't eat, and cannot otherwise drink. The French people bring coffee, fruit, and all sorts of things to them when we stop.

The number of casualties must be nearly into five figures this last battle alone; and when you think of the Russians, the Germans, the French, the Austrians, and the Belgians all like that, the whole convulsion seems more meaningless than ever for civilised nations.

Friday, 25 September

In train back to Le Mans, 9pm. We landed our tired, stiff, painful convoy at St Nazaire at 8.45 yesterday evening. The MOs there told us our lot made 1800 that had come down since early morning; one load of bad cases took eight hours to unload.

The Padre told me he was the only one at St Nazaire for all the hospitals and all the troops in camp (15,000 in one camp alone). He had commandeered the Bishop of Khartoum to help him, and another bishop, who both happen to be here.

Sunday, 27 September [Le Mans]

Went to the Voluntary Evening Service for the troops at the theatre at 5. The Padres and a Union Jack and the Allies' Flags; a piano on the stage; officers and sisters in the stalls; and the rest packed tight with men: they were very reverent, and nearly took the roof off in the Hymns, Creed, and Lord's Prayer. Excellent sermon. We had the War

Intercessions and a good prayer I didn't know, ending with 'Strengthen us in life, and comfort us in death.'

Friday, 2 October
I am frightfully attached to Le Mans as a place. The town is old and curly, and full of lovely corners and 'Places', views and Avenues and Gardens. The Cathedral grows more and more upon one; I have several special spots where you get the most exquisite poems of colour and stone, where I go and browse; it is very quiet and beautifully kept.

The Stationary Hospital is also set in a jewel of a spot. A Jesuits' College, full of cloisters covered with vines, and lawns with silver statues, shady avenues and sunny gardens, long corridors and big halls which are the wards; the cook-house is a camp under a splendid row of big chestnut trees, and there is of course a chapel.

Our occupation of it is rather incongruous; there is practically no furniture except the boys' beds, some chairs, many crucifixes and statues, terribly primitive sanitary arrangements and water supply. We have to boil our instruments and make their tea in the same one saucepan in the Officers' Ward; you do without dusters, dishcloths, soap-dishes, pillow-cases, and many other necessities in peace time.

They continue to die every day and night at both Hospitals, though we are taking few new cases.

On 10 October Sister Luard was sent from Le Mans to join an ambulance train at Villeneuve Triage.

Tuesday, 13 October
At last I am on the train, and have just unpacked. There is an Army Sister and two Reserve, a Major OC, and two junior officers. The train is one-third mile long, so three walks along its side gives you exercise for a mile. The ward beds are lovely: broad and soft, with lovely pillow-cases and soft thick blankets; any amount of dressings and surgical equipment, and a big kitchen, steward's store, and three orderlies to each waggon. Shouldn't be surprised if we get 'there' in the dark, and won't see the war country. Sometimes you are stopped by bridges being blown up in front of you, and little obstacles of that kind.

Saturday, 17 October [Braisne]
We are to stay here till Monday, to go on taking up the wounded from the 1st Division. They went on coming in all yesterday in motor ambulances. They come straight from the trenches, and are awfully happy on the train with the first attempts at comforts they have known.

10pm. Wrote the last before breakfast, and we haven't sat down since. We are to move back to Villeneuve tomorrow, dropping the sick probably at Versailles. Everyone thankful to be going to move at last. The gas has given out, and the entire train is lit by candles.

The patients are extraordinarily good, and take everything as it comes (or as it doesn't come!) without any grumbling. Your day is taken up in rapidly deciding which of all the things that want doing you must let go undone; shall they be washed or fed, or beds made, or have their hypodermics and brandies and medicines, or their dressings done? You end in doing some of each in each carriage, or in washing them after dinner instead of before breakfast.

The guns have been banging all the afternoon; some have dropped pretty near again today, but you haven't time to take much notice. Our meals are very funny – always candles stuck in a wine bottle – no tablecloth – everything on one plate with the same knife and fork – coffee in a glass, served by a charming dirty Frenchman; many jokes going on between the three tables – the French officials, the MOs, and us.

Monday, 19 October. Rouen, 9pm
Got here late last night, and all the wounded were taken off straight away to the two general hospitals here. One has 1,300 cases, and has kept two people operating day and night. A great many deaths from tetanus.

Tuesday, 20 October, 6pm. Just leaving Rouen for Boulogne
We have been busy today getting the train ready, stocking dressings, etc. All the 500 blankets are sent in to be fumigated after each journey, and 500 others drawn instead. And well they may be; one of the difficulties is the lively condition of the men's shirts and trousers (with worse than fleas) when they come from the trenches in the same clothes they've worn for five weeks or more. You can't wonder we made tracks for a bath at Rouen.

Wednesday, 21 October. Arrived at Boulogne 6am
Went on to Calais and reached St Omer at 2pm.

3.30pm. Off to Steenwerck, close to the Belgian frontier, N.W. of Lille. This feels like the Front again. Thousands and thousands of Indian troops are marching close to the line, with long fair British officers in turbans mounted, who salute us, and we wave back; transport on mules.

Thursday, 22 October. Steenwerk
Took on from convoys all night in pitch darkness – a very bad load this time; going to go septic; swelling under the bandages. There was a fractured spine and a malignant oedema, both dying; we put these two off today at St Omer. Now nearly back at Boulogne.

6pm. Hazebrouck again. We are said to be going to Belgium this time – possibly Ypres. There are a terrible lot of wounded to be got down – more than all the trains can take; they are putting some of them off on the stations where there is a MO, with a few men, and going back for more.

7pm. Ypres. Just arrived.

Sunday, 25 October [Ypres]
Couldn't write last night; the only thing was to try and forget it all. It has been an absolute hell of a journey – there is no other word for it. This big battle from Ostend to Lille is perhaps the most desperate of all, though that is said of each in turn – Mons, the Aisne, and this; but the men and officers who have been through all say this is the worst. The Germans are desperate, and stick at nothing, and the Allies are the same; and in determi-

nation to drive them back, each man personally seems to be the same. Consequently the 'carnage' is appalling, and we have been practically in it, as far as horrors go. Guns were cracking and splitting all night, lighting up the sky in flashes, and fires were burning on both sides. The Clearing Hospital close by, which was receiving the wounded from the field and sending them on to us, was packed and overflowing with badly wounded.

We had 368; a good 200 were dangerously and seriously wounded, perhaps more; and the sitting-up cases were bad enough. The compound-fractured femurs were put up with rifles and pick-handles for splints, padded with bits of kilts and straw; nearly all the men had more than one wound – some had ten; one man with a huge compound fracture above the elbow had tied on a bit of string with a bullet in it as a tourniquet above the wound himself. When I cut off his soaked three layers of sleeve there was no dressing on it at all.

They were bleeding faster than we could cope with it; and the agony of getting them off the stretchers and on to the top bunks is a thing to forget. We were full up by about 2am, and then were delayed by a collision up the line, which was blocked by dead horses as a result. All night and without a break till we got back to Boulogne at 4pm next day (yesterday) we grappled with them and some were not dressed when we got into Boulogne. The head cases were delirious, and trying to get out of the window, and we were giving strychnine and morphia all round. Two were put off dying at St Omer, but we kept the rest alive to Boulogne.

The outstanding shining thing that hit you in the eye all through was the universal silent pluck of the men; they stuck it all without a whine or complaint or even a comment. The bleeding made them all frightfully thirsty (they had only been hit a few hours many of them), and luckily we had got in a good supply of boiled water beforehand on each carriage, so we had plenty when there was time to get it. In the middle of the worst of it in the night I became conscious of a Belgian Boy Scout of fourteen in the corridor, with a glass and a pail of drinking water; that boy worked for hours with his glass and pail on his own. We took him back to Calais. He had come up into the firing line on his cycle fitted with a rifle, with tobacco for the troops, and lived with the British whom he loved, sharing their rations. He was a little brick.

There were twenty-five officers on the train. They said there were 11,000 Germans dead, and they were using the dead piled up instead of trenches.

It took from 4 to 10pm to unload our bad cases and get them into hospitals on motor ambulances: they lay in rows on their stretchers on the platform waiting their turn without a grumble.

There have been so many hundreds brought down this week that they've had suddenly to clear four hotels for hospitals.

We are now in the filthiest of sidings, and the smell of the burning of our heaps of filthy debris off the train is enough to make you sick. We all slept like logs last night, and could have gone on all day; but the train has to be cleaned down by the orderlies, and everything got ready for the next lot.

Monday, 26 October, 7am. Ypres

We got here again about 10pm last night in pouring wet, and expected another night like Friday night, but we for some reason remained short of the station, and when we found there was nothing doing, lay down in our clothes and slept, booted and spurred in mackintosh, aprons, etc. We were all so tired and done up yesterday, MOs, Sisters, and orderlies, that we were glad of the respite. There was a tremendous banging and flashing to the north about three o'clock, and this morning it was very noisy, like a continuous roll of thunder interrupted by loud bangs and shaking the train. Some of it sounds quite close.

This place is full of Belgian women and children refugees in a bad way from exhaustion.

A long line of our horse ambulances is coming slowly in.

Got leave to go into the town and see the Cathedral of St Martin. Town chock-full of French and Belgian troops, and unending streams of columns, also Belgian refugees, cars full of staff officers. The Cathedral is thirteenth century, glorious as usual. There are hundreds of German prisoners in the town in the Cloth Hall. It was a very warrish feeling saying one's prayers in the Cathedral to the sound of the guns of one of the greatest battles in the world.

Friday, 30 October. Boulogne

After filling up at Nieppe we went back to Bailleul and took up 239 Indians, mostly with smashed left arms from a machine-gun that caught them in the act of firing over a trench. They are nearly all 47th Sikhs.

Sunday, 15 November

The cold of this train life is going to be rather a problem. Our quarters are not heated, but we have 'made' (i.e. acquired, looted) a very small oil-stove which faintly warms the corridor, but you can imagine how no amount of coats or clothes keeps you warm in a railway carriage in winter. A smart walk out of doors would do it, but that you can't get off when the train is stationary for fear of its vanishing, and for obvious reasons when it is moving. I did walk round the train for an hour in the dark and slime in the siding yesterday evening, but it is not a cheering form of exercise.

Today it is pouring cats and dogs, awful for loading sick, and there will be many after this week for the trains.

Everyone has of course cleared out of beautiful Ypres, but we are going to load up at Poperinghe, the town next before it, which is now Railhead.

Monday, 16 November. Boulogne, 9am

We loaded up at Bailleul 344. The Clearing Hospitals were very full, and some came off a convoy. One of mine died. One, wounded above the knee, was four days in the open before being picked up; he had six bullets in his leg, two in each arm, and crawled about till found; one of the arm wounds he got doing this. I went to bed at 4.

Tuesday, 17 November. 3am

When we got our load down to Boulogne yesterday morning all the hospitals were full, and the weather was too rough for the ships to come in and clear them, so we were ordered on to Havre, a very long journey. A German died before we got to

Abbeville, where we put off two more very bad ones; and at Amiens we put off four more, who wouldn't have reached Havre. About midnight something broke on the train, and we were hung up for hours, and haven't yet got to Rouen, so we shall have them on the train all tomorrow too, and have all the dressings to do for the third time. One of the night orderlies has been run in for being asleep on duty. He climbed into a top bunk (where a Frenchman was taken off at Amiens), and deliberately covered up and went to sleep. He was in charge of 28 patients. Another was left behind at Boulogne, absent without leave, thinking we should unload, and the train went off for Havre. He'll be run in too. Shows how you can't leave the train.

Our load is a heavy and anxious one – 344; we shall be glad to land them safely somewhere. The amputations, fractures, and lung cases stand these long journeys very badly.

Wednesday, 18 November. 5pm

We are getting on for Havre at last. This long journey from Belgium down to Havre has been a strange mixture. Glorious country with the flame and blue haze of late autumn on hills, towns, and valleys, bare beech-woods with hot red carpets. Glorious British Army lying broken in the train – sleep (or the chance of it) three hours one night and four the next, with all the hours between (except meals) hard work putting the British Army together again; haven't taken off my puttees since Sunday. Seems funny, 400 people (of whom four are women and about sixty are sound) all whirling through France by special train. Why? Because of the Swelled Head of the All-Highest.

We had a boy with no wound, suffering from shock from shell bursts. When he came round, if you asked him his name he would look fixedly at you and say 'Yes.' If you asked him something else, with a great effort he said 'Mother.'

Wednesday, 25 November

Arrived at 11pm last night at a God-forsaken little place about 8 miles from the firing line. Found a very depressed major taking a most gloomy view of life and the war, in charge of Indians. Pitch-dark night, and they were a mile away from the station, so we went to bed at 12 and loaded up at 7.30 this morning, all Indians, mostly badly wounded.

Wednesday, 2 December. 9pm

We filled up at St Omer from the three hospitals there. A great many cases of frost-bite were put on. They crawl on hands and knees, poor dears. Some left in hospital are very severe and have had to be amputated below the knee. Some of the toes drop off. I have one carriage of twenty-four Indians.

1914
Serbia and Poland

Miss Flora Sandes

Serbian Military Hospital, Kragujevatz, Serbia

On 12 August 1914, the day that Austrian troops invaded Serbia and met with strong resistance from the Serbian army, Flora Sandes, accompanied by her violin, was travelling to Serbia with a St John's Ambulance Unit. She was not a trained nurse, but had been an active member of the St John's Ambulance Brigade for three years and had learnt the rudiments of first aid. She was one of eight women, five of whom were fully trained nurses. One, Emily Simmonds, had trained in England and then went to America where she became a theatre sister. The leader of the party was Madame Mabel Grouitch, an American married to the Serbian secretary of state for foreign affairs, who had gone to England urgently seeking doctors, nurses, medical supplies, and financial aid. When the unit arrived at the hospital in Kragujevatz they were given a small room and straw to sleep on. They had brought a few comforts with them – portable canvas wash stands, sleeping bags, hot water bottles and insect powder.

The journey to Serbia, in chaotic early wartime conditions, took over three weeks.

Madame Grouitch was financing the party, and she had not much money to do it on – we travelled most of the way third class – but she had what was very much more useful at that time at any rate – and perhaps always – she had very fascinating manners, and was extremely pretty. Everyone said that it was impossible to get a party of women across Europe at that time, France was still mobilising, all the trains were disorganised, and travelling was very difficult. We used to get stuck at some little wayside station, with nobody to meet us, and nowhere to go to, and Madame Grouitch used just to go up to the Military Commandant and smile at him, and in five minutes there would be motor cars to fetch us, and we would be taken up to the best hotel in the place, and everything done for us, and the next morning there would be the Military Commandant to see us off, all smiles and bows, and bouquets of flowers for Madame Grouitch. The station platforms used to be crowded with French soldiers on their way to the Front, who were much interested in our party.

We got on all right until we got to Italy, which was then a neutral country. Among other little things we had picked up in Paris thirty Serbian students, who were there studying law or medicine, and we took them through with us by way of being for the Serbian Red X, but in reality to fight in the Army, where every man was needed.

The Italians got wind of this, and we were all very nearly being locked up as spies, the whole party of us, in fact the last day of our journey through Italy we had an Italian soldier posted as sentry at the door of each of our railway carriages, with strict orders that none of us were to be allowed to move about anywhere. I had the presence of mind to give the sentry nearest to me a drink out of my emergency flask – after that I was allowed to move about wherever I liked. We finished up that journey with 36 hours on the deck of a Greek cattle ship, in a raging thunderstorm … but we did finally, through the pluck and perseverance of Madame Grouitch, arrive in Serbia.

We were sent straight to a large Military Hospital in a town called Kragujevatz. There were two big buildings in our Hospital, one holding about 500 wounded, and the other about the same number of sick, and there were only us seven (the eighth having gone somewhere else) to do all the nursing, under the Serbian doctors, and with Serbian orderlies to help. The wounded were pouring in then, the Serbs were repelling the first Austrian invasion across the Danube, and sometimes they used to arrive by train, at three o'clock in the morning, when we all had to turn out to receive them, but more often by bullock waggon, travelling three or four days from the Front on the floor of the bullock waggon with only their first bloodstained field dressings on their wounds. Many of the worst wounded died on the way, and those that did arrive were in a terrible condition.

We were very short of all hospital material, especially of chloroform, and only the very worst cases could be done with an anaesthetic, but the Serbian soldier prides himself on being able to stand an operation and he will draw himself up proudly, and say 'Ja sam Serbin' – that means 'I am a Serb' – by which he means to imply that he will go through anything without flinching. I have seen a soldier, after a very painful operation done without any anaesthetic, take a bottle of rakia, a kind of homemade brandy, from under his shirt and hand it to the operating surgeon with the remark, 'You will need a drink after that Brother'. Not he, the man who had stood the pain, but the operating surgeon who had been kind enough to do it for him. They have more endurance than any other race I have ever met.

We knew nothing of the language when we went, and our conversation had to be carried on almost entirely by means of signs, so of course we made many ludicrous mistakes in consequence.

Besides working all day, it came to each one's turn every sixth night to do night duty, and this meant 36 hours on duty without any sleep, as the hospital was crowded, and we all lived and ate and slept in one small room. It was very weird walking round those hospital wards all night, only dimly lighted by flickering oil lamps, and wholly and solely responsible for 500 badly wounded men, and it didn't make matters any easier because the Serbian soldier, like all soldiers, when he goes to sleep covers his head entirely over with the blanket, so that you could not tell by just glancing at a man whether he was dead or whether he was only asleep, and he was not at all pleased if you woke him up to find out either.

These men's mothers walked in long journeys over the mountains to see their boys in hospital. If you ask a Serb where his home is he will tell you 'three or four days away', and that means three or four days' march, as the little villages are not connected by the railway, there are no motor service cars, and the only way to get about was to walk. These women walked three or four days, carrying a great heavy basket of home-made provisions for their boys. When they found them they didn't cry over them, or ask if they were badly hurt, they went straight up to their bedside and said, 'My son, I congratulate you on being wounded in the defence of your country.' …

Sister Joan Martin-Nicholson

Military Hospital, Warsaw, Poland

After she was told to leave the Hôpital Militaire in Brussels, Sister Martin-Nicholson spent a little time with her friends in the city. The German authorities then sent her to the royal palace, which they had commandeered and turned into a Hospital. In September she was released and was sent, with a group of nurses under armed guard, through Germany by train and then by ship to Copenhagan, where they were given a wonderful reception. She offered her services to the Russian Red Cross and then continued, with a friend, on her journey to Petrograd. As there was very little extra nursing needed there they took another train to Warsaw where the population lived under the threat of German occupation.

Standing at the foot of the hill upon which Warsaw spreads, this hospital consisted of a number of separate buildings, each used for a special purpose, dotted about in large grounds.

We were received with open arms and taken across to the newest building, which had not as yet been occupied, and where men were still at work cleaning and polishing and furnishing. The steam heat was turned on, the luggage brought up, and, when we had changed into our most spotless uniform, we went across the grounds to lunch in the separate building for meals.

The Polish Sisters, who were already seated, rose in a body on the advent of the strangers, each one murmuring some courteous welcome. Many were the meals, with strange dishes and at odd hours, we were to eat with our Polish friends. Breakfast was from 8 to 9.30, with every kind of bread and cake, jam and preserved fruit; lunch at 12, with soup and queer-shaped fish, pickled cucumbers so strong they took away the breath, hot meat with extraordinary sauces, weird puddings, rank cheese, and the ever present kvass; tea at any hour all through the day for the nurse who had a moment in which to run across the usually sodden grounds to drink it; and supper at 8 if the work was done, but kept going till 11 if the nurses were late, as they usually were on account of the strenuous work.

A little group of nurses ran quickly from the mealhouse, as it was called, to the buildings which contained the principal surgical ward. They were all in white with white caps; but when they lifted their overalls to escape the mud, I noticed for the first time the much-to-be-deplored habit, practised throughout Russia and Poland, of wearing the ordinary dress underneath. Tweed, cotton, or silk skirts topped with lace, cotton, or satin blouses were to be seen, according to the wearer's station in life.

There are many items which should be remedied in the English hospital uniform, and in which the Danes are far ahead, such as the wearing of elbow sleeves, enabling the nurse to disinfect herself to the elbow if necessary, instead of the long tight sleeve either covered by another one in cotton which must get dirty and tainted with septic matter, or ending in a celluloid cuff which has to be removed and the sleeve turned up and pinned whenever there is the smallest dressing to be done.

We went up a flight of steps, with orderlies sitting or leaning on the railings, smoking, through a little anteroom into the ward. For a moment I paused to take in the scene, so different from anything I had ever seen before. In the enormous low-pitched room were four long rows of twenty beds and shorter cross-rows of six: at the end was a small room with eight beds in which were put the worst cases.

Every window was tight shut, and there were two blazing stoves. Orderlies sat on the beds playing cards with the patients. Every bed was one jumbled heap of sheets and quilt. Dirty basins, glasses, plates and mugs were scattered everywhere, and two orderlies were busy sweeping up the orange-peel, fruit-skins, cigarette-ends and matches lying on the floor. And over all hung a dense blue cloud of smoke, for, as I discovered later, no matter how ill a patient may be, he may smoke if he wants to, little children running in all day long with boxes of cigarettes for their beloved soldiers.

'When do you make the beds and wash the patients?' I asked after a tour of inspection.

Pretty little Sister Sokovono glanced up from an illustrated paper and smiled.

'They are all washed when they come in, and the beds will be made if they go down to be dressed!'

'You don't do the dressings in the ward, then?'

'Oh no! They either walk down or are taken on stretchers in the lift to the theatre. We begin in half an hour, and it's pretty hard work!'

'But the very bad cases – the man over there on the left, for instance?'

'Oh, they all go down …'

A ring of spurs, a subdued hum, and the senior surgeon entered, accompanied by a lady doctor and the head of the hospital, who was also a doctor, and who confided in me later that he often came and dabbled in dressings and smaller operations to keep his hand in.

The English Sisters were introduced, and after we had been put through a searching catechism on the prospect of peace in the West, the strength of the different countries' fighting forces, and the methods in the hospitals of various nations, we all descended, a cheery little party, into the theatre.

'You will find us rather different from yourselves. In fact, we are rather afraid of what you will think of us.' The lady doctor smiled as she put her hand on my shoulder.

'We are very thorough, but a little behind in many things. And, above all, don't give heed to the men if they scream. They will begin directly when they see you coming, and will continue crescendo until the end, but if you keep a packet of cigarettes in your apron pocket and give them one, or a sweet, when all is over they will be as content as a child. Will you take this case. He's bad, had his back clean stripped from neck to heel by shrapnel. It's a horrid sight, and I don't like to give it to one of the new girls. We dress five at a time. Sister Sokovono will assist you as she speaks English.'

I went up to my case, who was lying face down on the table, and placed my hand on his outstretched one. He was but an ordinary peasant, and yet he raised my hand very gently to his lips as he murmured in broken English, 'I am honoured to suffer pain at the English lady's hand.'

And then began a silent exhibition of endurance such as I shall never forget. The details are too ghastly to give here, and I decided that in all my travels this was the worst experience I had ever been through.

'Can't I dress him under an anaesthetic?' I asked hurriedly, when I saw that the man was on the point of fainting.

'No! No! He's used to it. He's splendid today; he usually makes an awful fuss.'

One after another the men passed under my hands. Dirty dressings were pulled off and thrown on the floor, and fresh ones wasted in every possible way. Doctor, orderlies, patients all smoked, whilst girls who had been perhaps only three weeks' training probed and swabbed the most excruciating cases. Screams rent the air, and great sobs shook the very tables the men lay on.

There was certainly some truth in what the doctor had told me, as I found out on approaching a little Siberian, suffering from some trivial wound in the arm. Whilst I had been occupied he had sat whistling contentedly; when I moved in his direction he just opened his mouth and screamed. An orderly cuffed him smartly on the head, but that did not stop him. It seemed as if nothing could. He shrieked even when I was not touching him. Then at last I had a sudden inspiration. I took two caramels and stuffed them into his mouth.

Silence! Then his eyes opened wide with content, and with a muttered 'Haracho!' ('Beautiful!') he sat happily sucking the mess until the bandage was on.

We became great friends, we two who could barely make each other understand. He insisted on being tucked up each night, and while I was tucking him in he would talk of the beautiful bed and covering. I suppose even these hospital mattresses, full of prickly straw, and these thin hospital sheets were luxurious to one who at home probably slept on the straw-covered ground.

There were operations at night to which we would be called, as though to something marvellous, only to find them something we had seen a hundred times before. But I confess that I found the women surgeons marvellously good and quiet, confident and undisturbed. They would carry on an ordinary conversation with those around even while engaged in the most dangerous work.

Asepsis was almost nil, but 99 per cent of the cases recovered, due to the hard and simple lives the patients underwent in normal times …

Sister Violetta Thurstan

Prince Volkonsky's Flying Field Ambulance Surgery, Lodz, Russian Poland

Prince Volkonsky's Flying Field Ambulance Surgery, Radzivilow, Russian Poland

Violetta Thurstan, a trained nurse, joined the Westminster detachment of the British Red Cross in 1913. She was called up at the beginning of August 1914 and asked to take a party of nurses to Brussels to work under the auspices of the Belgian Red Cross Society. After the Germans marched into Brussels she organised a hospital at a fire station and then, at the request of the Burgomaster of Charleroi, she went as matron to a hospital in the town. In mid-September the Germans ordered all English doctors and nurses to leave and Violetta Thurstan and her nurses were taken under armed escort by train to the Danish border. In Copenhagan the Dowager Empress of Russia arranged for Violetta Thurstan and three other nursing Sisters to be transferred to the Russian Red Cross. They arrived in Russia at the end of October. After a short time attached to the community of sisters at Smolney, where they underwent 'instructions in Russian and their methods of First Aid', they were sent to a hospital in Warsaw. In the middle of November they joined Prince and Princess Volkonsky's Flying Ambulance Surgery Service at the height of the battle for Lodz.

It took us a long time to get to Lodz, though it is not much more that 200 kilometres away. Russian roads are villainously bad anyhow, and the Germans, though their retreat had been hasty, had had time to destroy the roads and bridges as they went. Another thing that delayed us were the enormous reinforcements of troops going up from Warsaw to the front. It was very interesting to watch the different groups as we passed, first a Cossack regiment going up, then an immense convoy followed with about 200 wagons of forage. Just ahead of that we passed the remounts – sturdy, shaggy Siberian ponies. They are the most delightful creatures in the world, as tame as a dog, and not much bigger, and many of them of a most unusual and beautiful shade of golden cream. They had been brought from Siberia by the thousand, and most of the little things had never seen a motor car before, and pranced and kicked and jumped, and went through all kinds of circus tricks as we passed.

As we grew nearer to Lodz it was sad to see a good many dead horses lying by the roadside, mostly killed by shell-fire. The shells had made great holes in the road too, and the last part of the journey was like a ride on a switchback railway.

Lodz is a large cotton manufacturing town – sometimes called the Manchester of Poland – but now of course all the factories were closed, and many destroyed by shell.

We had to make a long detour and get into the town by an unfrequented country road, as Lodz was being heavily bombarded by the German guns. We were put down at a large building which we were told was the military hospital. Princess Volkonsky, Basil Petrov [the unit surgeon], and a Russian student were working hard in the operating-room, and we hastily put on clean overalls and joined them. They all looked absolutely worn out, and the doctor dropped asleep between each case; but fresh wounded were being brought in every minute and there was no one else to help. Lodz was one big hospital. We heard that there were more than 18,000 wounded there. Every building of any size had been turned into a hospital, and almost all the supplies of every kind had given out.

The building we were in had been a day-school, and the top floor was made up of large airy schoolrooms that were quite suitable for wards. But the shelling recommenced so violently that the wounded all had to be moved down to the ground floor and into the cellars. The place was an absolute inferno. It was fearfully cold, and the hospital was not heated at all, for there was no wood or coal in Lodz, and for the same reason the gas-jets gave out only the faintest glimmer of light. There was no clean linen, and the poor fellows were lying there still in their verminous, blood-soaked shirts, shivering with cold, as we had only one small blanket each for them. They were lucky if they had a bed at all, for many were lying with only a little straw between them and the cold stone floor. There were no basins or towels or anything to wash up with, and no spittoons, so the men were spitting all over the already filthy floor. In the largest ward where there were seventy or eighty men lying, there was a lavatory adjoining which had got blocked up, and a thin stream of dirty water trickled under the door and meandered in little rivulets all over the room. The smell was awful, as some of the men had been there already several days without having had their dressings done.

This was the state in which the hospital had been handed over to us. It was a military hospital whose staff had had orders to leave at four o'clock that morning, and they handed the whole hospital with its 270 patients over to us just as it was; and we could do very little towards making it more comfortable for them. The stench of the whole place was horrible, but it was too cold to do more than open the window for a minute or two every now and then. It was no one's fault that things were in such a horrible condition – it was just the force of circumstances and the fortune of war that the place had been taxed far beyond its possible capacities.

All night long the most terribly wounded men were being brought in from the field, some were already dead when they arrived, others had only a few minutes to live; all the rest were very cold and wet and exhausted, and we had nothing to make them comfortable. What a blessing hot water bottles would have been – but after all there would have been no hot water to fill them if we had had them. But the wounded had to be brought in for shelter somewhere, and at least we had a roof over their heads, and hot tea to give them.

At 5am there came a lull. The tragic procession ceased for a while, and we went to lie down. At seven o'clock we were called again – another batch of wounded was being brought in.

The shelling had begun again, and was terrific; crash, crash, over our heads the whole time. A clock-tower close to the hospital was demolished and windows broken everywhere. The shells were bursting everywhere in the street, and civilians were being brought in to us severely wounded. A little child was carried in with half its head blown open, and then an old Jewish woman with both legs blown off, and a terrible wound in her chest, who only lived an hour or two. Apparently she suffered no pain, but was most dreadfully agitated, poor old dear, at having lost her wig in the transit. They began bringing in so many that we had to stop civilians being brought in at all, as it was more than we could do to cope with the wounded soldiers that were being brought in all the time.

At midday we went to a hotel for a meal. There was very, very little food left in Lodz, but they brought what they could. Coming back to the hospital we tried everywhere to get some bread, but there was none to be had anywhere – all the provision shops were quite empty, and the inhabitants looked miserable and starved, the Jewish population particularly so. On our way back a shell burst quite close to us in the street, but no one was hurt.

It was more like hell than anything I can imagine. The never-ending processions of groaning men being brought in on those horrible blood-soaked stretchers, suffering unimagined tortures, the filth, the cold, the stench, the hunger, the vermin, and the squalor of it all, added to one's utter helplessness.

On the third day after our arrival a young Russian doctor and some Russian sisters arrived to relieve us for a few hours, and we most thankfully went to bed – at least it was not a bed in the ordinary sense, but a wire bedstead on which we lay down in all our clothes; but we were very comfortable all the same.

When we woke we were told that the military authorities had given orders for the patients to be evacuated, and the Red Cross carts were coming all night to take them away to the station, where some ambulance trains awaited them. So we worked hard all night to get the dressings done before the men were sent away, and as we finished each case, he was carried down to the hall to await his turn to go; but it was very difficult as all the time they were bringing in fresh cases as fast as they were taking the others away and many had to go off without having had their dressings done at all. The next afternoon we were still taking in, when we got another order that all the fresh patients were to be evacuated and the hospital closed, as the Russians had decided to retire from Lodz. Again we worked all night, and by ten the next morning we had got all the patients away. The sanitars collected all the bedding in the yard to be burnt, the bedsteads were piled high on one another, and we opened all the windows wide to let the clean, cold wind blow over everything.

We had all our own dressings and equipment to pack, and were all just about at our last gasp from want of food and sleep, when a very kind Polish lady came and carried the Princess, we two Sisters, and the surgeon off to her house, where she had prepared bedrooms for us. Our hostess simply heaped benefits on us by preparing us each a hot bath in turn. We had not washed or had our clothes off since we came to Lodz, and were covered with vermin which had come to us from the patients; men and officers alike suffer terribly from this plague of insects, which really do make one's life a burden. There are three varieties commonly met with: ordinary fleas that no one minds in the least; white insects that are the commonest and live in the folds of one's clothes, whose young are most difficult to find, and who grow middle-aged and very hungry in a single night; and, lastly, the red insects with a good many legs, which are much less numerous but much more ravenous than the other kinds.

After the bath and the hunt, we sat down to a delicious supper, and were looking forward to a still more delicious night in bed, when suddenly Prince Volkonsky arrived and said we must leave at once. We guessed instantly that the Germans must be very near. So we left our unfinished supper and quickly collected our belongings and took them to the hotel where our Red Cross car should have been waiting for us. But the Red Cross authorities had sent off our car with some wounded, which of course was just as it should be, and we were promised another 'seechas', which literally translated signifies 'immediately', but in Russia means today or tomorrow or not at all.

'Let us come into the hotel and get a meal while we wait,' suggested the Prince, mindful of our uneaten supper, and we followed him to the restaurant – still mourning those beautiful beds we had left behind us, and so tired we didn't much care whether the Germans came or not. A large hole was ripped out of the wall of the big restaurant, close to the alcove where the band used to play, while the smart people dined. An elaborate wine-list still graced each little table, but coffee made from rye bread crusts mixed with a little chicory was the only drink that a few white-faced waiters who crept about the room like shadows could apologetically offer us. We sat there till nearly 3am, and the surgeon, utterly worn out, was fast asleep with his head on the little table …

In the morning things began to look cheerful. The Germans had still not arrived, our own car turned up, and best of all the Prince heard officially that every wounded man who was at all transportable had now been successfully got out of Lodz. It was a gigantic task, this evacuation of over 18,000 wounded in four days, and it is a great feather in the Russian cap to have achieved it so successfully …

A few days after she returned safely to Warsaw, Violetta Thurstan left once more with Prince Volkonsky's Flying Field Ambulance to nurse wounded in a temporary hospital in the Tsar's private theatre at Skiernevice. In December the column was then evacuated to Zyradow, a few miles away.

The next morning we went up to Radzivilow. It is the next station to Skiernevice, and there was very heavy fighting going on there. The Russian battery was at that time at the south of the railway line, the German battery on the north of it – and we were in the centre of the sandwich. At Zyradow these cannon sounded distant, but as we neared Radzivilow the guns were crashing away as they did at Lodz, and we prepared for a hot time. The station had been entirely wrecked and was simply in ruins, but the station-master's house nearby was still intact, and we had orders to rig up a temporary dressing-station there.

Before we had time to unpack our dressings, a messenger arrived to tell us that the Germans had succeeded in enfilading a Russian trench close by, and that they were bringing fifty very badly wounded men to us almost at once. We had just time to start the steriliser when the little carts began to arrive with some terribly wounded men. The machine guns had simply swept the trench from end to end. The worst of it was that some lived for hours when death would have been a more merciful release. Thank

God we had plenty of morphia with us and could ease their terrible sufferings. One man had practically his whole face blown off, another had all his clothes and the flesh of his back all torn away. Another poor old fellow was brought in with nine wounds in the abdomen. He looked quite a patriarch with a long flowing beard – quite the oldest man I have seen in the Russian army. Poor Ivan, he had only just been called up to the front and this was his first battle. He was beautifully dressed, and so clean; his wife had prepared everything for him with such loving care, a warm knitted vest, and a white linen shirt most beautifully embroidered with scarlet in an intricate key-pattern. Ivan was almost more unhappy at his wife's beautiful work having to be cut than at his own terrible wounds. He was quite conscious and not in much pain, and did so long to live even a week or two longer, so that he might see his wife once again. But it was not to be, and he died early the next morning – one of the dearest old men one could ever meet, and so pathetically grateful for the very little we could do for him.

The shells were crashing over our heads and bursting everywhere, but we were too busy to heed them, as more and more men were brought to the dressing-station. It was an awful problem what to do with them: the house was small and we were using the two biggest rooms downstairs as operating and dressing-rooms. Straw was procured and laid on the floors of all the little rooms upstairs, and after each man's wounds were dressed he was carried with difficulty up the narrow winding staircase and laid on the floor. The day wore on and as it got dark we began to do the work under great difficulties, for there were no shutters or blinds to the upstairs windows, and we dared not have any light – even a candle – there, as it would have brought down the German fire on us at once. So those poor men had to lie up there in the pitch dark, and one of us went round from time to time with a little electric torch. Downstairs we managed to darken the windows, but the dressings and operations had all to be done by candle-light.

The Germans were constantly sending up rockets of blue fire which illuminated the whole place, and we were afraid every moment they would find us out. Some of the shells had set houses nearby on fire too, and the sky was lighted up with a dull red glow. The carts bringing the men showed no lights, and they were lifted out in the dark when they arrived and laid in rows in the lobby till we had time to see to them.

By nine o'clock that evening we had more than 300 men, and were thankful to see an ambulance train coming up the line to take them away. The sanitars had a difficult job getting these poor men downstairs and carrying them to the train, which was quite dark too. But the men were thankful themselves to get away – it was nerve-racking work for them, lying wounded in that little house with the shells bursting continually over it.

All night long the men were being brought in from the trenches. About four in the morning there was a little lull and someone made tea. We had it in the stuffy dressing-room where we had been working without a stop for sixteen hours with tightly-closed windows, and every smell that can be imagined pervading it, the floor covered with mud, blood and debris of dressings wherever there were not stretchers on which were men who had just been operated on. The meal of milkless tea, black bread and cheese was spread on a sterilised towel on the operating table, illuminated by two candles stuck in bottles. Princess Volkonsky sat in the only chair, and the rest of us eased our weary feet by sitting on the edge of the dressing-boxes. Two dead soldiers lay at our feet – it was not safe just at that moment to take them out and bury them.

At eleven o'clock in the morning another ambulance train arrived and was quickly filled. By that time we had had more than 750 patients through our hands, and they were still being brought in large numbers. The fighting must have been terrific, for the men were absolutely worn out when they arrived, and fell asleep at once from exhaustion, in spite of their wounds. Some of them must have been a long time in the trenches, for many were in a terribly verminous condition. On one poor boy with a smashed leg the insects could have only been counted by the million. About ten minutes after his dressing was done, his white bandage was quite grey with the army of invaders that had collected on it from his other garments.

Early that afternoon we got a message that another Column was coming to relieve us, and that we were to return to Zyradow for a rest. We were very sorry to leave our little dressing-station, but rejoiced to hear that we were to go up again in two days' time to relieve this second Column, and that we were to work alternately with them, forty-eight hours on, and then forty-eight hours off duty.

We had left Zyradow rather quiet, but when we came back we found the cannon going hard, both from the Radzivilow and the Goosof direction. It would have taken much more than cannon to keep us awake and we lay down most gratefully on our stretchers in the empty room at the Red Cross Bureau and slept.

I woke up in the evening to hear the church bells ringing, and remembered that it was Christmas Eve and that they were ringing for the Midnight Mass, so I got up quickly. The large church was packed with people, every one of the little side chapels was full and people were even sitting on the altar steps. There must have been 3 or 4,000 people there, most of them the people of the place, but also soldiers, Red Cross workers, and many refugees, mostly from Lowice. Poor people, it was a sad Christmas for them – having lost so much already and not knowing from day to day if they would lose all, as at that time it was a question of whether or not the Russian authorities would decide for strategic reasons to fall back once more.

And then twelve o'clock and the Mass began.

Soon a young priest got up into the pulpit and gave them a little sermon. It was in Polish, but though I could not understand the words, I could tell from the people's faces what it was about. When he spoke of the horrors of war, the losses and the deaths and the suffering that had come to so many of them, one woman put her apron to her face and sobbed aloud in the tense silence. And in a moment the whole congregation began sobbing and moaning and swaying themselves to and fro. The young priest stopped and left them alone a moment or two, and then began to speak in a low persuasive voice. I do not know what he said, but he gradually soothed them. And then the organ began pealing out triumphantly, and while the guns crashed and thundered outside, the choir within sang of peace and goodwill to all men.

Christmas Day was a very mournful one for us, as we heard of the loss of our new and best automobile, which had just been given as a present to the Column. One of the boys was taking it to Warsaw from Skiernevice with some wounded officers, and it had broken down just outside the village. The mud was awful, and with the very greatest difficulty they managed to get it towed as far as Rawa, but had to finally abandon it to the Germans, though fortunately they got off safely themselves. It was a great blow to the Column, as it was impossible to replace it, these big ambulance cars costing something like 8000 roubles.

So our Christmas dinner eaten at our usual dirty little restaurant could not be called a success.

Food was very scarce at that time in Zyradow; there was hardly any meat or sugar, and no milk or eggs or white bread. One of us had brought a cake for Christmas from Warsaw weeks before, and it was partaken of on this melancholy occasion without enthusiasm. Even the punch made out of a teaspoonful of brandy from the bottom of the Princess's flask mixed with about a pint of water and two lumps of sugar failed to move us to any hilarity. Our menu did not vary in any particular from that usually provided at the restaurant, though we did feel we might have had a clean cloth for once.

MENU
Christmas 1914

Gravy Soup
Roast Horse. Boiled Potatoes
Currant Cake
Tea. Punch

We were very glad to go up to Radzivilow once more. Our former dressing-station had been abandoned as too dangerous for staff and patients, and the dressing- and operating- room was now in a train about five versts down the line from Radzivilow station. Our train was a permanency on the line, and we lived and worked in it, while twice a day an ambulance train came up, our wounded were transferred to it and taken away, and we filled up once more. We found things fairly quiet this time when we went up. The Germans had been making some very fierce attacks, trying to cross the River Rawka, and therefore their losses must have been very heavy, but the Russians were merely holding their ground, and so there were comparatively few wounded on our side. This time we were able to divide up into shifts for the work – a luxury we were very seldom able to indulge in.

We had previously made great friends with a Siberian captain, and we found to our delight that he was living in a little hut close to our train. He asked me one day if I would like to go up to the positions with him and take some Christmas presents round to the men. Of course I was more than delighted, and as he was going up that night and I was not on duty, the general very kindly gave permission for me to go up too. In the end the surgeon and one of the Russian Sisters accompanied us as well. The captain got a rough cart and horse to take us part of the way, and he and another man rode on horseback beside us. We started off about ten o'clock, a very bright moonlight night – so bright that we had to take off our brassards and anything that could have shown up white against the dark background of the woods. We drove as far as the pine-woods in which the Russian positions were, and left the cart and horses in charge of a Cossack while we were away. The general had intended that we should see the reserve trenches, but we had seen plenty of them before, and our captain meant that we should see all the fun that was going on, so he took us right up to the front positions. We went through the wood silently in single file, taking care that if possible not even a twig should crackle under our feet, till we came to the very front trenches at the edge of the wood. We crouched down and watched for some time. Everything was brilliantly illuminated by the moonlight, and we had to be very careful not to show ourselves. A very fierce German attack was going on, and the bullets were pattering like hail on the trees all around us. We could see nothing for some time but the smoke of the rifles.

The Germans were only about 100 yards away from us at this time, and we could see the River Rawka glittering below in the moonlight. What an absurd little river to have so much fighting about. That night it looked as if we could easily wade across it. The captain made a sign, and we crept with him along the edge of the wood, till we got to a Siberian officer's dug-out. At first we could not see anything, then we saw a hole between two bushes, and after slithering backwards down the hole, we got into a sort of cave that had been roofed in with poles and branches, and was absolutely invisible a few steps away. It was fearfully hot and frowzy – a little stove in the corner threw out a great heat, and the men all began to smoke, which made it worse.

We stayed a while talking, and then crawled along to visit one of the men's dug-outs, a German bullet just missing us as we passed, and burying itself in a tree. There were six men already in the dug-out, so we did not attempt to get in, but gave them tobacco and matches, for which they were very grateful. These men had an 'ikon', or sacred picture, hanging up inside their cave; the Russian soldiers on active service carry a regimental ikon, and many carry them in their pockets too. One man had his life saved by his ikon. He showed it to us; the bullet had gone just between the Mother and the Child, and was embedded in the wood.

It was all intensely interesting, and we left the positions with great reluctance, to return through the moonlit pine-woods till we reached our cart. We had indeed made a night of it, for it was five o'clock in the morning when we got back to the train once more, and both the doctor and I were on duty again at eight. But it was well worth losing a night's sleep to go up to the positions during a violent German attack.

We finished our forty-eight hours' duty and returned once more to Zyradow. It was New Year's Eve and we found ourselves billeted in a new house where there was not only a bed each, but a bathroom and a bath.

Midnight struck as we were having supper, and we drank the health of the New Year in many glasses of tea …

1915
France and Belgium

Dr Hilda Clark

Maternity Hospital, Châlons-sur-Marne and Cottage Hospital, Sermaise les Bains, France

Dr Hilda Clark, an obstetrician, suffragist and Quaker, had become increasingly involved with researching ill-health in the working-class population when the war started. The following month, supported by the Friends War Victims Relief Committee, her friend Edith Pye, a midwife, went to Paris to offer assistance to the French authorities after the Battle of the Marne left devastation in the countryside. Refugees were fleeing from Rheims; mothers and children were stranded and helpless and there was no medical aid for their suffering after all the doctors had been mobilised to join the French army.

In November 1914 a team of three doctors, eleven trained nurses, one medical student, two chemists, one sanitary inspector and fourteen male chauffeurs and orderlies, arrived in France. Some remained in Paris and the others went to Châlons-sur-Marne, 15km behind the fighting lines. Mr Edmund Harvey, MP, was in charge of the party and Dr Hilda Clark was responsible for the medical organisation. Edith Pye immediately started to establish an emergency maternity hospital in a wing of a workhouse which stood on the extreme edge of the town. She wrote later:

> *Built in separate blocks, of an ugliness almost unbelievable, like match-boxes set up on edge, within, the wards were light and lofty, ventilation good and adaptation seemed possible. The one offered to us had been the epileptic block, and so the ten-feet windows were caged in with wire netting, but they opened inward, and only to the discontented occasionally suggested a prison.*
>
> *The Director of the Asile (corresponding to the Master of an English workhouse) received us all with great kindness, and if he was surprised, and perhaps displeased at the invasion of a dozen men and women curiously dressed, speaking an unknown language (and very few spoke any other), with curious ways and customs, he never showed it, but only grieved for the displacement of his epileptic women, who with tears made up their little bundles and were driven off elsewhere …*

Downstairs there was a dining-room, cubicles for the nursing staff, and dormitories for the families of the women patients. Upstairs there was a ward of twelve beds and twelve cots for mothers and babies. A labour ward was partitioned off. There was also a waiting and convalescent ward of twelve beds, an isolation room, a dispensary, and a small kitchen. The sanitary arrangements were primitive and hot water had to be boiled on stoves. The 'least incapable of the female imbeciles' of the workhouse provided the domestic staff.

Over the following months pregnant women arrived in their hundreds to the maternity hospital. These included unmarried mothers, young wives expecting a first baby and older women already with a family. One was 'accompanied by eight children and a silent, black-bearded, horny-handed husband belonging to a sturdy farming class'.

The nursing staff at the hospital rarely had to call on medical help. If this was needed, and Dr Clark was at one of the other two hospitals she set up, a French army doctor was found on the station where train loads of troops were constantly arriving and departing.

Once the maternity hospital at Châlons was running smoothly Dr Hilda Clark started to plan the building of a small cottage hospital at Sermaise les Bains, and opened a home in a Château near Bettancourt, for refugee children from Reims.

January 1915
We really want the cottage hospital very badly, and I hope to put it in hand now, just one block here, and then try to get a château for a convalescent home.

There is very heavy firing up this way again. We mostly expect the Germans any day. At night the horizon is very gay with exploding shells and searchlights. Another taube came very near a few days ago, and we have discovered that very fine big guns have now been mounted close to us for defence against aircraft.

February 1915
I must try to see the Prefect of the Meuse this week, and also get a car permit to go further north than we were able to go today. Most of these villages are entirely destroyed or at any rate more than half; we chatted to people in about half a dozen, and were interested to find a rather different type. They were not at all oncoming at first, so I do not think they will be spongers. They had a poor physique but they said the general health was very good. Sommeille is one of the worst. It stands on the brow of a hill with a glorious view – a population of about 370, and at first we could not find a home standing – just the church which was little damaged, and we found two or three houses down the hill. There were very few people about and they seemed hopelessly depressed and apathetic. It is very sad to see these poor things for whom nothing has yet been done.

Châlons, March 1915
This week we have been out to Nancy to find out if we ought to prepare to work there and decided it would not be necessary for the present, and we have asked for ten more women and thirty more men, and hope to get the work in the Meuse started in a fortnight.

The women are already working there as the distribution of garden seeds is very urgent, and I mean to spend next week there to help. We feel that if we have enough men to get this whole district done in 2–3 months, we shall be ready at a time when one trusts it will be possible to extend further north.

There is no doubt we have got the district of the greatest distress to work in, and one where French help is least available.

In Meurthe and Moselle and Nancy people are able to do a great deal. It is a modern, well-organised town – a brave and energetic people; the Germans have not been in it, and they have organised help for the refugees from the beginning, and though they have been slow in putting up shelters on account of the scarcity of workmen, they are getting it done by degrees.

I came back here this morning by train and go to Fère Champenoise for Sunday to settle about the little hospital which we are to put up at Sermaise. There is a pleasant countess here this afternoon who is having a stolen interview with her son in the Army. We invite these people to come and see us and then they can see their sons in peace in our sitting-room. They send us clothes and subscriptions.

Châlons is much quieter than it was and troops are pouring away. I don't know where to. There is little firing going on.

The energies of the party are just now being concentrated on garden seeds – kitchen garden – which we find tremendously appreciated and do much to cheer and help people.

One gets more and more overwhelmed by the horror of the war. The very success of these little efforts to help the material losses makes the awful suffering that everyone is going through from the loss of their menfolk more emphasised.

Sermaise les Bains, March 1915
I write sitting on the doorstep of the little wooden house which has been erected in the field beside the wood at La Source, watching a great red sun go down while the birds sing all around one and the continual background of cannon rumble heavily as usual. Today has been perfect, spring rushing on, and the birds singing as if possessed. It was exquisite this morning. I could look down the field through the open door of my room to a soft blue mist entangled in the poplars below.

Today we have had a sad journey, to explore the neighbouring part of the Meuse. There is a district there where the line of battle turned northwards in a line parallel to, and west of that joining Bar-le-Duc to Verdun, where the fighting was tremendous, and where savage destruction of villages occurred – first much destruction by bombardment and then the Germans set fire to them as they retreated.

At Sermaise we now have a little cottage hospital with two wards and a verandah. Administration is rather difficult there but we can manage any urgent case.

April 1915
I am now trying to organise a convalescent home in this château, that has been lent to us, between Sermaise and Bettancourt. We think that we shall be able to fit it with Reims, Châlons and Bar-le-Duc patients. The difficulty is to know beforehand whether the patients who ought to come will be willing to!

I spend a weary time talking and trying to be nice to people. I never see anything of the refugees themselves. It is rather harassing and one can never be the least put out or moody except in the most private moments which results in great depression sometimes when by oneself. We are all a little too intense.

Châlons, April 1915
It is the essential spiritual difficulties – the standing up for peace in the midst of the machinery of war, while owing our lives and our scope for work to those who are fighting, the strain of work in the midst of intense personal sorrow and anxiety, of wondering whether it would be better to enlist, of a hundred doubts – it is all this that is at the bottom of difficulties which on the surface appear to be superficial practical ones that someone is to blame for …

Paris, April 1915
The Prefect told us that the F.150,000 which was voted for us by the Conseil General the other day, is definitely for the wooden huts – for the wood, and if we choose, for furniture. It is to be entirely in our hands and may possibly be actually paid over to us. He was quite emphatic that it was not to be handed over to the Paris ladies who have offered to furnish the huts, and we soon realised that an unfortunate mistake had been made by them and that they were counting on this to carry out their promise! There is not enough money to do more than pay for the wood of the huts and some of the fixtures that can be included, and we are getting rather anxious whether we shall really get the rent which Mme de G. so glibly promised. Thinking that all this furniture was being provided we have undertaken to use the money voted by the Committee for it, to provide 400 beds for the sinistres (burnt out families) of Sermaise and have used this offer as a lever to get the Prefecture to give the other 400 beds which were necessary in order that a grant of one bed might be made to each burned out family. This will cost us £1,000 and the Prefecture a similar amount.

Reims, May 1915
We have arranged with the Civil Hospital at Reims to take any women and children (except infectious diseases) that are willing to be sent away from danger of further shells.

There are less than 30,000 people left in the town now out of 120,000 and the whole place is shattered and shuttered – like a city of the dead. Still there is a surprising amount of life here and there – newspaper boys, a few voitures de place, flowers and fruit, a few shops open – some good ones, and prices hardly raised.

We keep very busy at Châlons, but are better staffed now. Getting the Reims children for evacuation is a big job. We have had thirty this week, sending twenty-four to Paris today and six to Sermaise and Bettancourt. There will be four more car loads today, tomorrow and Friday, bringing ten each time. They have to be fitted out in clothes, medically examined and allocated to different places.

How stifled by lies and hatred one feels, especially in all the news from England. Here one could easily forget the most trying parts – one lives so much in the present, and the psychology of our lives and those around us seems more simple. I sometimes wonder if we shall have rather a shock when the weather changes. It is still glorious and the country is ablaze with flowers, sometimes, alas, the result of land being uncultivated. The colours are as splendid as in the Alps, and the sweeping lines and queer broad check patterns of the rolling hills are just wonderful, and give one a new and living idea of post-impressionism.

I have been motoring steadily day after day – sometimes in other cars but generally driving myself in the Belsize – rarely less than 40 miles a day and often more.

July 1915
If one did not feel so entirely remote from the earth it would make one very homesick. I sometimes wonder if one will ever really feel anything at all or always be numb. The saving mercy I find in the companionship of such splendid people as we have working here …

Miss Pat Waddell

First Aid Nursing Yeomanry Corps, Lamarck Hospital, Calais, France

Pat Waddell, who was training to become a professional violinist, joined the First Aid Nursing Yeomanry (FANY) before the war and continued her training until she was called up in February 1915. She was sent to the Lamarck Hospital, a convent school, opposite Notre Dame Cathedral in Calais, which had been commandeered by the Belgians. The first contingent of the FANY had arrived there four months previously.

There were three wards for the wounded in the main hospital and in another building across the yard typhoid patients were nursed.

Pat Waddell had expected to be an ambulance driver but as there was a shortage of nursing staff she was sent to work in the wards. The storeroom, full of 'tins of biscuits and pots of jam', was her haven where she practised on her violin.

A few weeks after her arrival Pat Waddell and three other girls set off in an ambulance to deliver stores to advanced dressing-stations. They spent part of the day avoiding shells during a bombardment and then reported to the Belgian headquarters at Ramscapelle where they sorted out stores, including socks and mufflers, to take to Belgian soldiers in trenches on the Yser. They had to wait until it was dark before they set off.

When all was ready, we were given our final instructions – we were to keep together till we had passed through the village; the doctor would meet us and with a guide conduct us to the trenches; we were to proceed one after the other at twenty-pace intervals, no word was to be spoken, and should a Very light show up, we were to drop flat.

Off we set and my heart was pounding pretty hard. It was nerve-racking work once we were beyond the village, straining our eyes through the darkness to follow the figure ahead. Occasionally a sentry appeared from apparently nowhere. A whispered word and on we went. I cannot say how far we walked, it seemed miles. Suddenly a light flared in the sky, illuminating the surrounding country in an eerie glare. It did not take me many seconds to drop flat! Luckily it was pavé, but I would have welcomed mud rather than stand silhouetted within sight of the German trenches on that shell-riddled road.

At last we saw a long black line running at right angles and the guide in front motioned me to stop while he went on ahead. I had time to look round and examine the place as well as I could and also to put down my bundle of woollies which had become extremely heavy. These trenches were built against a railway bank, the railway lines having been long since destroyed or torn up, and just beyond ran the famous Yser and the inundations which the Belgians had brought about by breaking the canal banks, thus helping to stem the German advance.

A touch on the shoulder, and we clambered into the trench along a slippery plank. The men looked very surprised to see us. I crawled into one of their dug-outs, little larger than a rabbit-hutch, on my hands and knees, the door being very low. The two occupants had a small brazier burning; straw was on the floor. The sight of a new pair of socks cheered them tremendously.

We pushed on as it was getting late. I shall never forget that trench. It was the second line, the first line consisting of 'listening posts' somewhere in that watery waste beyond, where the men wore waders reaching well above their knees. We squelched along a narrow strip of plank with the trenches on one side and a sort of cesspool on the other – sanitary arrangements seemed non-existent, no wonder they got typhoid – and I prayed that I would not slip.

Farther on we could walk upright without our heads showing above the parapet, which was a relief as it was extremely tiring to walk for long in a stooping position. Through an observation hole we looked out across the inundations to where the famous 'Ferme Violette', which had changed hands so often and was at present German, could plainly be seen. Dark objects sticking up in the water were pointed out to us. They, the sergeant cheerfully observed, holding his nose meanwhile, were 'sales Boches' [filthy Germans]. The stench was not pleasant.

We hurried on to a bigger dug-out and helped the doctor with several blessés injured that afternoon, and later we helped remove them to the village and thence to a field-hospital. Just then, the 75s which we had seen earlier began bombarding. The row was deafening – first a terrific bang, then a swishing through the air with a sound like a sob, then a plop at the other end as it exploded – somewhere. At first, as with all new-comers in the firing line, we ducked our heads as the shells went over, to a roar of delight from the men, but in time we gave that up. During this bombardment, we went on distributing our woollies along the line; I thought my head would split, the noise was so great. I asked one of the officers, during a pause, why the Germans were not replying, to which he answered that we had just got the range of one of their positions by 'phone, and as these guns we were employing had just been brought up, the Boche would not waste any shells until he thought he had our range.

Presently we came to the officer's dug-out, and, incredibly, he had small windows with lace curtains! They were the size of pocket-handkerchiefs, still, the fact remains, they were curtains. He showed us two bits of a shell that had burst overhead the day before and made the roof collapse, but since then the damage had been remedied by a stout beam. He was a merry little man with twinkling eyes and very proud of his little house.

Our things began to give out and we were not at the end of the line by any means. It was heart-breaking to hear one man say, 'Une paire de chausettes, mees, je vous en prie; il y a trois mois depuis que j'en ai eues' ('A pair of socks, miss, I beseech you; it's three months since I had any'). I gave him my scarf which he put on immediately, cheerfully, accepting the substitute. 'Ah-ha!' he cried to his friends, 'it's still warm. This will bring me luck. A thousand thanks, mademoiselle.'

There was no reason for us to go any farther, so we bade them good night, trying not to see the rows of hands stretching out beyond. If the knitters could have seen how much their work was appreciated, they would have been rewarded. We passed the word along that more would be forthcoming another night and their turn would come.

One by one we crawled out of the trenches on to the road and began the perilous journey homewards with the blessés, knowing that at any moment Very lights might go up. As we were resting, the captain of the battery joined us, and in the semi-darkness I saw that he was offering me a bunch of snowdrops! It certainly was an odd moment to receive a bouquet, but I tucked them into my tunic and treasured them for days afterwards – snowdrops that in spite of war had flowered in the garden of some cottage long since destroyed.

Arrived once more at headquarters, we were pressed to a petit verre of some very hot and raw liqueur, but nevertheless very warming and very good. We had got terribly cold in the trenches. Taking leave of our kind hosts, we set off for the hospital.

It was now about 1.30am and we were stopped no less than seventeen times on our way back. As it was my job – 'me with my French' – to lean out and whisper into the sentry's ear, I was rather tired by the time I had passed the seventeenth 'Gustave'.

The blessés were taken to a Casualty Clearing Station, and the Mors [ambulance], rid of its wounded load, sped through the night back to Lamarck …

Miss Eleonora B. Pemberton

No. 1 British Red Cross VAD Unit Dressing Station and Canteen at Abbeville Railway Station attached to No. 5 Stationary Hospital (B Sector), Abbeville, France

During the six months Eleonora Pemberton and the No. 1 British Red Cross VAD Unit worked at the Gare Centrale, Boulogne they gave food to almost 80,000 sick and wounded soldiers and some 2,000 men were treated in the dispensary; 40,000 magazines and papers were distributed to patients. The member who drove the unit's ambulance took 1,677 cases to hospitals and hospital ships. Early in 1915 the unit opened a club with a lending library for nursing sisters and a small branch feeding station at Hesdigneul Junction which fed 6,000 men between February and April 1915. On behalf of the Army and British Red Cross Post Offices the members of the unit also traced the owners of many hundreds of misdirected letters and parcels.

At the end of February 1915 Eleonora Pemberton and five other VADs were sent to form a small rest station at Gournay-en-Bray for sick and injured men of the convalescent horse

Depot. In May 1915 she was transferred to set up a dressing-station and canteen at Abbeville railway station. She continued to write letters home.

15 May 1915
No. 5 Stationary Hospital
L.of C. BEF
The place as we took it over consisted merely of a large piece of platform in the goods station roughly screened off with tent canvas hung by cords and all sagging and dirty and disreputable looking. Inside there were six benches and one long, old and dirty tressle table. Outside there were three Sawyer boilers for hot water and near by on the platform was a little cabine with windows on three sides and a door which locked. This was our entire nucleus and foundation and I don't mind telling you that, coming from Gournay where we had made everything so nice and complete, my heart rather sank at the prospect of dealing successfully with such scant material.

That is a fortnight ago and today my dressing-station (oh, the excruciating pride and joy of that personal pronoun!!!) is really rather a picture.

The very first thing to be done was to get the canvas stretched on to battens top and bottom, with a wooden outline for the doorways: then the canvas had to be thoroughly washed down on both sides. We have four orderlies and they did this, and helped with the wood work. (Pause, while I am called away to prescribe for a man with bad toothache). One of our party, Miss Barber, is a great carpenter and we have to thank her to a very large extent for the transformation in our abode.

Once the canvas was stretched it looked a different place; then we proceeded to matchboard in the space between the cabine and the wall – about 6ftx10ft, and this makes us a store and place to put our own things in during the day.

The store now has a cupboard of 4 shelves and a canvas curtain in front of which are tinned milk, jam, soup, matches, tobacco, tea, etc., a set of lockers also with a canvas curtain for our personal belongings, and a thing to hang coats on, and it is a picture of neatness, small though it is. All the cupboards, shelves, and lockers are made out of packing cases, and you have no idea what an ornamental thing a packing case can be when it is thoroughly scrubbed and provided with shelves, doors, hinges and a padlock! (The man with the toothache has just come beaming to say that the iodine has done the trick; but he must have the tooth out tomorrow as it is thoroughly rotten.)

The Surgery looks awfully nice. We covered the long table with white oilcloth, and it has arrayed upon it enamel and tin bowls (all turned upside down because of the smuts), a brown earthenware jar with a cover, labelled 'Swabs', four large square biscuit tins, all polished up and labelled respectively Bandages, Wool, Boric Lint, White Gauze, and in the centre is a tray with a methylated spirit lamp and bowl and saucepan (small) for fomentations and sterilising instruments; safety pins, strapping and matches and a fomentation wringer etc. At one end is a bowl of prepared iodine swabs, and at the other cyanide gauze in carbolic, which are the two chief lotions we use. Under the table are pails for dirty dressings and slops. One of our orderlies is by trade a sign painter and with the aid of a little red paint he has worked wonders, and everything is labelled in large letters. The little table is supplied with requisites for the doctors to wash their hands; the others are for us to work at. I have the one in the middle of the long side and on it I have set out everything I am likely to require for dressings, including my instruments and torch. Our work is nearly all at night.

In our large enclosure which we call the 'Surgery' we have now six cupboards of different sizes, and as soon as we can get hold of more cases we are going to make still more. Having got our Store, my next craving was for some place where we could with decency muddle! The surgery is too big to do odd jobs in; also it must not be made untidy and the store is too small, though we all four had tea there very happily several times. There was however a large corner between the surgery and the boilers and this seemed to ask to be enclosed and made into a ward-scullery.

The canvas all along one side of the surgery which was against the wall seemed superfluous, so down it came, and with a certain amount of planning and shifting and contriving, it made the two remaining walls of the scullery and then we were very happy. We are right inside the goods shed so are under cover, which is a good thing.

My patients sit on the bench to the left of the table and as one is finished another moves up.

Greg, the other nursing member, works at the table by the scullery door and the MOs work at the big table and the one in the corner, or anywhere they feel inclined.

We are going to have proper tressles for a stretcher as soon as the REs have time to make them, but until then we have piled up ration boxes to act as supports. Anything really does, the only point is to raise the stretcher, as it is both back-breaking and not over clean, kneeling about on the floor.

We work here directly under No. 5 Stationary Hospital, which is an RAMC one. Major Meadows the CO and all the staff have been most awfully kind to us, have helped us in every possible way. They come down when a train comes in, but otherwise leave us entirely alone (except for friendly visits), and I am left an absolutely free hand to make what preparations I think best; and indent for what dressings, lotions, etc. I think we ought to have in stock. There is a glorious independence about it which really seems quite strange after six months 'in the ranks' so to speak.

The actual procedure is as follows: when any kind of 'improvised' train of wounded is announced the RTO sends us round a notice, sometimes stating the number on board, and sometimes not. We then proceed to make cocoa which means opening about 16 tins of that and 42 of condensed milk, as 1 tin of cocoa is supposed to do 64 men. Then just before the train is due Greg and I uncover everything in the Surgery, prepare the lotions and set the Primus going on a bench between the cupboards with a dixie of boiling water on it.

The first night, which was 1 May, a Sister came down with the Medical Officer, but the next time Major Meadows asked whether we could do without her, and since then only the MOs have come, usually 2 or 3, or sometimes even 4 of them.

As soon as the train is actually in the Voie Sanitaire, which is a siding kept for French and English trains of wounded, the feeding parties set out. They consist of the other two members, Barber and Saunders, who start at opposite ends of the train, each with an orderly to collect mugs, and one to fetch cocoa, which they do in enamelled pails. We almost always have to borrow one more orderly, either from the BRC or No. 5 as we have to leave one at the boilers to keep the fires up and deal out the cocoa. Sometimes we are asked to issue Army rations – a loaf of bread to each carriage and a tin of bully beef, or 3 tins of jam, and then one boy does this entirely, and they have to work with 3 at the train and not 4.

Meanwhile we are not idle, as any men whose dressings are through, or who want them renewing, are sent to the Surgery. One of the MOs always meets the train MO, and consults with him. We do not have anything to do with the regular Ambulance Trains, as they are fully equipped both for feeding and dressing on board, but the improvised trains consist merely of ordinary carriages with men sitting up, or lying on the floor, and in the racks, and anywhere else, and as they are not corridored, no dressing can be done on board.

We had a really turbid time from Sunday evening till Wednesday, and I am thankful it has slacked for the last two days, as we could not have gone on much longer at that pressure.

On Saturday night Greg had a wire to say that her brother was in hospital in Boulogne, wounded, so as an Ambulance was going in on Sunday from No. 3 BRC Hospital I arranged for her to go in for the day; this reduced us to 3.

It was nearly 6 and as the two others were very anxious to go to church, and there had been no word of a train, I let them go, and also sent an orderly for their rations, leaving just one on duty (the other two form the night shift, and were asleep in their tent). Of course just after they had all departed word came that a train of 1,000 was to be expected at eight o'clock!

For a moment I was as near a panic as I ever have been as it takes a good long time to get everything ready, even with all of us on, and now there was only Hodgson and myself. Panic was, however, the last thing to help one, so we just set to and worked. I telephoned up to No. 3 for the loan of three orderlies as Greg was still away, and lived in hopes that Barber and Saunders would soon return. They did in due course but none of us got any dinner that night – there was no time. Luckily all went well, and there were about 50 dressings to be done by two MOs and myself.

When all was over Greg turned up, and just as we were finishing Miss Macarthy the Army Matron-in-Chief stalked in. We had been expecting an inspection by her, but not at midnight, and I do hope she didn't think the place always looked like that. You know what a room looks like after a party, and you can perhaps imagine a little of what it looks like after a rush of dressings – not beautiful.

She came to ask us to look after 3 Army Sisters whom she was expecting to arrive during the night. We were not really intending to do night duty, but as the motto of the VADs is never to say no to anything, and as we also wished to stand well in her eyes, I did not let this on, but said we would certainly look after them, and thought with a sigh of my comfortable bed! Greg not having been working all day was quite fresh, and said she would stay too, so the others went off to bed, and I also lay down for an hour in the cabine. It was really very lucky we did stay up, as word came that another train was expected about 4.45am, so we turned again to preparing cocoa, and at 4 had to go and rouse the others, poor things. (I really think it is worse to go to bed and be dragged out than not to go at all!)

Soon Captain Hughson (a very nice MO From No. 5) and Mr Gordon who is attached to the RE who are building sidings here, arrived, and then we had a time and a half. They simply poured in, and from time to time we looked despairingly round, and wondered how on earth we were going to get through. We ran out of wool and bandages, and almost all the dressings, and had to send post haste up to the hospital for more and yet more. It took us till nearly 8 to get through, even with the help of three RAMC nursing orderlies, and (towards the end when the feeding was finished) of our own orderly Clough and Barber and Saunders who in reality know very little and really only listen. There were some awfully heavy cases too, and Captain Hughson reckoned that we did about 200, and this was working full steam ahead the whole time.

When we first started I thought we should simply wait on the MOs, but I soon found that we should never get through at that rate, nor was it what they expected, so now I just go ahead with whatever I can, and if there is something doubtful I call one of them. Nearly always one simply puts on a fresh dressing of whatever they had before and it is the freshness and coolness instead of the stiffness which comes from clotted blood, which relieves.

Well, by the time we had cleaned up and had breakfast it was 9.30am and I was quite ready for bed, so I went off till 12.30 when Greg and Saunders went. Barber having had some sleep in the night, stayed on till tea time, and hardly had she gone when the notice of another train came. It was however not to arrive till 8pm, but was said to be followed by others at intervals of 3 hours during the night!

This time Mr Gordon, Mr Douglas and Mr Wilson from No. 5 came down, and an Army Sister, who was waiting for a train to go up to a Clearing Hospital, was sent round by the RTO to see whether she could help. It was rather funny having her there, as of course she was our superior in every way, and yet it was our show, and we had to tell her where everything was, and how everything was done!

Again it was a big train, and heavy dressings – very – about 150. Afterwards we all had tea, including the RTO and an engineer officer (there are swarms of them about). The next train was expected about 2am and Captain Hughson came down instead of Mr Douglas, but it didn't come, and didn't come, and finally Barber and I who were in the scullery came into the surgery, and found Mr Gordon huddled up asleep on the reserve dressings hamper; Captain Hughson asleep on a form, and at the other end Greg and Saunders asleep on stretchers! So we did likewise in the scullery. The train never came at all, and about 6am we set to work to do the morning cleaning, and I had to think out schemes for providing everybody with some rest and sleep and yet have enough on duty.

Mercifully I arranged for Barber and Saunders to go to bed till lunch time as, about 10am, when Greg and I had got everything looking spick and span, who should stroll in but General Wodehouse and his ADC. He expressed great pleasure, and said the place was a totally different one from when he last saw it. Just then the RTO sent round to say that an empty supply train with 150 wounded on board was expected in half an hour, and as the Voies Sanitaires were both occupied with French ambulance trains, it would come in right the other side of the station. Nothing could have been more unfortunate, as General Wodehouse was there to see our success or failure, and as we had never yet had to carry the cocoa right over there I quite thought it would be the latter, especially as there were only two boys on. To add to everything they said it was too far for any wounded to come, and the dressings must be done on the train.

Greg had run a nail into her foot, and was limping, so I handed over the dressing part to her, and took over the cocoa (as neither of the feeding members were on). Luckily it all went very easily, as the trucks were all provided with their own mugs and the cocoa simply had to be poured out.

The train consisted of cattle trucks, but awfully well fitted up: there were ten men in each, each on a straw palliase with blankets. Each truck had an orderly and a table, mugs, water and all necessary arrangements. By this time Captain Hughson and Mr Gordon had started doing dressings, and Greg worked with the former while I accompanied the latter. I did not attempt to do any on my own, as it was, as you may well imagine, fearfully difficult and inconvenient, and I thought it would probably go quicker if I just helped him and handed him things. Before this train was finished another 200 cases came in, and then shunted on to the same line. This time the RTO had sent over for Barber and Saunders so they were able to do the feeding entirely. Also Captain Hughson said it was utterly impossible to do everything on the train, and all the men who could must come to the Surgery whither two Red X Sisters from No. 3 had also been summoned. He therefore with the Sisters and Greg carried on there, while Mr Gordon and I took on the cases that were too bad to leave the train, or could not walk.

It was a wonderful sight that morning: the whole station seemed to be given up to soldiers and wounded and people carrying food and dressings and stretchers. The two French trains had Turcos and Algerians and all sorts on board, and there were altogether hundreds swarming over the station. It reminded me of that first rush at Boulogne.

It also made me realise what a tremendous lot I had learnt since that time. Those were the first wounds I had seen, and they filled me with horror, though I never felt in the least degree bad. I felt, however, very uncertain of handling them, whereas now I feel quite different, and far more sure of myself …

Miss Olive Dent

Race Course Hospital, Rouen, France

Olive Dent went on courses in hygiene and psychology and worked with the St John's Ambulance before the war. She served as a VAD in the same hospital for 'twenty strenuous and crowded months' between September 1915 and May 1917.

The first day's duty in a camp hospital is a perplexing, nonplussing affair. Primarily, I wasn't certain where I was. For a bird's eye view of the camp would have revealed a forest of marquees and a webbing of tent-ropes. The marquees sometimes clustered so close that the ropes of two roofs on the adjoining side were not pegged to the ground, but were tied overhead, the one to the other, so supporting each other and saving space. Between such dual marquees was a tarpaulin passage, usually spoken of as a tunnel.

Each row of marquees was known as a 'line' and named as a letter in the alphabet. Thus 'A' line consisted of eight or nine tents, known as A1, A2, A3, and so on. All these marquees were exactly alike, and as we nurses passed from one to the other several times in the morning, it was at first a little difficult to know whether one was in A1, A3, or A5.

The early morning's work consisted of making twenty beds, dusting twenty-four lockers, taking twenty-four temperatures, and tidying the wards. Then came a snack lunch, and a change of apron followed by the giving of the necessary medicines, a couple of inhalations, the applying of two or three fomentations, a small eusol dressing, the dispensing of one or two doses of castor oil, and the cleaning of a linen cupboard.

Then came the boys' dinner, for which most of the up-patients went to the (marquee) dining-hall, leaving only two boys sitting at the ward table. In the afternoon, more medicines were to be given, the washing of patients was to be done and the beds made. At five o'clock came tea and off-duty.

The newcomer to a camp hospital finds matters very different to what she has been accustomed in England; no hot water, no taps, no sinks, no fires, no gas-stoves. She probably finds the syringe has no suction, that all the cradles are in use, and there is none for the boy with bad trench feet, that there are only six wash-bowls for the washing of 140 patients, and that there is nothing but a testing stand and a small syringe with which to help the medical officer through a dozen typhoid inoculations.

'Pinching' is always quite an accepted condition of affairs. Meeting an orderly carrying some planks of wood on his shoulders the other morning, I said in somewhat slip-shod fashion, 'And what are you making yourself, Smith?' 'As usual, sister, I'm making myself a thief,' came the unhesitating reply. All the consolation the late owner of any article may receive is the overworked tag, 'You're unlucky, mate. You shouldn't have joined.'

The nursing quarters of most of the camp hospitals in France consist of a wooden hut for the mess-and-sitting-room – by the way, it is almost solely the one and very rarely the other – a shed of some kind for the cook's kitchen, and bell tents, marquees, Alwyn huts, Armstrong huts, and wooden huts for the housing of the staff.

In the early days, some of our nursing sisters had improvised bedrooms from the loose boxes which were near us, in virtue of our being on a racecourse. Later, when tents and huts materialised at a quicker rate, these were left for the accommodation of the batmen. Bell tents and marquees were always very popular, being absolutely delightful in summer and very cosy in winter with the aid of stoves.

It was wonderful how pretty and comfortable bunks and bell tents could be made. All the furniture was of the packing-box variety. Chests of 'drawers' were built from small boxes on the cumulative principle and by the system of dovetailing. Then a chintz curtain was hung in front. Another chintz curtain served as a wardrobe. Indeed, chintz like charity covered a multitude of sins, the greatest of these being untidiness.

Most ambitious dressing-tables and writing-tables were evolved by standing a sugar-box on end, knocking out the lower side, and nailing on top at the back a small narrow box. These made a brave show stained with permanganate of potash, or, later, when this got rare, with solignum. A camp-bed, too, is easily convertible into a 'Chesterfield', flanked at either end with one's pillows pushed into pretty cushion-covers. An admirable 'Saxon stool', too, most of us possessed, fashioned from three sides of a box and stained.

A 'canvas existence' is great fun. It has its pros and its cons, but the pros are so delightful as to outweigh the cons, especially when these latter are made light of with true active service philosophy. The dog walks into the bell-tent in the middle of the night and rudely awakes one by vigorously licking one's face, and exhibiting other unseemly symptoms of canine affection. The bantam proclaims about 3am that he is roosting on the foot of one's bed, by violently crowing in a piercing falsetto an unappreciated solo, from which he refuses to desist even though he has hurled at him a damp sponge, a rolled-up knot of a handkerchief, a comb, an orange, and many a 'Shoo, Christopher, shoo, you little wretch!'

Field mice scuttle across the doors on early morning travels as we dress, insects always and perpetually hold high revel, earwigs are discovered holding a confab in the folds of one's apron, while one nurse is found asleep with a lighted candle in her tent. No, she isn't ill, only left on the light to scare the rats.

It is not quite so delightful, however, to be awakened in the wee, small hours by the rain pattering on one's face, to be obliged to get up hurriedly, scramble into slippers and raincoat, and go out sleepily and stammeringly into the darkness to fumble and fasten down tent ropes and tent flaps, which latter have been well turned back because the evening was originally so warm.

Leaves, spiders and wood bugs in one's wash and bath water are frequent occurrences, while overnight the acacia leaves flutter upon one's face and hair with persistent babes-in-the-wood effort. Towards creeping things one grows to an amazing tolerance, indeed, to a live-and-let-live nonchalance, a mild interest which would have astounded one in pre-war days.

Three of us – all VADs – ran the home and mess, which at the time consisted of between sixty and seventy nurses. We were helped by batmen, all PB men, who cleaned the huts and tents, swept and washed floors, attended to our supply of drinking, cooking and washing water – taps and sinks were unknown luxuries – mended fires, washed dishes, cleaned and cooked vegetables, cut up and cooked meats, and generally did the heavier work.

We planned the menus, laid the tables, carved, served out the different meals, cooked certain dishes, did the shopping, dusted, had the management of the home quarters, e.g. preparing rooms for newcomers, tending indisposed sisters, and were generally responsible for the hundred and one little trifles necessary to the smooth running of affairs.

Our mess kitchen is an example of the utilisation of existing buildings. It consists of two, open-fronted, loose boxes formerly used for horses. One acts as larder, while in the other are accommodated a stove, table, and a boiler for hot water. The boilers are busy night and day not merely boiling water, but also acting as porridge pots, stock pots, soup pans and pudding pans. The kitchen is the scene of much crowded activity, for here thousands of meals are cooked per day, hundreds of men supplied with porridge and tea for breakfast, a certain number of eggs cooked and rashers of bacon fried, several hundreds of pints of soup made for dinner, meat and fresh vegetables prepared and cooked, milk or suet or bread pudding cooked for some hundreds of men, a great quantity of 'milk-rice' boiled for the 'milk-diet' patients, a certain number of minced and boiled chicken diets supplied, a certain number of custard puddings made, probably a number of fish diets prepared, and several pints of beef tea made. In the afternoon barley water, more cooked fish, cooked eggs, and some hundreds of pints of tea will be supplied, while in the evening a similar quantity of cocoa will be in demand. Meantime, preparations for the next morning's breakfast and dinner will be proceeding apace, while emergency meals for convoy patients – stews, soups, tea or cocoa – may be required at very short notice.

The responsibility for securing supplies rests with the quartermaster. His is the task of ensuring the presence of great quantities of tins of milk, tins of jam, chests of tea, boxes of sugar, bags of rice and cereals, thousands of loaves of bread, tins of beef and vegetables, baskets of fresh vegetables, rounds and joints of fresh meat, gallons of fresh milk, stones of fresh fruit, boxes of dried fruits, tins of butter, crates of fresh eggs, and a whole host of other things.

Camp housekeeping in France quickly proved itself to be quite an arithmetical affair. Thus if one decided on making scones, immediately there was a little mental arithmetic to be done in ratios and substitutions, with the home quantity as a basis. For example, if half a pound of flour makes sixteen scones, how many are required for sixty people – with camp appetites – a quantity which must then be calculated in demi-kilos, those being the weights we had in the kitchen. Then the quantity of butter, sugar, cream of tartar, etc., must be calculated. Similar arithmetical tussles were necessary before making, say, a custard, and sending for the milk.

Bully beef made excellent curry, good shepherd's pie and most appetising rissoles, particularly when served with tomato sauce made active-service style from a tin of tomatoes, heated, sieved, and thickened with a little flour. Ration biscuits, otherwise irreverently known as dog biscuits, only required considerate treatment to be responsible for quite agreeable puddings and porridge …

I dreaded the very thought of night duty with its tense anxieties, its straining vigilance, its many sorrows. The weather is a very important factor during night duty in a camp hospital. We have had nights when wind and rain have raged and lashed, when our hurricanes have blown out directly we have lifted the tent flaps to go out, when we have been splashed to the knees with mud, when even our elastic-strapped sou'westers have blown off, when the rain has stung our cheeks like whipcord. The normal outfit of a night nurse on winter duty consists of woollen garments piled on cocoon-like under her dress, a jersey over the dress and under the apron or overall, another jersey above the apron, a greatcoat, two pairs of stockings, service boots or gum boots with a pair of woolly soles, a sou'wester, mittens or gloves (perhaps both) and a scarf.

My introduction to active service night nursing was a small hut under the same roof as the theatre, a few of the more anxious cases being brought there for special watching.

Poor boys, almost every patient in addition to other wounds and injuries, had had a leg amputated, and I used to go round from one to another in the dimly-lighted ward with an electric torch, and flash on the light to see that each stump was correct and there was no sign of haemorrhage.

With regard to work on 'the lines', so far from being dull, one is kept ceaselessly busy, for, in addition to dressings, many four-hourly foments, four-hourly charts, periodical stimulants and feeds – the latter including jaw-cases where the mouth must be syringed and washed and the india-rubber tube attached to the feeding-cup cleaned and boiled – there comes the unending, infinitely pathetic call of 'Sister, sister, may I have …': a drink, my pillows moved, my heel rubbed, now my toe, my splint moved, my bandage tightened, my bandage slackened, the tent or the window closed – or opened – a blanket off, a blanket on, a hot water bag, a drink of water, of lemonade, of hot milk, of hot tea, now a cold drink, sister, to cool my mouth, a crease taken out of the under-sheet, the air-pillow altered, my hands and face washed, my lips rubbed with ointment, my fan, that fly killed, a match, a cigarette lighted, another drink, some grapes, my apple peeled, a cushion under my arm, under my back, a pad of cotton-wool under my heel, knee, arm, a bed sock put on, the bed-clothes tucked in, I feel sick, I can't go to sleep …

Naturally, we have had nights never-to-be-forgotten, nights of aching anxiety and grim, gruesome tragedy, nights that have seared themselves into our brain for as long a time as we shall possess human knowledge and human understanding, nights when we have shared and suffered with delirious patients the stench, the choking thirst, the sound of groans – all the devilish horror and racking torture of living again the eternal age with its waiting, waiting, waiting in No Man's Land, nights when a dying man on whom morphia has had no effect has persistently cackled ragtime while another – one of the very, very few who have realised they are in the Valley of the Shadow – reiterated again and again, 'I'm dying, I'm dying, I'm dying.' …

Miss Dorothy Brook

No. 18 General Hospital, Camiers, near Étaples, France

Dorothy Brook was at the Wagner Festival in Bayreuth when Germany and Austria declared war on Serbia on 28 July 1914. Immediately the opera house was closed and all cars in the town were commandeered. Everyone rushed to get out of Bayreuth and Dorothy Brook and her Austrian friends managed to catch an already overcrowded train. Most of the stations they passed were packed with troops ordered to the front. Although her friends were very pro-British and she stayed at their home, she had no means of communication with her family for over nine weeks until the US consul in Vienna got in touch with the mayor of her home town. As she had neither passport nor identification papers, Dorothy Brook had to visit the police station each day and life became increasingly difficult for her. Towards the end of November 1914 she was told she must leave as she was the only enemy subject in the district. She had to go over the frontier to Dresden, where she had been at school for two years, and had learnt to speak German fluently. After getting papers from the US consul signed at the police headquarters she embarked on a 'nightmare journey' via Magdeburg and Hanover. At one station British wives of men interned in Ruhleben Camp were put into her compartment. She reached home on 25 November.

She enrolled with her local VAD and worked in a small hospital for a few weeks before responding to an urgent appeal from the British Red Cross for VAD volunteers to serve in France. She arrived at the huge camp hospital of marquees and bell tents at Camiers in October 1915.

The Sisters' Mess was a small marquee with two long scrubbed wooden tables and wooden forms. Outside this were four grim-looking Sawyer stoves with their long black chimneys. All our food was cooked on these and all water for tea and hot drinks boiled on them. We had 126 Sisters and Staff Nurses and VADs. Staff Nurses and VADs went on duty 7.30am and the Sisters at 8. The night staff had their breakfast at 9. Porridge was cooked for breakfast on the Sawyer boilers and now and again we had eggs – boiled in a large net – or kedgeree boiled rice with tinned fish mixed with it. Corned beef and pickles for lunch and onion stew in the evening. Water was very scarce. There were no sluices and we had no running water in the wards so orderlies had to fetch it from the workhouse or doctors' or sisters' messes. All water was chlorinated and our tea and coffee had a weird taste – especially if the water had also got the onion flavour after the stew. We used to say if it looks like tea and tastes like coffee, it is cocoa! We were often too tired or too hungry to care, but there was always a jolly atmosphere in the mess for we were all in the same boat. We loved our work.

Our bell tents were not exactly spacious with 2 camp beds, 2 trunks, 2 lockers – folding washstands and chair, and tent pole serving as wardrobe with the outdoor and indoor uniforms of 2 VADs hanging from hooks strapped to the top of the pole. A small metal mirror dangled from a string.

Mice were a nuisance. They found anything edible and would gnaw through boxes to get it. One of the VADs was leaving to get married and had bought some lovely nighties at Paris Plage for her trousseau. Unfortunately there must have been a piece of chocolate biscuit in her locker before she put in the boxes containing her undies. In order to get at the eatables the mice had gnawed through boxes and the VAD was horrified when she took out her nighties, now very well ventilated, to show her pals.

Rats, too, were a menace. As our unit had recently been erected a lot of digging had had to be done – and the rats 'quarters' disturbed and they were very hungry. One orderly came on duty one morning with the skin off the end of his nose. He had been very fast asleep wearing a woollen Balaclava to keep his head warm and a rat had had a nibble! At intervals village men would be asked to bring their dogs, duck boards lifted and rats killed one marquee at a time.

On night duty there would be a VAD and an orderly in one marquee – in the next there would be a Sister, a VAD and an orderly and in the next just a VAD and orderly, so that the Sister could easily be called to either ward if required. Night duty seemed weird at first. The Tommies snoring or having nightmares and 'going over the top' and the rats scurrying down from one end to the other. If the patients couldn't sleep the only help we could give them was 2 aspirins and some evaporated milk and hot water heated on a Beatrice stove, but it worked quite often. Later in the war Glaxo appeared and the men preferred that.

When the big battles were raging we frequently had sudden orders to clear the wards of as many patients as possible to make room for a big convoy from the front. A Doctor would go round each ward marking the charts of the men. 'A' was for helpless stretcher cases – 'B' for sitting cases – 'C' for walking cases. The remainder went to convalescent camp. The nurses on night duty had to dress the 'A' cases in warm clothes – long socks and wrap army blankets over them. It was such a joy to see the happy faces of men marked for 'good old Blighty'. We gave them hot drinks before they were taken to the ambulance by the stretcher-bearers and then they were driven to the hospital train at the siding en route for the hospital ship. When they had all gone we had to start immediately getting beds ready for new arrivals. Usually we put a blanket on the top – for many of the new patients were in a very dirty state after being in the muddy trenches and not having their boots off for many days. Before a convoy we nurses were given long calico overalls – with high collars and short sleeves slotted with tape so that they could be drawn up tightly and prevent the nasty 'grey backs' (lice) from crawling underneath. The overalls tied at the back. When we took off the cotton wool from dressings we used swabs with carbolic to kill the insects.

The trouble with marquees is that they are dark, no light coming in from outside and in the early days we had only storm lamps. We had only enough time to get off the worst dirt before the doctor came to examine the patients and put on fresh dressings. Then we put blankets over patients and left the dog-tired men to have a much needed sleep, and cleaning up was continued in the morning. The men used to say they felt in heaven to be clean and in a bed after the mud and dangers of the trenches. That made our hard work so very worthwhile.

It got around that there was gas and we looked down the very long camp road. The ambulances were bringing the very bad cases up the road. Some of them just about made it and that was all, but the ones who could walk but couldn't see were sent in front of one man with sight and he took six with him, with their hands on his shoulders. The road was filled with these men.

All VADs had to do a spell in the Mess. Two had volunteered to be the regular cooks as they couldn't stand ward work. Others did 6 weeks as kitchen helpers or waitresses. One evening Matron told me that I was to be head cook from the next morning and my friend was to be my assistant. When I told her I couldn't cook she said, 'Nurse, there is no such word as can't'. One of the regular VAD cooks had measles and the other was due to go on leave next day. I had to go to her tent to get instructions about quantities, etc. The Sawyer stoves were used only for water.

By now there was a long hut which was divided into a small sitting room, the long mess room and kitchen. The kitchen stove had a half flat top and the chimney was very smoky. Often I had five clean aprons in a day. I had to be on duty at 6am in order to get first breakfast at 7. The porridge was made in a huge brown glazed bread crock and it was really hard work stirring such a quantity and preventing it burning. The rations for the day arrived about 9.30. A huge lump of frozen stiff meat was dumped on the wooden table and I had to cut it as well as possible for the evening stew. At the end I felt as though I had frostbite. Sugar was strictly rationed. Everyone had a small labelled box (often a tobacco tin) and each morning 2 teaspoonfuls were put into each and that was all we had to last the day. Sometimes we had plain boiled puddings – rolled in long pieces of lint – and boiled in the Sawyer boilers. We were allowed plum and apple jam (the Tommies called it 'poggy') with these and we really enjoyed them.

Although some distance away we could hear the noise of the guns and at one time when the Germans were advancing the noise got louder each day. Then one day in December the Colonel gave the order that the wards should be evacuated except the very serious cases and most of the equipment packed and stacked ready to be moved at short notice. When this was done we just waited – not allowed far out of the camp …

Mrs Elsie Fenwick

Belgian Red Cross Hospital (Hôtel de l'Ocean), La Panne, Belgium

There were very few trained Belgian nurses at the outbreak of the war, and the British Red Cross sent a number of trained nurses and some VADs to the Belgian hospital at La Panne, a seaside resort and fishing village. Dr Depage was the senior physician. He was a well-known Brussels doctor before the war – a skilled surgeon and an exceptional organiser. Elsie Fenwick, a forty-two-year-old married woman, arrived at the hospital as a probationer in February 1915. At this time in La Panne the Court of the King and Queen of the Belgians lived in six small villas, and the British Mission had established its headquarters. Elsie Fenwick moved in social circles at home – her father was a banker, her brother and her husband were Etonians – and she was the lady of a fine manor house in Rutland. She therefore knew members of the Royal Family and many senior diplomats and officers who were stationed or passed through the British Mission, and in their company, she enjoyed a lively social life. This acted as a necessary panacea to the tough nursing conditions and suffering she witnessed daily.

Wednesday, 17 February

At last we arrived at La Panne, a fair-sized town about the size of Buckingham, crammed full of Belgian and French soldiers. We drove up to the Hospital, a large good hotel, covered everywhere with Red Cross. I was terrified pretending to be a nurse and felt such a humbug, but anyhow the Matron [Miss Winch] knows we aren't so that's something. Anyhow we were ushered into her offices and she was quite charming and showed us over the Hospital – nice big clean passages, but of course only small rooms with about two patients in each – which makes it hard work to nurse.

Then she took us over to the villa we are to live in, about five minutes' walk and tucked away in the sand dunes, with some refugees from Ypres to look after us – a shoemaker, his wife and two tiny children, and we were shown our rooms, all four together and then we tidied up and went to lunch at the Hospital. What an awful moment it was, about forty nurses all having a look at us, but anyhow we had a good meal and then went and undid our packing. It was funny to think we're only 7 miles from the firing line and we had boy scouts and a carpenter to arrange our room and hang up things as we wanted, and altogether everybody was very nice and except for masses of soldiers everywhere and three mitrailleuses placed outside our villa and the sounds of guns booming in the distance, which is too thrilling, one would think one was at just an ordinary French seaside place with lovely sands and sand dunes.

Thursday, 18 February

A lovely day, but cold, and we were up early and very punctual to eat our breakfast and then Aline [Aline Cholmeley] went on to the Second floor and I went on to the Third floor, and felt very bewildered not knowing where anything was kept, any names of the sisters or numbers or wounds of the men. Anyhow I worked hard at housemaid's work and helping everyone and the men all seemed very nice, poor fellows, some are so bad. One poor fellow had his leg cut off high up after awful haemorrhages and another with an arm off.

It's lovely looking out of the hospital over the sands, seeing hundreds of soldiers drilling and the horses being exercised and the gun carriages washed in the sea.

Tuesday, Wednesday, Thursday, 23, 24 and 25 February

Went to the British Mission to find out how to get parcels out here as not a thing ever arrives and all the good things I have ordered from Fortnum and Mason have never arrived.

Found Prince Alexander of Teck and the Duke of Sutherland there. What they are working at I am not quite sure.

Friday, 26 February

Woke up to a lovely, frosty, calm day which turned out anything but calm as the German aeroplanes were round and over us at intervals all day.

A poor woman was brought into our ward and had her head trepanned and I was with her all the evening. Also a child of ten was killed and two women.

A lot of wounded were brought in last night, about forty. There has been a lot of fighting near Nieuport – 6 miles off here.

Saturday, 27 February

I am now happy in a ward with Sister Ashford and we run it all to ourselves. She is so nice, and I like it.

We've got a poor little nun who was wounded by a shell while she was walking alone in the convent garden at Furnes. It cut her arm clean off by her shoulder and broke the other, which is quite useless to her and so poor little thing she has to be fed and everything, and thirty shrapnel wounds on her body, and she is so good.

We've got nine soldiers, two women and a little girl to look after. I am no more treated like a bit of dirt.

Wednesday, 10 March
A nice day and we had our second half-day since we've been here, and we were glad of it. We spent most of it tidying up and then we went to tea at the Mission with the Duke of Sutherland, Prince Alexander of Teck and Mr Johnnie Baird, and a nice sailor (Shoppee) [Lieutenant Denys Charles Gerald Shoppee, Royal Navy]. We had a jolly good tea and tried to find out what news they'd got, but they were very British Missionish and didn't tell us much, except that the English are coming this way and Nieuport is being violently bombarded with the big guns. The nearest German trenches are 6 miles off, so when they want to turn their attention on us, they very easily can!

We walked off with an oil stove much to our delight, as we have been icy the last few nights and even two blankets, a sleeping bag, a dressing gown and flannel pyjamas didn't keep me warm.

Friday, 19 March
Madame de Glos (a dear little Russian lady who helps in the Hospital in the afternoons), took Aline and I to see Sarah Wilson at Maxine Elliott's barge [Maxine Elliott was a well-known American actress]. Just a flat black ugly thing with the American flag flying, but inside too nice. Miss Elliott has done the whole thing, fitted it up with gas, water and stoves and it was perfectly lovely getting warm by a real coal stove again. The barge consisted of a very nice sitting room, dining room, cabins, kitchen in one – a huge store room for all the clothes and food they give away – masses of clothes, sacks of flour, potatoes and onions and they feed the unfortunate refugees for miles around. They've got a family of five living in a cart and another nine living in a greenhouse.

Monday, 22 March
Our floor had such a hard day's work we didn't get off all day from eight until 8.30 as the 'trepanned' woman and another man on our floor have got Scarlet Fever, so the whole ward of fifty beds had to be evacuated and disinfected during the day.

Wednesday, Thursday, 24, 25 March
Both fairly quiet days, no fresh cases of Scarlet Fever, but some wounded civilians came in from Pervyse which the Germans were shelling. A whole family – the father died on the way, the mother died on the operating table – they never gave her chloroform, cut off her hair, left her waiting over half an hour, then searched for the bullet without anything. They left a baby of three weeks old with its foot blown away.

Prince Alexander and Major Baird came to see me and asked us to dine. I absolutely refuse to turn out when I am tired for anyone.

Friday, 26 March
Aline and I went to lunch at the British Mission, quite amusing as Prince Alexander thawed and we fairly teased them for being pompous and telling us nothing and being so important! Major Baird, Prince Alexander, the Duke of Sutherland, Captain Tyrrell, Mr Shoppee and another man were there: they live in great comfort – an excellent cook, two refugees to mend their clothes and six menservants!

Prince Alexander, Major Baird and the Duke of Sutherland took us for a walk on the beach, much to my disgust as I had my best shoes on!

More civilians brought into the Hospital as they are shelling Furnes again, one was a woman who is going to have a baby in a month.

Sunday, 4 April. Easter Day
We had a charming service in the salon, a parson from Dunkirk and all the English nurses and British Mission were there. The Matron had made such a pretty altar, out of tables and boxes with a white sheet over it and lots of white flowers in green vases and a cross with yellow flowers.

Sunday, 11 April
Worked hard all the morning at dressings, etc., and then about lunch time poor Colonel Bridges [Head of the British Mission with the Belgian Army in Flanders] was brought in wounded by a shell at Nieuport this morning. He was brought to our floor and after having sworn never to nurse an officer I knew, I was promptly told to take his clothes off and put on his pyjamas! Anyhow I did it, but won't have anything more to do with him as I think he'd hate it too. Very bad luck, a shell burst close to him and Mr Shoppee and it caught him in the cheek and on his shoulder.

Monday, 12 April
In the afternoon Maxine Elliott came and gave lovely clothes to all the refugees on our floor. Awfully kind of her. She told me she hasn't had one word of thanks for all the work she has done from the Queen or anyone. I don't think there is much gratitude left in this country.

Wednesday, 14 April
Four new patients in our Annexe. One nice young boy with all his knee-cap shot through and most of it away and he is so patient. They bombarded Furnes all the morning and most of the afternoon. I watched it from the hospital. Great puffs of smoke in the air and one just wondered who and how many were killed.

Thursday, 15 April
Sister Ashford and I had a patient sent up with the most awful smashed leg I have ever seen, all pulp from knee to ankle and gas gangrene as well. We had to put the leg in a peroxide bath. It was hard work and we did get hot and tired.

Saturday, 17 April
We lunched at the 'Mish' – Colonel Fairholme was there, he is Military Attaché to the Belgians and I knew him in Marienbad. The war has made him no thinner! Prince Alexander, Captain Bridges, Major Baird and his brother were there – had plovers' eggs and a jolly good lunch and then went back to duty.

Then the King [King Albert of Belgium] came and decorated one of my men in the Annexe. No fuss, he just came with one ADC and pinned it on and said a few words.

Then all the English came to see Colonel Bridges who is nearly all right now. The Duchess of Sutherland [qv], Captain FitzGerald and Diana Wyndham and Major Tyrrell all came, one after another, and each I had to take round my Annexe and they were all very nice. I took Prince Alexander round too. I think my patients are rather surprised at the very ordinary nurse's friends!!

Friday, 23 April [Second Battle of Ypres]
So cold, windy and sand-storms – beastly.

As soon as I got on duty we began receiving wounded and all day long it went on. Then rumours things were going badly for us, that the French had retreated and we had to fall back to help them and the losses were awful.

Saturday, 24 April
All night long and all day the guns were at it the whole time. Wild rumours all day and wounded coming in. Our Annexe is full up. A poor man came in early and nearly died on the stretcher in his room, but Dr Jansen tied him up with a tourniquet and sent him down to the theatre and he returned minus an arm. It was so sad in the evening when I was washing him, he asked me if I wasn't going to wash his left hand. I simply couldn't tell him.

Wednesday, 28 April
So busy, no time to think. We've got a man with a bullet in his brain and he lies all day unconscious and they are leaving him to see what happens. Another had his leg cut off at the hip joint today. I had to hold him. They cut him just as if he was a joint of meat. Dr Depage is a butcher, but he did it as well as possible. Another with a bullet in his neck. It's all awful, and they call us civilised.

Thursday, 29 April
Still terribly busy as the wounded keep on coming in and so many shot through the head.

Friday, 30 April
Awfully busy in hospital and I'm afraid our poor man is going to die with his leg off and he is so very brave.

Saturday, 1 May
Our poor man with the leg off seemed better, but in the afternoon he collapsed and died soon after we went home at night. I'm so sorry, he was such a brave fellow and so keen to live.

Sunday, 2 May
Much colder and still very busy as the wounded still keep on coming in and we've got two men with bullets in their heads – both alive but one has hardly spoken and the other speaks, but his left side is paralysed, so in the evening he was taken to the theatre and I had to go with him. The operation was too big and while digging in his

brain they cut the artery and he just died on the table. It was horrible and while I was with him poor Sister Ashford had the other head case die with her upstairs, and so it was all very depressing.

In the evening, when it was calm we saw two taubes come over. They'd been to Dunkirk. Wild rumours of how we are cut off from Dunkirk and supplies will be difficult to get. They killed forty in Dunkirk the other night and destroyed a lot of houses.

Thursday, 6 May

We can't do anything against these beastly gasses. We've lost Hill 60 and they say we shall lose Ypres in another week.

Saturday, 8 May

Everybody rather wondering whether we shall be bombarded or not.

Nothing but depressing news all day. A report at lunch that the *Lusitania* had been sunk as the Germans said they were going to. She went down with 1,600 souls on her off Queenstown at 2.30 yesterday afternoon. Then a good cruiser of ours the *Myra* was sunk 10 miles up this coast last night by a mine, but the crew is interned in Holland. All disgusting and depressing.

Monday, 10 May

A lovely day, but found wounded had been received all night and I went up as quickly as possible to find we'd got three new ones. One awfully bad, shot through the neck, his head nearly off. It was awful and thank goodness he died in about an hour. The other two aren't bad.

We spent the morning sending off six wounded from our Annexe, hardly fit to go some weren't, but we must have room for all the wounded coming in.

Tuesday, 11 May

A very busy day and two of our head cases died and the beds were hardly made before they filled again and all was forgotten. It's very horrible. They keep on coming in and so now we've got fifty-five beds full and only Sisters Allan, Ashford, Harrison, Wallace and myself. It's real hard work and none of us sat down all day, except for meals. It's the same on all the floors and everybody is dead tired.

Wednesday, 12 May

A man, Leopold, came to our Annexe today shot through the body and Dr Jansen sent him up from the operating room as sure to die! But we worked hard with *huile camphre, caffeine and salines,* until I'm sick at the sight of them, but he's doing all right.

An officer was brought up, shot through his eye, the whole of the side of his face gone, his shoulder out, his arm broken and a wound on his leg. He died, thank goodness. Another with both legs broken and amputated – he died too. We had two bad haemorrhages in the evening, but going on all right. We've got a room of three with gas gangrene. One had his leg off and I'm afraid the others will too.

Friday, 14 May
Poor Madame Depage was drowned in the *Lusitania* having gone over to America to collect money and nurses. Such a tragedy and poor old Dr Depage had gone to meet her and now is coming back tomorrow, with her body.

Tuesday, 18 May
Leopold is getting on, but we've got a gas gangrene case the worst that's been in the hospital and not died immediately. They operated on him today, it was horrible, but necessary to save his life, and he is such a fine young fellow and suffers awfully. There is very little chance for him.

Wednesday, 19 May
Twenty-five American nurses and ten doctors have arrived and so I hope now we shall have more duty off.

Thursday, 20 May
A glorious hot summer day, the first we've really had. We had a terrible day of it as Madame Depage's funeral took place. First we had to walk 2 miles to the Church and go through a service for an hour. Poor Dr Depage and the boys looked too awful and the Queen came looking neat and housemaid-like in black, and her lady-in-waiting in black with white boots! Lots of Generals and soldiers there and it was all very sad. We all went in our indoor uniform and veils and made a sort of guard of honour, about fifty of us and we had to carry all the wreaths and walk back in lines of six, all the way to this villa, as she was going to be buried on the dune just behind. It is a solitary spot right on the top of a sand dune and the idea is she is to be moved to Brussels later. The wreaths were lovely, but it was awfully hard work carrying them for at least half an hour and I was dead tired and so we all were.

Then back on duty directly afterwards and an hour off later.

Our wounded are very bad and our two show cases of the hospital Leopold and the gas gangrene, are both worse and never gave us a minute's peace. Poor gas gangrene had to be moved from our Annexe as he kept the others awake and he was so miserable and so was I.

Friday, 21 May
A lovely day and we started off with the most sad thing as all of us that had carried wreaths had to go to Dr Depage's villa and he made a little speech thanking us. He broke down and it was so sad.

Poor gas gangrene was much worse and I went to see him, though he wasn't any more my patient, so nearly got myself disliked! But I didn't care and he was taken down to have the dressing done and they found his leg so bad, they settled to cut it off. Poor man he was practically dead and he died under chloroform. He was such a fine grenadier and I was more miserable at losing him than anyone – he died so hard.

Leopold was better and so we had a much easier day.

In May, Elsie Fenwick went home on leave. She returned to find that Sister Ashford, with whom she had worked in harmony for nearly five months, was leaving to take up another post. The hospital was still very busy coping with a constant intake of casualties.

Friday, 25 June
A terrible scandal and excitement in the hospital as a nurse on our floor was assaulted in the night!! She was in a villa close to ours and alone in a room. A soldier climbed up the balcony, got in, knocked her down because she screamed, and tried to gag her. Luckily the nurses next door heard and got into the room. He hid under the bed and was caught! The poor nurse is the ugliest in the hospital, and is suffering from terrible shock! I think the man will get several years as he is going to be tried by court martial. What dangers we go through, and Aline and I have lived for weeks in a night villa all alone, not even a caretaker living in it.

Tuesday, 29 June
A very sad day, as Miss Winch [the Matron] went off and it all seems so blank without her. Half an hour before she left the Queen sent for her, and of course we were delighted and thought she was going to get something nice. I was disgusted when she came back with a signed photo of the Queen, unframed – when she's given all her wits and body to work for these Belgians for seven months and done wonders – ungrateful people – and all for nothing.

Friday, 9 July
A lovely day and not much to do, until this afternoon when another abdominal case was brought up, awfully bad. Sister Campbell and I worked at him hard all the evening and got him a tiny bit better.

Saturday, 10 July
Our man no better and I hardly was off all day, trying to save him, but I'm afraid it's a hopeless case as gas gangrene has started.

In the afternoon an English officer, Captain Knight, was brought up to the corridor with an awful wound in the hip. He was in charge of an anti-aircraft gun at Nieuport and a shell burst close to him.

Prince Alexander and Major Baird came to see us and asked us to dine tonight, and it's the best thing to get hospital horrors out of one's head, so off we went. Prince Alexander, Major Baird, General Bridges and the head officer Commander Halahan of the big gun at Nieuport [in command of the Naval Heavy Batteries attached to the Belgian Army] and the Duchess of Sutherland motored over from her hospital between Dunkirk and Calais – it's in a ploughed field, only tents, but she lives in a house herself.

Sunday, 11 July
A beastly day of horrors. First of all my nice man who I've worked so hard for died, the whole time begging me to keep the Germans off – too sad – then our English Officer has got such bad gangrene he can't do any good.

Monday, 12 July

Our poor Captain Knight died on the operating table, the only chance was to amputate his leg and he died under it, too sad.

Tuesday, 13 July

A nice cool day, which was lucky, as all the English nurses had to go to Captain Knight's funeral and walk to Adinkerk, 3 miles on cobble stones. The Service was in the salon and the coffin in the middle draped with a Union Jack and his Khaki coat on the top, lovely wreaths all round from the Belgians and English. The English Chaplain from the Dunkirk Aero ground did it, and it was very nice, and then we marched in procession to Adinkirk – all his regiment, the anti-aircraft corps from Nieuport, and the coffin on a gun carriage. He was buried with all the other soldiers that have died in hospital – rows and rows and rows of tiny black crosses with just the name – and some not even that.

Then Maxine Elliott was very kind and sent her car for us, and we took the Matron, Miss Hughes, and Faber to tea on her barge, and they were quite delighted.

Thursday, 15 July

A nice day and nothing doing and so Aline and I had our half day off, and Maxine Elliott was awfully kind and came and picked us up in her motor.

We went to Steenkirk where Mrs Knocker [qv] and Miss Chisholm [qv] live in a wooden hut, such a place!! So dirty; unfortunately they were not in, but we went in to the camp. I've never seen anything so untidy and they'd got several soldier servants too. Their idea is to look after about five blessés, ones that aren't bad enough to go away, but they were packed into a tiny room. Her bedroom was tiny, with both beds unmade and not even a looking-glass, but I hear they have a very good time as they are attached to the Belgian Army. As they've been there for months I should have thought they could have got it nicer.

We came back by Furnes, which is a bit more knocked about than when we were there last. We saw Lady Dorothie Feilding, rather a pretty little thing, and she had on a skirt!! She lives in Furnes, with no other woman, so they say!!

We went back to tea at the barge and just home in time for dinner.

Saturday, 31 July

Just before lunch an English aviator called Captain Liddell was brought in with a bad smashed leg. I saw the observer with him, Mr Peck, such a bounder, but they did a wonderful plucky thing and had a marvellous escape. They were flying over Bruges and a German aeroplane had got above them, and so they couldn't see it and they shot him in the leg. He lost consciousness and the aeroplane made a nose dive for about 1,000 feet, which apparently pulled him together enough to make him realise the danger. He worked the leg lever with his hand and looped the loop downwards. The observer told him he saw a flying ground, and he made for it and arrived at Furnes, landed safely, did up his own leg in splints and then was brought on here. He is very bad, but they hope he'll be all right.

Thursday, 5 August
I received in the worst case we've had in yet. I went to the operating theatre and found his legs smashed to bits by an 'aubu' and they had to cut them both off as high up as possible. He had the stuff injected into the spine and no chloroform, but he suffered a good deal and called the whole time for his mother, and it was heart-rending, and then to take that shapeless bundle up on the stretcher. Only a little boy of 19, the only child, and his parents with the Germans.

Friday, 6 August
The poor little boy, Alfred, was going on well, but it was too pitiful all day long asking me what was the matter with his legs and why they hurt him so much and when he'd be able to go back to his regiment. We must leave him to find it out for himself, poor boy. Another awful evening in the operating theatre when his legs were dressed. He yelled with the pain and I don't know how he bears it.

Sunday, 8 August
A lovely day and I sat on the sands all the morning and it was delicious. In the afternoon I had to go down to the theatre for an awful case, shot by shrapnel through the thighs and abdomen and Dr Deparge operated for two hours and then the poor man was brought up most awfully bad. He lived from about 6 till 9 at night and I never wish to have a more ghastly three hours, dying all the time, and fighting.

The poor little boy with the amputations is going on well and is so good and brave.

Thursday, 12 August
I was talking to Prince Alexander and Major Baird and up came Sister Campbell to say there was an awful abdominal case in the theatre and I was to go down. I stood in the heat down there for 2½ hours while Dr Antoine did the most awful operation. He was shot through and through. He never had a chance and died on the table. I was tired and never got home till after 9 and went to bed thoroughly sick with life and the war.

Friday, 13 August
A lovely day, but I hated everything and felt thoroughly depressed and wished I was home.

I'm afraid Captain Liddell's leg is doing badly and will have to be cut off after all, but we still hope not.

Saturday, 14 August
In the afternoon, a German aeroplane dropped four bombs in the town and wounded two soldiers, killed one, and killed a mother and two dear little girls. They were all brought into the hospital and died. One poor little girl had both her legs off and it was too pitiful to see the doctor carrying her in his arms in her little white frock drenched with blood and rushing her to the theatre.

Monday, 16 August
My little double amputation is a little sweet and so good and brave.

Poor Captain Liddell is not doing well.

Tuesday, 17 August
Poor Captain Liddell is much worse and they settled to have his leg off tomorrow morning. It's too sad, after a fortnight's pain for nothing.

In the afternoon Prince Alexander came up to say he'd been given a VC. It's splendid, but it was very sad going to congratulate him, knowing that his leg was doomed and he didn't know it. One felt such a humbug, but he was so happy.

Thursday, 19 August
A sad day as Captain Liddell had his leg off. It's the only thing that may save him, but he is very bad – poison all over his body, and there is not much chance for his life.

Friday, 20 August
Captain Liddell very bad.

Saturday, 21 August
Captain Liddell so bad that the Mission wired for his mother. I do hope he will live, he's such a nice young fellow … [Captain Liddell died on 31 August.]

Miss Edith Cavell

L'École Belge d'Infirmières Diplômées, Brussels, Belgium

In 1907, Edith Cavell, a forty-two-year-old trained nurse, was asked by the distinguished Belgian surgeon, Dr Antoine Depage, to become matron of Belgium's first teaching hospital for nurses in Brussels. He saw the need for qualified nurses to replace nuns, who until then had been responsible for the care of the sick. The clinique, l'Ecole Belge d'Infirmières Diplômées, in the Rue de la Culture, consisted of four adjoining residential houses and opened in October 1907. Five years later, Dr Depage, spoke at the International Congress of Nurses in Cologne and told them that the Belgian school of nursing had been a great success. 'It now provides the nurses for three hospitals, three private nursing homes, twenty-four communal schools and thirteen kindergartens in Brussels'. In addition to training young women to become nurses, the hospital had its own nursing staff and patients.

When war was declared, Edith Cavell was at home in Norfolk but returned to Brussels immediately. She sent the Dutch and German nurses home and as the clinique became a Red Cross Hospital, she told the remaining staff that the first duty of a nurse was to care for the wounded irrespective of their nationality.

The Germans marched into Brussels on 20 August 1914. A few English nurses were sent home but Edith Cavell remained with some members of her staff, including two French-speaking Sisters, Elisabeth Wilkins and Millicent White.

On 1 November 1914 Herman Capiau, a member of the Belgian resistance, brought two British soldiers, Colonel Dudley Boger and Sergeant Frederick Meachin, to the clinique. They had been wounded during the Battle of Mons. Edith Cavell agreed to shelter them and many more hunted men who found their way to the clinique over the next nine months. By this time at the Château of Bellignies, a few kilometres from Mons, Princess Marie de Cröy was nursing wounded German and British soldiers. Very soon an underground movement was established by the Princess and her brother, the Prince de Cröy. Other members of the group, organised by Philippe Baucq, an architect, guided the disguised soldiers to safety across the Dutch frontier. The password used by the members of the resistance was 'Yorc' (Cröy backwards).

After the Germans had taken over Brussels, Edith Cavell's letters home were wisely restrained. Only eighteen of these written to her family between August 1914 and June 1915 have survived. However, she wrote a diary between April and May 1915 and hid it in a cushion. It was not discovered for over thirty years.

27 April: This month during which I have been unable to keep a diary has been full of interest and anxiety. Yesterday a letter from M. Cap [Herman Capiau], who has gone to G [Germany] voluntarily to inspect at Essen! With some other B [Belgian] engineers. The letter came through a young Frenchman who with 7 others had come from N. France to escape and hopes to get over the D [Dutch] frontier in a day or two. The frontier has been absolutely impassable the last few days. G [Germany] and H [Holland] have been on the verge of war over the sinking of the *Catwyk* [a Dutch ship carrying a cargo of grain which was torpedoed near Flushing on 14 April]. The Dutch refused to allow anyone to cross and had massed their troops and laid mines all along from Maastricht to Antwerp, a sentinel on the D [Dutch] side was posted every 15 metres and all the young men who had left to try and cross were stuck or came back – 5 of ours were heard of at Herrenthall yesterday morning and the guide left to bring them back. Last night great numbers of G [German] wounded passed thro' the city; the Gare de Schaerbeck was cleared of the public to let them thro' – all the Dutch newspapers were burned at the G. du Midi. None from France or Eng. Have come through for some days. The Gs post a victory on the Yser – but rumour ascribes it to the B and E [Belgian and English] armies aided by the Hindous …

Fr [Monsieur Fromage – Philippe Baucq's nom de guerre] brought me word from the town authorities that the house is watched and several attempts I think have been made to catch me in default – several suspicious persons have been to ask for help to leave the country either in the form of money, lodging or guides. People have been taken in this way several times. Today a doctor was had up because a guide who was caught carried a letter on him for post in Holland; he also had one for me, but as yet I have heard nothing of this. A young girl of 22 Cte [Comtesse] d'Ursel is condemned to one year's fortress in G. She has been allowed to return for a week first, perhaps with the idea of allowing her to escape and then making her family pay a heavy fine. Charles [Charles Vanderlinden, an escape route guide] is here with plans which he has tried to use, but was obliged to return; he tries again in a day or two, acting as friend to four young Belgians. People are wonderfully generous with their loyal help – I went to a new house and there secured the services of a man who comes to take our guests [allied soldiers] of Café Oviers to safe houses where they can abide till it is time for departure. A little widow with a big house gives shelter to some and does all the work without a servant, waiting on and cooking for them with the best courage and good will in the world.

One of our guides Nom de guerre V. Gilles helped greatly in an ambulance at Mons at the beginning of the war. Miss Hosier [sister-in-law of Winston Churchill] was there, she spoke French like a Parisienne – and made friends of the common people – eventually she decided to send Gilles to London with letters to bring back money …

Baroness de Cromburgghe came to tea last Friday. She and N. Cambridge [Sister Kathleen Cambridge, a member of the Belgian Red Cross] told many things of interest concerning the battle of Mons and the 10 wounded they received in the Baroness's house – one of the 2 Gs told them that 9 officers of his regiment were killed, 'but not with Eng. Bullets'. …

31 April 1915, Friday: Glorious and warm e. wind … 2 guides left this morning – Charles Vanderlinden with 3 FX and 2 BE … last 2 paying 60 francs each. This boy of 23 is one of a family of 9 sons, all strong and fighters. 3 are colonial volunteers and 1 is in the reg. Army, 2 little ones are dying to pass the frontier and enlist. Charles says he will take them if it becomes easier. This fellow is a fine type – about 5ft 6 or 7, slightly made but very strong and muscular. He amused himself when small with boxing a great sack of sand or corn which swung forward and butted him in the face if he failed to hit it in the right place. He afterwards got some lessons in boxing and obliged me with a description of the right way to catch a man's head under the arm and 'crack' his neck or to give him a back-handed blow and destroy the trachea or larynx. He is also a poacher in time of peace and sets lassoes in rows so that hares racing to their feeding grounds are bound to be caught in one of them. He and 3 friends will catch from 20 to 30 in 2 or 3 days. The gamekeeper's dogs they hang to a tree when they get a chance. He is nearly always sober but when on the drink will be drunk for 10 days on the stretch. He and his brothers, men equally strong and pugilistic, would fight at times, but when they entered a cafe together no one would dare say a word to any of them. He has one blind eye smashed in a fight with a boxer.

He has travelled far oftener on foot than otherwise and has many trades to which he can turn his hand. He is extremely intelligent and has a good memory. He has ideas of justice and straight dealing and is very anxious to repay any money given him. He boasts in the most open manner and enjoys to talk of himself and his prowess. Withal he is, at least here, a gentleman and well-behaved in the house and gives us no trouble, also his conversation is clean and quite pleasing. He has crossed the line once and taken his news and been back for more, which he has started again to deliver. He is very scornful over the young men with no pluck and has a grand contempt for the Gs. He is a repoussé [one unfit for military service] – unwillingly, on account of his eye, he can swim and walk great distances, and knows how to pass a leisure day sound asleep on our garden grass. He wears grey corduroys, a rough tweed jacket, and a grey muffler, a cap, shoes which he exchanges for sabots when necessary in the country. He wears his trousers tied in at the ankle and under the tie places his letters – or ours. He will be caught one day and if so will be shot, but he will make a first class bid for life and freedom …

On Monday night over 8,000 blessés were brought into Brussels all Gs M. Victor tells me. He is a tradesman of 60 or thereabouts with a pale and puffy face, bald-headed, fat and short. He has a benevolent smile and spends his days in going from place to place to look after our guests. He too holds the Gs in complete contempt and does his best for the patrie.

Edith Cavell kept her underground activities from her nursing staff so they could not be incriminated, but by June 1915 the net was closing. Although she also eliminated all possible evidence the clinique was searched by the German authorities after a Belgian 'collaborator' passed through. The next day the Château of Bellignies was also under suspicion. Five days later, after two members of the escape route team were captured, Edith Cavell was arrested. By then she had assisted in the escape of many hundreds of allied soldiers. She was taken on 5 August to the Kommandantur and on 7 August to a cell in the prison of St Gilles. On 14 September she wrote to her nurses.

Your delightful letter gave me great pleasure, and your lovely flowers have made my cell gay, the roses are still fresh, but the chrysanthemums did not like prison any more than I do – hence they did not live very long.

I am happy to know that you are working well, that you are devoted to your patients and that you are happy in your services. It is necessary that you should study well, for some of you must shortly sit for your examinations and I want you very much to succeed. The year's course will commence shortly, try to profit from it, and be punctual at lectures so that your professor need not be kept waiting.

In everything one can learn new lessons of life, and if you were in my place you would realise how precious liberty is, and would certainly undertake never to abuse it.

To be a good nurse one must have lots of patience – here one learns to have that quality, I assure you.

It appears that the new school is advancing – I hope to see it again one of these days, as well as all of you.

Au revoir, be really good.

Your devoted Matron, E. Cavell.

Some members of the resistance organisation escaped arrest, but on 7 October 1915, after ten weeks in prison, Edith Cavell and thirty-four others accused of sheltering or assisting the escape of allied soldiers, went on trial in the senate chamber. The list included Princess Marie de Cröy, Herman Capiau, and Philippe Baucq. After four days of cross examinations the sentences were read out. Herman Capiau was sentenced to fifteen years' hard labour. Princess Marie de Cröy to ten years' imprisonment. Comtesse Jeanne de Belleville, a French woman; Mlle Louise Thuliez, a schoolmistress from Lille; Louis Severin, a chemist; Philippe Baucq and Edith Cavell were all sentenced to death.

On 11 October, the evening before her execution, the English chaplain, the Reverend Stirling Gahan, visited Edith Cavell in her cell. She told him that her trial had been fairly conducted and that she was not surprised at her sentence. Her ten weeks' imprisonment had been like 'a solemn fast from all earthly distractions and diversions'. 'I have no fear nor shrinking', she said.

> *I have seen death so often that it is not strange or fearful to me … This I would say, standing as I do in view of God and Eternity. I realize that patriotism is not enough. I must have no hatred or bitterness towards anyone.*

Stirling Gahan later wrote:

> *There was no moveable table in the cell but we sat upon the edge of the bed with the one chair between us. This served as our Communion table, and I placed the vessels with the bread and wine upon it. Then we partook of the Lord's Supper together …*

One of Edith Cavell's last letters was to her staff.

My dear Nurses,

This is a sad moment for me as I write to say good-bye. It reminds me that on 17 September I had been running the School for eight years.

I was so happy to be called to help in the organisation of the work which our Committee had just founded. On 1 October 1907 there were only four young pupils, whereas now you are many – fifty or sixty in all I believe, including those who have gained their certificates and are about to leave the School.

I have often told you about those early days and the difficulties we met with, even down to the choice of words for your on-duty hours and your off-duty hours.

For Belgium, everything about the profession was new. Gradually one service after the other was set up; nurses for private needs, school nurses, the St Gilles Hospital. We have staffed Dr Depage's Institute, the Sanatorium at Buysingen, Dr Mayer's clinic, and now many are called (as perhaps you will be later) to tend the brave men wounded in war. If our work has diminished during the last year, it is because of the sad time we are passing through; when better days come our work will grow again and recover all its power to do good.

If I have spoken to you of the past, this is because it is a good thing sometimes to stop and look back along the path we have travelled to take stock of our progress and the mistakes we have made. You will have more patients in your fine house, and you will have everything necessary for their comfort and your own.

To my sorrow I have not always been able to talk to you each privately. You know that I had my share of burdens. But I hope that you will not forget our evening chats.

I told you that devotion would bring you true happiness and the thought that, before God and in your own eyes, you have done your duty well and with a good heart, will sustain you in trouble and face to face with death. There are two or three of you who will recall the little talks we had together. Do not forget them. As I had already gone so far along life's road, I was perhaps able to see more clearly than you, and show you the straight path.

One word more. Never speak evil. May I tell you, who love your country with all my heart, that this has been the great fault here. During these last eight years I have seen so many sorrows which could have been avoided or lessened if a little word had not been breathed here and there, perhaps without evil intention, and thus destroyed the happiness or even the life of someone. Nurses all need to think of this, and to cultivate a loyalty and team spirit among themselves.

If any of you has a grievance against me, I beg you to forgive me; I have perhaps been unjust sometimes, but I have loved you much more than you think.

I send my good wishes for the happiness of all my girls, as much for those who have left the School as for those who are still there.

Thank you for the kindness you have always shown me.

Your Matron,
Edith Cavell

1915
Russia, Serbia, Egypt and Dardanelles

Miss Florence Farmborough

1st Letuchka (Flying Column)

Red Cross Unit of the 10th Field Surgical Otryad of the Zemstvo of all the Russias

Florence Farmborough was twenty-one when she first went to Russia in 1908. After spending two years in Kiev she moved to Moscow and lived with Dr Pavel Sergeyevich Usov, an eminent heart surgeon, and his family. She taught English to his two daughters, Asya and Nadya.

When Germany declared war on Russia in August 1914 Florence Farmborough and the Usov family were on holiday in their country dacha. A few days later they returned to Moscow.

Dr Usov was appointed to the medical staff of a Red Cross hospital under the patronage of Princess Golitsin and he persuaded the Princess to take Florence, Asya and Nadva as members of the Russian Red Cross Voluntary Aid Detachment. The three young women nursed the wounded in the medical and surgical sections of the hospital and although Florence's spoken Russian improved during this time she found the theoretical language hard to master. She learnt whole chapters 'parrot-fashion' and at the end of six months passed the Red Cross examination.

A special church service was held to celebrate the promotion from VAD to qualified Red Cross nurse.

Before each jewelled icon the lampada glowed with a ruby light. On the altar the high brass candlesticks held steadily-shining candles; near them stood a silver chalice containing holy water, with the Book of Books alongside; a silver plate, heaped with red crosses, had been placed in the centre of the Holy Table. In front of the congregation, standing side by side, were sixteen young women, the first draft of nurses from a class of nearly 200. They were wearing the light grey dress, white apron and long white head-veil of the hospital nurse. A priest, in full canonicals, entered and slowly made his way towards the altar. Soon his rich, resonant voice was heard reciting the beautiful Slavonic prayers of the Greek Orthodox liturgy. Heads were reverently bowed; a murmur of voices rose and fell. The censer was swung lightly to and fro, emitting trembling breaths of fine grey, fragrant smoke.

Finally there was silence. The golden-robed priest rose from his knees and faced the congregation crucifix in hand. At a sign from him, the nurses moved slowly, in relays, to kneel at the altar. The priest then pronounced God's blessing on the red crosses and on their recipients and, taking the crosses in his hand, moved towards the kneeling nurses. Bending down, he asked each one her name … Over each he intoned a prayer, placed the red cross on her white apron and held his crucifix to her lips …

Now he was standing before me. 'Your name?' 'Florence,' I answered. The priest paused and whispered to his deacon-acolyte. A book was brought and consulted, then he consulted me: 'Of the pravoslavny [Orthodox] Church?' 'No,' I whispered, 'of the Church of England.' Again the whispered consultation, again the book was referred to. I felt myself growing cold with fear. But he was back again and resumed the prescribed ritual, his tongue slightly twisting at the pronunciation of the foreign name:

> To thee, Floronz, child of God, servant of the Most High, is given this token of faith, of hope, of charity. With faith shalt thou follow Christ the Master, with hope shalt thou look towards Christ for thy salvation, with charity shalt thou fulfil thy duties. Thou shalt tend the sick, the wounded, the needy; with words of comfort shalt thou cheer them.

I held the red cross to my breast and pressed my lips to the crucifix with a heart full of gratitude to God, for He had accepted me.

One by one, we moved back to our appointed places. On our breasts the Red Cross gleamed. I looked at my Russian sisters. We exchanged happy, congratulatory smiles. As for me, I stood there with a great contentment in mind and spirit. A dream had been fulfilled: I was now an official member of the great Sisterhood of the Red Cross. What the future held in store I could not say, but, please God, my work must lie among those of our suffering brothers who most needed medical aid and human sympathy – among those who were dying for their country on the battlefields of war-stricken Russia.

Florence was determined to serve on the front and in January 1915 she was enrolled as a surgical nurse in the newly formed front line unit, the 10th Field Surgical Otryad of the Zemstvo of all the Russias. This was divided into three parts: the 1st and 2nd Letuchkas (flying columns), mobile units, each with a staff of forty-four, which could be called at any time to any part of the front. Each Letuchka had twenty-four light, two-wheeled carts, with a large red cross painted on each canvas hood, twenty-four horses, grooms and drivers, two motor cars and several large drays (drawn by two horses). The third unit formed the base, where several supply officers looked after the stores of food and Red Cross material.

At this time the Russians were successfully pushing the Austrians back over the Carpathian mountains. On 11 April Florence Farmborough and members of the 1st Letuchka finally arrived at Gorlitse, East Galicia on the Russo-Austrian front after travelling by train from Moscow for over four weeks. They set up a hospital in a large house. In addition to her nurse's dresses, aprons and veils, Florence was equipped with a flannel-lined, black leather jacket and a sheepskin waistcoat for the winter months. As the only means of communication in this mountainous region was by riding, high boots and black leather breeches were also added to her wardrobe.

Florence Farmborough's handwriting was very small and she wrote her pencilled diaries in notebooks and on scraps of paper, intermittently between April 1915 and April 1918.

Wednesday, 22 April. Frishtak
So much has happened. I am dreadfully tired. We are retreating! In that one word lies all the agony of the last few days. We were called from our beds before dawn on Saturday 18th. The Germans had launched their offensive! Explosion after explosion rent the air; shells and shrapnel fell in and around Gorlitse. The roar of the rival cannons grew increasingly intense. Rockets and projectors were at work. Patches of lurid, red light glowed here and there where fires had been kindled by shells. Our house shook to its very foundations, its windows rattling and quivering in their hinges. Death was very busy, his hands full of victims. Then the wounded began to arrive. We started work in acute earnest. At first we could cope; then we were overwhelmed by their numbers. They came in their hundreds, from all directions; some able to walk, others crawling, dragging themselves along the ground. We worked night and day. And still they came! And the thunder of the guns never ceased. Soon their deadly shells were exploding around our Unit; for hours on end, the horror and confusion continued. We had no rest and were worn out with the intensity and immensity of the work. The stream of wounded was endless. Those who could walk were sent on immediately without attention. 'The Base hospitals will attend to you,' we told them; 'Go! Go! Quickly!' The groans and cries of the wounded were pitiful to hear. We dressed their severe wounds where they lay on the open ground; one by one we tended them, first alleviating their pain by injections. And all the time the bombardment of Gorlitse was continuing with brutal ferocity.

On Sunday, the violence of the thunderous detonations grew in length and strength. Then, suddenly, the terrible word *retreat* was heard. At first in a whisper; then, in loud, forceful tone: 'The Russians are retreating!' And the first-line troops came into sight: a long procession of dirt-bespattered, weary, desperate men – in full retreat! We had received no marching-orders. The thunder of the guns came nearer and nearer. We were frightened and perplexed; they had forgotten us! But they came at last – urgent, decisive orders: we were to start without delay, leaving behind all the wounded and all the equipment that might hinder us. A dreadful feeling of dismay and bewilderment took possession of us; to go away, leaving the wounded and the Unit's equipment! It was impossible; there must be some mistake! But there was no mistake, we had to obey; we had to go.

Snatching up coats, knapsacks, any of our personal belongings which could be carried – we started off quickly down the rough road. And the wounded? They shouted to us when they saw us leaving; called out to us in piteous language to stop – to take them with us; not to forsake them, for the love of God; not to leave them – our brothers – to the enemy. Those who could walk, got up and followed us; running, hopping, limping, by our sides. The badly crippled crawled after us; all begging, beseeching us not to abandon them in their need. And, on the road, there were others, many others; some of them lying down in the dust, exhausted. They, too, called after us. They held on to us; praying us to stop with them. We had to wrench our skirts from their clinging hands. Then their prayers were intermingled with curses; and, far behind them, we could hear the curses repeated by those of our brothers whom we had left to their fate. The gathering darkness accentuated the panic and misery. To the accompaniment of the thunder of exploding shells, and of the curses and prayers of the wounded men around and behind us, we hurried on into the night.

We had hoped to stop in Biyech, if only for an hour or two, but it was quite impossible. Infantry, cavalry, artillery were pressing forward. This was no place, or time, to think of rest or food. The enemy was close behind; his shells were falling ever nearer and nearer, claiming many victims.

We reached Yaslo on Monday morning, but there, too, were confusion and chaos; and with that huge wave of retreating men and vehicles we were swept forwards, ever eastwards. There was no alternative … Retreat had us in its grip.

We came to a place called Skolychin and, miraculously, an empty house was found to be available.

We were ordered to halt and open a dressing-station immediately. I don't know where the food came from, but even while we were unpacking some of the bales which contained first aid equipment, a cup of hot tea and a slice of black bread and cheese were put in our hands. Mechanically, we ate and drank, then, refreshed, we prepared to receive our wounded. They were already at our door, clamouring for help and food. Many there were who could no longer walk, and could scarcely speak, their bodies sorely wounded and their minds numbed by the severity of those wounds, yet their strength of will had been such as had enabled them to traverse many painful versts [one *verst* is a little more than 1 kilometre] in those first tragic hours of retreat.

It is only today that we have heard that the bombardment of Gorlitse was quite unequalled as yet in the present War's history. But our men have suffered enormous casualties; it is said that our 3rd Army has been cruelly decimated and that the 61st Division, to which we are attached, has lost many thousands of its men.

Monday 20 April. Skolychin

Weary and dust-laden we looked at each other, conscious of the calamity at our Front. There was no time for questions, or for explanations; the sullen and continuous tramping of retreating feet on the roads told it own tale. What is happening there? What will soon happen here? The stricken faces and frightened eyes of the wounded told us. They were exhausted beyond words, too exhausted to groan as their wounds were dressed. Gun-carriages, batteries, motor lorries lumbered in and out of the streams of marching soldiers. Dust hung about the road in a thick grey mist; the sun beat down mercilessly. Now and then ambulance vans would pull up in front of our house and the orderlies would hastily drag the occupants out and deposit them on the ground near the entrance. Cries and groans accompanied this performance, but we were too busy to leave our posts and, beyond a much-needed admonition to the orderlies to use their hands more gently, the newcomers and their sufferings had, for the time being, to be ignored. The wounds were dreadful: bodies and limbs were torn and lacerated beyond repair. Those in a hopeless condition were set apart and not sent on with the more promising cases to the Base. All those who could still walk, unless obviously in need of treatment, were dismissed at once without examination. But there were few of these, for the 'walkers' preferred to walk on. Not even a mug of tea could tempt some of them to turn off from the road for a few minutes' rest. This was no time for resting, with the enemy at one's heels.

Into our 'dressing-room' rushed the tall figure of Alexander Mikhaylovich, one of the divisional surgeons. His usually care-worn face had taken on a more serious expression, but he was silent and we went on working. After a few minutes, he looked up and said: 'In half an hour's time, I want two sisters to be ready to return to Biyech. There are many wounded there and we must open a dressing-station at once. Sister Florence and Sister Anna will be ready to leave at 6.30pm, that is in half an hour.' I could scarcely refrain from crying aloud my thanks to him. Anna seized me and together we rushed off to the wagon on which our stores of material for dressings were packed. Hastily collecting several large drum-shaped, air-tight boxes, which held our sterilised dressings, we placed them, with bundles of wadding, bandages and the like, on two large sheets and tied them all together. We packed, too, the most necessary liquids, instruments, candles, gloves, splints. Our equipment complete, we donned our leather coats and clambered into a huge, dirty-looking lorry which was waiting for us …

Alexander Mikhaylovich came out of the house. His first glance told him that we and our equipment were ready; he nodded approval and carefully, but with some difficulty, because of his stoutness, climbed up and took his seat. The divisional officer suddenly appeared and jumped in, followed by two orderlies. During the journey there was no conversation, only a few instructions given by the divisional surgeon to the chauffeur in an undertone. We were far from comfortable; the straw upon which we were sitting was coarse and scanty. Alexander Mikhaylovich, too, was not happy; every time the car bumped and jolted, which was often, he was tossed up and down like a rubber ball. The evening was growing cool and a keen east wind was rising. We saw innumerable soldiers; their faces all turned in one direction and wearing grim, dogged expressions. Some were hurrying, others stumbling. Many of them looked at us in amazement, wondering what was impelling us to return to the scene of disaster. Small bands of wounded, with blood-stained bandages round head or arm, met us. There were those, too, who were limping painfully, who, noticing the kosinka [head veil] of a Sister, would stop, and with inarticulate sounds point beseechingly to their wounded limbs. But we could not stop and explanations in that continuous din were of no avail; we could but point towards the road we had traversed, trying to make it clear to them that help was at hand if they would only continue their journey. Saddest of all sights was to see wounded men exhausted, lying by the side of the road – unable to drag themselves any further. We saw, too, how more than one soldier would stop to speak, to try to assist them to rise; then, finding that it was useless, would look awhile, sorrowing, and pass on.

Nearing Biyech, we met a hooded van containing wounded and our car drew up for a moment while the divisional doctor interrogated the driver. It seemed that all was quiet in the town save for an occasional shell from the enemy; the inhabitants were sheltering in their cellars, but many badly wounded men were there, unable to leave owing to lack of Red Cross assistance and transport.

At last we pulled up at the gate of a large white monastery. Alexander Mikhaylovich, considerably shaken after his rough ride, hastily got down from the lorry and, passing down the small front garden, disappeared through the white doorway. After a few minutes he beckoned us to follow him. In the doorway stood a black-robed priest; his face was stern and very pale, but so calm and passive was his manner, it was evident that this was not the first time that he had encountered a uniformed contingent.

We followed him from room to room as he explained, in broken Russian, that we were at liberty to make what use we pleased of the monastery with its scanty supply of furniture. We told him that only water and basins were necessary and he at once brought in a bucket of water and three small tin pans. The large room, chosen for the dressing-room, was devoid of furniture, but some benches dragged in from an adjoining one were easily transformed into a table, on which we arranged our equipment. All this was done in feverish haste, Alexander Mikhaylovich having impressed upon us the fact that we might have to leave at any minute, and therefore, could not afford to waste a single moment.

Before we had had time to put on our white khalati [overalls], the wounded were in the room – all stretcher cases, all in a terrible state of suffering and exhaustion. To enquire as to when and how the wounds had been inflicted was impossible; in the midst of that great wave of suffering, the acuteness of which was plainly visible and audible, we could but set our teeth and work … and work. The orderlies would carry them in on improvised stretchers, would lift them on to the floor and would return for others. Where they found them, God only knows – but there was no dearth of them – and they carried them in, one after another until our room and the adjoining ones were full of them; and the stench of the wounds and the unsanitary conditions of many of the sufferers filled the place with a heavy, oppressive atmosphere. By this time, several ambulance vans of our Transport, together with some half-dozen from the divisional vehicle-column, had arrived and, with the help of a few divisional orderlies, we packed many of the wounded into them and sent them off to the Base. Now and then there was a shrapnel scare, but it caused little or no confusion. As the day drew on, however, the bombardment became more severe and, after 9 in the evening, heavy shells began to fall.

In the next two hours we worked blindly and feverishly, knowing that many lives depended on the swiftness and accuracy of our handiwork. 'Water,' gasped parched lips, but we dared not break away until the bandaging of the wound was complete. Hearing, yet as with deafness, we listened to the entreaties of those agonised souls. 'Give me something to ease my pain; for the love of God, give me something, Sestritsa.' With cheering words we strove to comfort them; but pain is a hard master; and the wounds were such as to set one's heart beating with wonder that a man could be so mutilated in body and yet live, speak and understand.

The priest gave us what little help he could: supplying us with fresh water, carrying off receptacles of blood-stained clothes and bandages. In and out among the wounded he walked; placing more straw under one man's head, raising a leg into a more comfortable position, holding, now and then, a cup of water to thirsty lips. His lips were compressed, his face drawn, but only once did I notice that he was affected by the sights around him. A soldier was lying in a corner, breathing heavily, but otherwise quiet. It was his turn now; I went and knelt down on the straw at his side. His left leg and side were saturated with blood. I began to rip up the trouser-leg, clotted blood and filth flowing over my gloved hands. He turned dull, uncomprehending eyes towards me and I went on ripping the cloth up to the waist. I pushed the clothes back and saw a pulp, a mere mass of smashed body from the ribs downwards; the stomach and abdomen were completely crushed and his left leg was hanging to the pulped body by only a few shreds of flesh. I heard a stifled groan at my side and, glancing round, I saw the priest with his hand across his eyes turn and walk heavily across the room towards the door. The soldier's dull eyes were still looking at me and his lips moved, but no words came. What it cost me to turn away without aiding him, I cannot describe, but we could not waste time and material on hopeless cases, and there were so many others … waiting … waiting …

From one room to the other we went always bandaging and, when darkness fell, bandaging by the flickering light of candles. Those whose wounds were dressed were carried off immediately to the Transport vans or cars awaiting them, and orders were given to the drivers to make their way as quickly as possible to the Divisional Base lazarets [hospitals], and to send back any other vans or cars available without delay. Shrapnel was falling thickly now, but the monastery did not alarm us over much. If only the wounded could be sent away to a place of safety in time, that was the problem which worried us.

I think that, by now, some curious change had come over both Anna and me. Anna's face was stony, quite expressionless, and while she worked, the same words came from her lips every few moments. 'Nichevo! nichevo! golubchik, skoro, skoro!' [It's nothing! It's nothing! My dear, quickly, quickly!] Suddenly with a shock I realised that I, too, had been repeating similar words, repeating them at intervals when the groans and cries of my patients had been too heart-rending. I caught a glimpse of my white overall, covered with blood-stains and dirt, but this was no place to probe my feelings, or to ask myself what were my impressions, my sympathies. It was as though I had become blunt to the fact that this was war, that these were wounded. Mechanically my fingers worked: ripping, cleaning, dressing, binding. Now this one was finished, another one begun; my heart seemed empty of emotion, my mind dull, and all the time my lips comforted: 'Skoro, golubchick, skoro!'

I was bandaging a young soldier, shot through the lung, when the first heavy shell fell. He was sitting up sideways against the wall, a wound the size of a small coin on his right breast and a wound big enough to put my hand into in his back. His right lung had been cruelly rent and his breath was coming out of the large back-wound in gurgling, bubbling sobs. The wounds had been quickly cleaned; the larger one filled with long swabs, a pad tightly bound over it, when an angry hiss was heard, grew louder and louder and then the explosion! The roar was deafening, the room shook and there were frightened noises of splintering, slicing masonry and of glass breaking and falling. A great silence followed, but the room continued to shake and tremble; or was it, perhaps, our own limbs? The soldier in front of me was shaking as with ague. 'Chemodan! [heavy shell!]', he whispered hoarsely. I turned towards the table for a new roll of bandage. When I returned my patient had disappeared. In his half-bandaged condition he had run off, not caring for aught else and possessed with the one wild desire to escape to a safer place. Strangely enough, the rooms had emptied themselves of several of their wounded occupants; many of those whom we had thought too weak to move had, under this violent shock, been imbued with supernatural strength, as it were, had arisen and crawled away out into the night.

After this, the work seemed to slacken. The remaining wounded were in a terrible, nervous state; the new ones brought in begged only to be sent on; no need for bandaging now, they urged. Almost every five minutes the explosion would be repeated, sometimes more distant, sometimes very near, so near as to seem on our very roof-top.

The divisional surgeon had taken his leave and had retired with his men. Alexander Mikhaylovich told us to prepare to leave in about a quarter of an hour; one of our light cars had been detained for us. The last vans had left; all the wounded had been safely despatched, with the exception of those who were nearing death's door. Our stained overalls off and folded up, we stood by the door, waiting for orders. Outside the night was dark.

The priest came round the corner of the house. 'There are three craters in the back garden,' he said in a muffled voice, 'and the outhouses have been destroyed.' 'Shall you stay here?' I enquired. 'Mademoiselle,' he answered slowly, 'I am in charge of the monastery. I cannot leave my post. And why should I leave when my flock remains?' 'Are there many people here?' 'There are many,' he replied, 'old men and many women and children.' He was silent and, in the half light, I saw that his eyes wandered towards the monastery windows, as if hoping to see some signs of life. I realised then that the house was a refuge for numberless poor people sheltering from the violent storms outside; and there might have been others in those 'outhouses' so lately destroyed.

'Pardon me,' the priest was saying, 'but Mademoiselle is not Russian?' 'No,' I answered, 'I am English.' 'Ah! English!' his voice took on a more animated tone. 'I knew that Mademoiselle was not Russian, for you have the look of the Western world. I, too, have been in France.' He broke off suddenly, the familiar hiss was in our ears and, once again, earth and air seemed convulsed with hideous noise in a world which swayed and rocked.

There were faint cries from within the monastery. I turned from the doorway and stepped inside over the littered floor and paused by that row of silent figures stretched out on their straw beds. Two were already dead, one with eyes wide open as though looking attentively at something – or someone; I closed them and laid his hands on his breast. To his left a man was lying; great convulsions ran every now and then down his long frame and a queer gurgling noise was audible in his throat. Death had taken his hand, too. And he – in the corner – was lying as before, with strangely contracted limbs and eyes still dull and glazed, but his lips had ceased to move.

There were unaccountable noises outside – a sudden rush of sound, the buzz of many voices hushed and subdued, the tramp of many, hurrying feet, and then Alexander Mikhaylovich's voice – loudly, peremptorily. I turned to go, but, before I went, I moved towards the corner and laid my hand on the clammy forehead and seemed to hear once again his inarticulate entreaty. 'Skoro, golubchik, skoro,' I whispered.

'Florence! Florence!' Anna called. I stumbled down the steps into the garden and followed her hurrying figure. There was tumult in the air and tumult in my heart. 'I will do what I can for them,' I heard the priest's voice say and then, to me: 'Adieu! Mademoiselle.' Shrapnel was crackling in the air every now and again with a fierce, metallic menace. We huddled together, Anna and I, in the car.

Outside the gate, we found our own car and two large Red Cross lorries. The lorries were packed with wounded. The drivers and Alexander Mikhaylovich were doing their best to send off those soldiers who, at the last moment, sought to climb on to them: 'Nelzya! Nelzya!' [Keep off!] The men, desperate to get away, began tugging at the lorries, shouting and climbing over each other to obtain a firmer grip. Then another shell boomed out its savage warning from behind the monastery. It helped us in that critical moment more than anything else could have done. In the hush that followed the explosion, one heard only the clatter of feet hurrying and stumbling away; running figures were faintly seen in the distance. 'Sestritsa!' the wounded called to us again. 'Sestritsa! Take us with you; we can't walk.' But the authoritative voice of Alexander Mikhaylovich came to our ears: 'To your car at once!'

The driver was in a dreadful state of excitement; but he drove well, though at a higher speed than usual. We huddled close to each other in the car and Anna whispered in my ear: 'They say that the Germans are entering Biyech at the other end.' The road-sides were strewn with wounded and exhausted men; they called to us as we rocked past, but we could not heed them. We could not have saved them all; there was other important work waiting for us to do. We drove on, but my heart seemed turned to stone and the weight of it was almost unbearable. Alexander Mikhaylovich had pulled his military cap far down over his eyes; Anna's face was hidden by her veil; and still we drove on. For all of us the evening's work had ended with nightmare-like horror. The remembrance of those dreadful curses thrown at us by desperate, pain-racked men could never be obliterated or forgotten.

Long after midnight Anna and I arrived back at our headquarters at Skolychin, too tired to eat or speak. At 8am we were back on duty attending to newly arrived wounded.

Biyech was now in German hands. Our Letuchka had lost contact with the General Staff of our Division and were at a loss to know what to do. News came that the Germans were still advancing rapidly, and we were told to move on within the next two hours. After a hasty meal and packing the wounded into the last few vans, we moved to Przhiseki where we halted and set up a dressing-station …

Miss Sarah Macnaughtan

Anglo-Russian Hospital, Petrograd, Russia

Red Cross Ambulance Unit, Tiflis, Russia

In January 1915 Sara Macnaughtan's soup kitchen moved to Adinkerke Station, sixteen miles from Dunkirk. She lived in an hotel at La Panne. In April she arrived at the station to find civilian casualties from Ypres and Poperinghe.

> *One whole ambulance was filled with wounded children. I think King Herod might have been sorry for them. Wee things in splints or with their curly heads bandaged; tiny mites, looking with wonder at their hands swathed in linen; babies with their tender flesh torn, and older children crying with terror. There were two tiny things seated opposite each other on a big stretcher playing with*

dolls, and a little Christmas card sort of baby in a red hood had had its mother and father killed beside it. Another little mite belonged to no one at all … I'm afraid many of them will never find their relations again … If this isn't frightfulness enough, God in heaven help us.

On the platform was a row of women lying on stretchers. They were decent-looking brown-haired Matrons for the most part, and it looked unnatural and ghastly to see them lying there …

At the hospital it was really awful, and the doctors were working in shifts of twenty-four hours at a time …

At the end of May she went to Steenkerke to call on Mrs Knocker [qv] and 'saw a terrible infirmary which must be put right. It isn't fit for dogs.'

Sarah Macnaughtan returned to England in June 1915 and for the next four months gave a series of lecture tours in England, Scotland and Wales. During the summer she was created a Chevalier de l'Ordre de Leopold for her services to Belgium.

On 16 October 1915 she left London for Russia with Mrs Wynne and Mr Bevan, 'two free-lance philanthropists'. The Russian wounded were suffering under terrible conditions and there were very few doctors and nurses near the battlefields. While the Red Cross group waited for permission to take their ambulances to the front they were attached to the Anglo-Russian Hospital at Petrograd.

24 November

Now I have got to work at the hospital. There are 25,000 amputation cases in Petrograd. The men at my hospital are mostly convalescent, but of course their wounds require dressing. This is never done in their beds, as the English plan is, but each man is carried in turn and laid on an operating-table and has his fresh dressings put on, and is then carried back to his bed again.

This war is the crucifixion of the youth of the world.

Yesterday one saw enough to stir one profoundly, and enough to make small things seem small indeed!

We had to be at the Finnish station at 10am, and my horse, with a long tail that embraced the reins every time that the driver urged speed, seemed incapable of doing more than potter over the frozen roads. I picked up Mme Takmakoff, who was taking me to the station, and we went on together.

At the station there was a long wooden building and, outside, a platform, all frozen and white, where we waited for the train to come in. Mme Sazonoff, a fine well-bred woman, the wife of the Minister for Foreign Affairs, was there, and 'many others' as the press notices say. The train was late. We went inside the long wooden building to shelter from the bitter cold beside the hot-water pipes, and as we waited we heard that the train was coming in. It came slowly and carefully alongside the platform with its crunching snow. Then it stopped. Its windows were frozen and dark, so that one could see nothing. I heard a voice behind me say, 'The blind are coming first,' and from the train there came groping one by one young men with their eyes shot out. They felt for the step of the train, and waited bewildered till someone came to lead them; then, with their sightless eyes looking upwards more than ours do, they moved stumbling along. Poor fellows, they'll never see home; but they turned with smiles of delight when the band, in its grey uniforms and fur caps, began to play the National Anthem.

These were the first wounded prisoners from Germany, sent home because they could never fight again – quite useless men, too sorely hurt to stand once more under raining bullets and hurtling shellfire – so back they came, and like dazed creatures they got out of the train, carrying their little bundles, limping, groping, but home.

After the blind came those who had lost limbs – one-legged men, men still in bandages, men hobbling with sticks or with an arm round a comrade's neck, and then the stretcher cases. There was one man carrying his crutches like a cross. Others lay twisted sideways. Some never moved their heads from their pillows. All seemed to me to have about them a splendid dignity which made the long, battered, suffering company into some great pageant. I have never seen men so lean as they were. I have never seen men's cheek-bones seem to cut through the flesh just where the close-cropped hair on their temples ends. I had never seen such hollow eyes; but they were Russian soldiers, Russian gentlemen, and they were home again!

In the great hall we greeted them with tables laid with food, and spread with wine and little presents beside each place. They know how to do this, the princely Russians, so each man got a welcome to make him proud. The band was there, and the long tables, the hot soup and the cigarettes.

All the men had washed at Torneo, and all of them wore clean cotton waistcoats. Their hair was cut, too, but their faces hadn't recovered. One knew they would never be young again. The Germans had done their work. Semi-starvation and wounds had made old men of these poor Russian soldiers. All was done that could be done to welcome them back, but no one could take it in for a time. A sister in black distributed some little Testaments, each with a cross on it, and the soldiers kissed the symbol of suffering passionately.

They filed into their places at the tables, and the stretchers were placed in a row two deep up the whole length of the room. In the middle of it stood an altar, covered with silver tinsel, and two priests in tinsel and gold stood beside it. Upon it was the sacred ikon, and the everlasting Mother and Child smiled down at the men laid in helplessness and weakness at their feet.

A General welcomed the soldiers back; and when they were thanked in the name of the Emperor for what they had done, the tears coursed down their thin cheeks. Quietly and sweetly a sister of mercy went from one group of soldiers to another, silently giving them handkerchiefs to dry their tears. We are all mothers now, and our sons are so helpless, so much in need of us.

Down the middle of the room were low tables for the men who lay down all the time. They saluted the ikon, as all the soldiers did, and some service began which I was unable to follow. About their comrades they said that 25,000 of them had died in two days from neglect. We shall never hear the worst perhaps.

There were three officers at a table. One of them was shot through the throat, and was bandaged. I saw him put all his food on one side, unable to swallow it. Then a high official came and sat down and drank his health. The officer raised his glass gallantly, and put his lips to the wine, but his throat was shot through, he made a face of agony, bowed to the great man opposite, and put down his glass.

Some surgeons in white began to go about, taking names and particulars of the men's condition. Everyone was kind to the returning soldiers, but they had borne too much. Some day they will smile perhaps, but yesterday they were silent men returned from the dead, and not yet certain that their feet touched Russia again …

Sarah Macnaughtan left Petrograd five days later and went to Moscow where she stayed for a few days before travelling on to Tiflis. She was hoping to take her ambulance to Persia, where there was fighting, or to join American missionaries helping Armenian refugees who had escaped from the terrible massacre they had suffered at the hands of the Turks. By September 1915 a million Armenians had been slaughtered in acts of genocide. A further 200,000, members of the Orthodox Church, were forced to convert to Islam.

She was not feeling well and sufferered from the bitterly cold weather and a bad, persistent cough. 'I believe I am looking rather a poor specimen, and my hair has fallen out.' The ambulance cars then became frozen in the river at Archangel. On Christmas Day she was invited to breakfast with the Grand Duke Nicholas at his palace in Tiflis.

A Court function in Russia is the most royal that you can imagine – no half measures about it! The Grand Duke is an adorably handsome man, quite extraordinarily and obviously a Grand Duke. He measures 6 feet 5 inches, and is worshipped by every soldier in the Army.

We went first into a huge anteroom, where a lady-in-waiting received us, and presented us to 'Son Altesse Imperiale' and then to the Grand Duke and to his brother, the Grand Duke Peter. I had a vision of a great polished floor, and many tall men in Cossack dress, with daggers and swords, most of them different grades of Princes and Imperial Highnesses.

A great party of Generals, and ladies, and members of the Household, then went into a big dining-room, where every imaginable hors d'oeuvre was laid out on dishes – dozens of different kinds – and we each ate caviare or something. Afterwards, with a great tramp and clank of spurs and swords, everyone moved on to a larger dining-room, where there were a lot of servants, who waited excellently.

In the middle of the dejeuner the Grand Duke Nicholas got up, and everyone else did the same and they toasted us! The Grand Duke made a speech about our 'gallantry', etc., etc., and everyone raised glasses and bowed to one. Nothing in a play could have been more of a real fine sort of scene. And certainly S. Macnaughtan in her wildest dreams hadn't thought of anything as wonderful as being toasted in Russia by the Imperial Staff. It's quite a thing to be tiresome about when one grows old! …

Miss Flora Sandes

Serbian Military Hospital, Valjevo, Serbia

After working for three months at the Serbian Military Hospital in Kragujevatz, Flora Sandes realised there were no medical supplies left and the wounded men could not be treated. In December 1914 she returned to England and, as a result of her lecture tour and campaign for contributions to a relief fund, the plight of the people of Serbia caught the pity and imagination of the English public. After the Daily Mail *printed Flora Sandes' appeal she collected £2,000 for the relief fund in three weeks. The British Red Cross also contributed generously and enabled her to return to Serbia with more than 110 tonnes of vital necessities – gauze, cotton wool, iodine, and medicines. She was now working for the Serbian Red Cross and travelled by sea with Emily Simmonds, who had been to America to gather equipment and medical supplies. As every country was very short of hospital material the two women sat on the cases at each port of call so no one was able to commandeer a single item of their precious cargo. They arrived back in Serbia at the beginning of February 1915.*

When Miss Simmonds and I got the stuff up to Nish the President of the Serbian Red X asked us to take it to Valjevo, a town in the north of Serbia, because he did not know what was going on there, except that typhus fever was raging, and the town was entirely cut off. No one would go into it, and no one was allowed out of it, and they had no hospital supplies there. We had read vague rumours in the English papers of this typhus fever, but had no idea of the state the country was really in. While I had been at home the Austrians had invaded all the northern half of Serbia, been driven out again by the Serbs with fearful losses, and left behind them as a legacy in Valjevo 60,000 prisoners, and typhus fever. The fever quickly raged like a plague over the whole country, claiming thousands and thousands of victims, among them many English and American doctors and nurses fighting their lone hand heroically against desperate odds.

We went and saw the British Consul in Nish, and he absolutely forbade us to go. We took a walk round, discussing it, and met an American doctor who said he would give us just one month to live if we went to Valjevo, which he called the death trap of Serbia. But when we went back to the British Consul we were handed a letter from Sir Edward Grey to all the nurses working in Serbia, saying that whatever we did to help Serbia was helping Britain and the Allies, and was of inestimable benefit to the common cause. That settled the matter. A man can only die once anyhow, so we got a truck and took the material straight up to Valjevo, though at many of the stations the people begged us to stay, saying they had not a single doctor or nurse.

When we got to Valjevo we found an indescribable condition of things. It is a small town, and there were over 5,000 down with typhus. There was not nearly enough hospital accommodation, not nearly enough beds, and soldiers were lying in their dirty uniforms, straight as they came from the trenches, swarming with lice, all over the floors of the hospitals, on the floors of the hotels, in the shops, out in the streets, lying on the bare boards or a little filthy straw, with no blankets, in the depth of the rigorous Serbian winter. There was no one to nurse them, no nursing could be attempted. The only thing that was being done was to sort out the dead from the living in the mornings, throw the dead into carts, and take them out and bury them in shallow trenches. There was no one to make coffins for them, and no time to make them, for they were dying at the rate of 200 a day, and the mortality among those that got it was 70 per cent. They were so sure that if a man got sick with typhus he would die. We heard of a couple of American doctors lying sick in a hotel. We went at once, and found that one doctor had died the day before and been taken away, and at the same time as they carried him out they brought in the coffin for his pal and laid it down beside his bed ready for him, and he was lying there with his coffin beside him having completely given up all hope of ever seeing America again. However, we cheered him up, and he eventually did get well.

There was not nearly enough hospital accommodation for the soldiers, and none at all for the civilians. The women and children used to come in in ox waggons from the outlying villages, and the doctor, if he had time, would go out and prescribe for them in their ox waggon, and then they would go back to their village, thus spreading the typhus all over the country. They lost twenty-one doctors in Valjevo in three weeks. As fast as a doctor was sent into the town he fell sick, and when we got there the first week in February 1915 there were only one or two doctors on their feet working frantically.

They received us with open arms. The mere fact of any English people being willing to share their troubles seemed to buck them up and put new life into them. The Serbian doctor in our hospital, the largest in Valjevo, who was working day and night like the little hero he was, told us the way we could help him most would be by taking charge of the operating room, and that would leave him more free to attend the typhus patients all over the town as well as in the hospital. So we got the operating room scrubbed out; licked the Serbian orderlies into shape, two of whom were very good at bandaging but needed supervising; unearthed an old steriliser from under a bed, and got everything ready for the operations. Then we were faced with something that we had never even contemplated before – that there was not a surgeon to do them. Miss Simmonds is not a surgeon, though she is a very clever surgical nurse and taught me nearly everything I know. I most certainly am not, but it was a case of doing something for these men, or see them die before our eyes without lifting our little finger to help them. Because, besides the sick, there were a great many men with badly frozen feet, frozen in the trenches in the snow, which had been neglected and gangrened, and had to come off. And no end of other wounds besides.

So as there was nothing else for it we screwed up our courage and bit by bit we finally ended by doing the operations ourselves. We were very short of anaesthetics, what we had we kept for the worst cases. Besides which, we were so overwhelmed with work that the cases had to be got through without any unnecessary delay. As I said, the Serb prides himself on being able to stand any amount of pain, and especially were they too proud to make a fuss before an Englishwoman. Besides that, I used to bribe them with cigarettes.

I had taken up 10,000 cigarettes to the hospital for the wounded. I was the only person in the whole of Valjevo almost who had one, you could not buy a cigarette or an ounce of tobacco in the whole town. In fact, for over a month you could not buy any tea, sugar, butter, vegetables, or anything at all like that. For a long time there was no meat, and everything was at famine prices. I used to stick up a box of cigarettes in a conspicuous place, and tell each man if he was good and didn't make a fuss I'd give him a cigarette when it was all over. They would go through almost anything, and then go off on their stretchers smiling and joking and smoking their cigarettes. In fact, I found they were beginning to play me up, and were coming in two or three times in the same day to get their dressings done. They didn't mind a little extra pain for the sake of the extra cigarette. As we had not time for that, we had to make lists of them, and only do each man every second day.

One day I had just finished an operation, and the man was coming to from the chloroform Miss Simmonds had given him when the Chief Military Surgeon for the whole of Serbia chose that very inopportune moment to walk in on a visit of inspection to all the hospitals. He happened to know me previously in Kragujevatz. He looked round and said 'Who is the Surgeon here?' And I, feeling very small indeed, said, 'I am Sir'. He just crossed himself three times without a word, and then said, 'Carry on, do the best you can, there's no one else to do it.'

So we did the best we could, and the men had such faith in us because we were English, that I really think we cured them more by faith than skill, but the main thing was they seemed to recover.

We ran an amateur dispensary too, with a well stocked medicine chest an English explorer had sent me and people used to come from all round to be doctored. Fortunately there was a book of the words with it, so I don't think I poisoned anybody.

We had our meals with the Serbian Doctor, and the other officials of the hospital, and there were fourteen of us at that Mess to start with, and over the head of each one of us as we sat at our place at table, hung the large black edged Funeral Notice of the man who had sat in our place before and had since died of typhus. But we never looked at these notices, we were on our feet in the operating room from eight o'clock in the morning till eight o'clock at night, and after supper it was the strict rule that nobody was to talk shop, nor mention the word 'typhus'. We used to sing (nearly all the Serbs have beautiful voices) and amuse ourselves and forget the Shadow of Death hanging over everyone. If we had not done that we could never have carried on from day to day.

As it was, if anyone ever did suggest going to bed early, the others used to say, 'Ah, don't go to bed too early, tonight may be your last night, for all you know, and what's the use of wasting time in bed.' It was very true, for we dwindled down one by one, till at the end of a month, out of those fourteen there were only left the Doctor, one other man, Miss Simmonds, and myself. Then Miss Simmonds got sick, and three days after I got typhus, just the month the American doctor had given us. We had been working against time because nothing short of a miracle could have stopped us getting it. Miss Simmonds got well first, but the doctor said I couldn't live. However, I was nursed by my batman, an Austrian prisoner. There was no one else to nurse me, and he pulled me through.

When I got back to the hospital after a couple of months, I found things were getting a bit better. The warm weather was coming on, and typhus is a winter disease usually, nearly everyone had had it, and the worst was over, so we worked for another three months or so, first in Valjevo, and then in a Field Hospital, and then decided to go home and have a rest. I went to London and Miss Simmonds to New York.

I had hardly been home six weeks when I saw by the papers that the Bulgarians had attacked. I went straight back to Serbia the quickest way [by sea on board the ship *Moussoul*], expecting to rejoin a Serbian Hospital as I had done before, as before I left the Hospital Authorities had asked me to come back. When I got to Salonika [3 November 1915] I found the town full of English doctors and nurses trying to rejoin their hospital units – there were a good many English hospitals in Serbia by this time – and no one could get up into Serbia because the line had been cut by the Bulgarians. Everything was in a state of chaos, and the Serbs were cut off from us. I asked where I could join up with the Serbs and everyone told me it was impossible – people do love to tell you you can't do things. However, I found by going on a branch line to Monastir, about 120 kilometres north of Salonika, and 25 kilometres north of that to Prilip, on a motor lorry, that I did get in touch again with the Serbs. I took my camp bed and blanket with me in case I stayed, and went to work in a Serbian hospital in Prilip. But it was no use staying there, as they were preparing to evacuate the hospital any night. So hearing that a couple of Serbian Infantry Regiments were fighting in the mountains about 12 miles north of Prilip, and being anxious to get near the Front, I applied to go to one of the Regimental Ambulances.

Under ordinary circumstances women are not allowed to go to the Regimental Ambulances – because it is only the First Aid Dressing Station, is frequently shelled, and there are only men up there – but they knew me very well already, so they gave me my Official Military papers, and sent me to the Ambulance of the Second Infantry Regiment, as a dresser.

The Regiment was fighting at Baboona Pass, near Monastir, or Bitol to call it by its Serbian name, in Southern Macedonia, and trying to hold the road open to Salonika for the refugees.

My education in the various aspect of War was proceeding with a vengeance. What I had previously imagined to be a hard, rough life in Kragujevatz Hospital – living seven in one small room and sleeping like the soldier on a straw mattress with one army blanket – I now looked back upon as absolute comfort in comparison to a bed of hay in a Regimental Ambulance in winter, close up to the Front.

The Serbian Army was slowly being driven back by overwhelming numbers. The Germans and Austrians were pressing them from the north, the Bulgarians from the east; and the south being blocked by Greece, still neutral, the only way of retreat lay through the Albanian mountains.

The soldiers in the Ambulance seemed to take it for granted that anyone who could ride and shoot, and I could do both, would be a soldier, in such a crisis.

So, when the brigade holding Baboona Pass began slowly to retreat towards Albania, where there were no roads, and we could take no ambulances to carry the sick, I took the Red Cross off my arm and said I would join the 2nd Infantry Regiment as a private …

Mrs Mabel Dearmer

Stobart Field Hospital, Kragujevatz, Serbia

By the end of 1914 the medical authorities in Serbia were in desperate need of hospitals and trained nurses. The Austrians had been defeated at the Battle of the Ridges, but they left behind filthy hospitals overcrowded with thousands of their own and Serbian wounded soldiers.

On 26 March 1915 a service was held at St Martin-in-the-Fields church in London to say farewell to Mrs Mabel Stobart [qv] and members of the Third Serbian Relief Fund Hospital Unit who were to leave for Serbia when transport was available. The preacher was the Reverend Percy Dearmer, the newly appointed chaplain to the British units in Serbia. At the end of the service his wife, Mabel, a well-known writer of plays, novels and children's stories, asked Mrs Stobart if she could join the unit. 'What are you trained for?' asked Mrs Stobart. 'Nothing,' replied Mabel Dearmer, 'but I am an ordinary sensible woman and can learn quickly.' Mrs Stobart looked at her elegant friend dressed in a green silk dress and a fur coat and wearing long earrings, and told her she must leave all pretty clothes at home and be prepared to accept discipline. When Mabel Dearmer agreed she was told that she could go with the unit as a hospital orderly.

Three weeks after her interview with Mrs Stobart the unit arrived in Kragujevatz and, over the next two months, Mrs Dearmer wrote of her experiences in letters to Stephen Gwynn, a close friend of the family.

Tuesday, 27 April

The place looked desolate and poverty stricken, with hospitals on all sides. Every big building is a hospital. The Serbians are kindness and gratitude itself – both officers and men.

It was wonderful to get into the air after the stuffy trains and filthy, filthy sanitary arrangements of Salonica. A good deal of our sickness on the way was due to foul smells and want of air. Now we are on a sort of plateau, not shut in and yet with mountains on all sides and wonderful sunshine and wonderful evening skies.

We get up at six o'clock – breakfast at seven – and our lights are out at ten o'clock. I find the sleeping-bag deliciously comfortable and have three blankets as well. I share a tent with three others but it is a sort of palace – 20ft by 18ft.

I suffer from foot-soreness more than anything else and change my shoes three or four times a day. It is so funny going to dinner with one's own plate and mug and knife and fork and washing them up afterwards.

We are taking our first patients on Friday – 50 wounded from another hospital. The camp arrangements are perfectly wonderful, and it is all made so that we can pack up and be off wherever we are needed in a few hours. There are two kitchens – a camp kitchen and a staff kitchen – and at present only four cooks.

We have really delicious food. The government here feeds us – they give a grant and we buy the stuff. We get heaps of vegetables, and have stews and salads. We don't get butter, but we have boiled eggs and buttered eggs, etc. for breakfast.

Percy had three services here on Sunday, an early one in the tent and mattins and evensong in the open air. The Serbians and Austrians were tremendously interested. Some of the Austrian prisoners who come to dig our trenches round the tents and our pits and things are very nice, and some can speak a little English, and they all laugh and joke and will do anything for us.

I have been put in charge of the linen tent for the whole camp, and am, in addition to this, doctor's orderly – although I don't quite know what this last may mean. The linen tent, which is getting into delightful order, is proving an immense success.

There are sixty-two tents in all, and now we have hospital tents all ready for patients.

Percy and I are in quite different classes. Percy sits with the great – the doctors and Mrs Stobart, and I with the common orderlies – that fills me with joy.

Friday, 30 April

Our first twenty-five patients come today, and the nurses are just passing my tent in their pretty blue dresses and white army caps. Mrs Stobart and the others who are going into the receiving-room are wearing their rubber suits – top-boots and oilskin hats.

Now I must go back to my linen tent – which has now expanded into three tents – as soon all the nurses will be clamouring for things.

1 May

As I am writing at the door of my clothing tent at 5.15 I can see the stretchers coming over the grass in the distance. The patients all have red flannel coats, so they are very conspicuous.

The routine of the hospital is sometimes rather funny. Before a patient is admitted he is washed, paraffined and shaved by the Austrian orderlies. Now, all these patients who have come straight out of a hospital have already been done – they are spotless, but they have to be done all over again. You never saw anything so clean in your life as these men.

The authorities won't let us take typhus here, so these wounded are coming to us to make room for the typhus patients in the town.

I have been told that I am responsible for the linen of the entire hospital and the clothing of the 200 patients and orderlies, and the tent and boxes in which it is stored – and that in the event of marching orders coming I must be ready in six hours. I have immense stores of clothing here, and a house is being disinfected for me today so that I shall pack most of my stuff in readiness. I have learned how to strike and pitch my own tent – (the clothing tent is a kind of Marquee!) – and what guy lines are – and also that I am much stronger in the arms than I thought I was, and that I can hammer in my own tent pegs and lift packing-cases that a month ago I shouldn't have dreamt of touching.

My synovitical knee is rather a nuisance, but I steadily decline to be influenced by it. It doesn't get painful, only puffed.

Later. News has just come from Headquarters that we travel with the Serbian Army. So when they go, we go.

I am taking my first night watch, and that is a great excitement. Two of us take it until one o'clock, and then we are relieved and two more come on. We have to walk round the entire camp every half hour. It takes nearly a quarter of an hour to do this, so I suppose it must be at least a quarter of a mile round.

Well – we have been and come back, and it has taken us half an hour, for we had many adventures. The nightingales were singing one against the other, frogs croaking, cocks crowing – and a continual noise coming from the direction of the town. The noise comes from a camp of soldiers that are looking after transports – great wagons go out every day full of guns – the soldiers seem to be a little drunk.

We have done another round – the sentries are wide awake, but our own men orderlies are sleeping all over the place, wrapped in blankets – four in the second dispensary, one in the kitchen. All these are Austrian prisoners – and there are two more men who are sent up from town to help us who refuse to go back because of the typhus. So we made them a jug of tea and took them up bread and marmalade, for they had had no food because they would not go near the typhus hospital to get it. However when we got back to them we found them fast asleep, and as we simply could not wake them we put the jug down beside them and left it there.

The cuckoo has now begun to cuckoo – the soldiers have stopped singing and shouting, and there is only one nightingale.

Sunday, 9 May

I am afraid that I rather overworked when I first came out, for my knee suddenly got worse, and on Thursday I found I could not walk at all without agony, so now I am a poor thing, crawling and lying about when there is so much to be done.

The hospital is nearly full now, and work is in full swing. A wayside dispensary has been started, to which people come from all parts, sometimes walking from twenty-five to 40 miles. The most common complaints are typhus, scarlet fever, and diphtheria. They also have an awful disease – a sort of fever which shows itself in huge glandular swellings of the neck and is contagious. There is no law here whereby they must be isolated, and they associate the word hospital with death. The only thing which can be done is to send them home with medicine and advice. Two more dispensaries are to be opened on the way to Belgrade at a distance of 10 miles apart. This seems to me to be the most splendid and most needed work.

11 May

Percy has just come back from Belgrade, where he has seen his first firing. Part of the hotel where he stayed has been destroyed.

My life is very quiet and happy. Part of the clothing bales has been sent down to a house near, and I go there every day and pack and sort. I begin about seven o'clock (we are up at five – breakfast at six) and go on till twelve, then rest until three and begin again.

We would give anything here for a pack of cards. The patients have nothing to do and simply beg for them.

My knee is nearly well and I can nearly walk again.

It has been pelting and pouring rain. The mud is ankle-deep.

13 May

This heavy rain continues. You would laugh at my costume – breeches and the heavy rubber boots, which are not one bit too heavy. I wear my macintosh over this, which has been shortened to the knee and girt round the waist with a luggage-strap.

16 May

I have not written for two days, and that is because I am happy. I am so much happier here than I could be anywhere else in the circumstances that I am more than glad I *came.*

I have a new job – to prepare the outgoing patients' clothes and supplement them with new. A man went out yesterday and two this morning. The thing they value of all others is shoes – these funny Serbian shoes that are made of narrow strips of leather interlaced – and *there are no shoes:* their own are useless, worn through and through. Percy and I brought out £50 that was sent us to spend, and we have already spent £20 of it on shoes. When I brought my poor man his clothes last night, he nearly cried when he saw the shoes. I like taking them these things, for I see so little of the patients, and it is only because of them that we are here.

Everything is so curiously mixed up. We are friends and enemies all together – half our wounded are Austrian – and strangest of all, the head doctor of the Serbian Hospital is an Austrian prisoner. He is a wonderful man, and looked after and treated 200 wounded all alone. He was taken prisoner, and never stopped his work of saving life – first as an officer of his own army, then as a doctor among the Serbs. There is an Irishwoman – named Wetherall – working at the Serbian Hospital. She is all alone, and has been here during all the awful time. In the Serbian Hospital the windows are never opened, and this nurse had to fight all the doctors to get any kind of decent sanitary arrangements. She says the nurses were bathed and soaked in typhus, and that it would have been a miracle if they had not got it. Somehow it seems quite wrong of us to be so flamboyantly well and healthy; but if we are to be a field hospital we must not have typhus and we must just learn to wait. We have all our tents full and send men away every day, so I don't think we have much to complain of. Still, when the death-cart goes past our camp (as it still does every day) – with the white cross painted on the side and the big wooden gold cross perched up high in front – we feel that we ought to be bearing more and helping more, and that it is the fever units who are having the work and the struggle.

19 May

We have had more than 100 patients a day at the wayside dispensary – ill with typhus, scarlet fever, intermittent fever, and diphtheria. We are going to have six of these dispensaries between this and Belgrade, and what is more, a hospital of 150 beds for any cases that need operation or who are too ill to return. At that hospital we shall take anything and everything. We are also adding another 100 beds to this hospital.

22 May
It is 7.30 now on this Saturday evening. I am sitting in front of my tent in a sea of mud – the little drain round it and the other that leads into the middle of the Broadway (which I have planked over with two stolen bits of wood) are like roaring rivers of brown water. I am dressed in breeches and top-boots (muddy to the knee nearly) and a shortened macintosh. Two cooks, a Serbian sergeant, the X-ray man, the Sanitary Inspector, and two nurses are playing at ball and shouting in French, German, and English. It is an awful thing if the ball falls because of the mud, and if it hits anybody excitement runs high. It is all soft grey all round, and the mountains are blue. The long lines of barracks (now a typhus hospital) are like a white line. It is getting dark, and the Austrian orderly is coming round to fill our tent lamps. I have now retired to the inside of the queer little tent, and the brown river is running round me. The hospital tents with some happy men and more suffering ones are behind me. By half-past eight the tents will be drawn, and all quiet by nine o'clock, except for night nurses and the night watch.

Whit Sunday
It has been rather a trying day, full of hard work, but also of foolish little difficulties and tryingnesses. They are not worth writing about. On the whole, I think this is a very united unit – there are no cliques, and everybody is fairly on an equality. If something terrible happened there are women here who would do splendid things – and the truth is that we are all rather positive in type, as is natural for people who have volunteered for this sort of work, and that makes it a little difficult for us to live together at close quarters.

Whit Monday
The 'enemy' came to tea today – the Austrian doctor who is a prisoner here and has worked for the Serbian wounded so nobly that he is head of the Military Hospital – and a prisoner – Oh, isn't it strange? He has in bad times dressed 500 wounds a day – besides operations – sleeping for a few hours at a time and eating when he can – and this for the enemy. Greater love hath no man than this, that a man lay down his life for his enemy. He only spoke German and a few words of English. Of course people are raving over the horror of the *Lusitania* – but was there ever any real gilt on war? If I never saw you or Geoffrey or Christopher [her two sons on active service] any more, I could no more be angry with the men or the nation that had taken you all from me than I could with an earthquake. It is all ignorance and folly, and we are working out through it to ordinary sense.

The only way to see war is from a hospital.

26 May
The storms have been simply terrific. I was nearly blown out of my bed last night. It was miserably depressing to crawl out in the mud and loosen ropes and get soaked through – especially as I had been having a stupid fit of depression – silly things that one can't write about and that one has no business to mind.

I see the papers ringing with the *Lusitania* disaster – and other things. Here we never talk of them – we only say 'it is war'. Still, one feels bound with a burden of unknown tragedy and desolation.

Our patients are so happy here, except, of course, those who are dangerously ill.

The men who are getting better are always singing and dancing. They dance in a ring, doing a sort of step all the time, and they sing too, long, long sagas of past wars in the strangest harmonies that are very beautiful. One begins and he holds the tune all the time, and then at the third and fifth line all the others join in, giving a sort of bass accompaniment to the notes, yet showing that all know the words.

3 June
I have not written for three days – there has been so much to do, and I have been very tired …

I am greedy for sleep, and when the work is heavy I sleep in my off time. The reason that my work has been heavy is that the dreaded typhus has come into the Camp. Our little Serbian interpreter – the 'Narednik' he was called (that means sergeant-major), a boy of twenty-two – was the first to get it – then Nurse Read, our theatre or operation nurse – and yesterday Mrs Stobart and Dorothy Picton were isolated. If I get it, will you always remember that I am very strong with a terrific constitution, and most tremendously alive and well from my life in the open, so that there is every chance of my pulling through. One has to stop some day, and personally I would rather 'stop' here, doing this work, than anywhere else in the world. There is nothing terrifying or agonising in typhus – you sleep most of the time, and just drift away into the unknown quite quietly.

I am suffering from prickly heat which, I understand, is a common complaint in these parts. We have all got it, and it is the most unbearable and tiresome thing you can imagine and takes away one's sleep.

4 Jun
You make me laugh when you talk of my linen cupboard; think of a tent – a sea of thick mud on the floor (in spite of most careful trenching) with rough packing-cases and crates on their sides all round – filled with things that are nearly always wet, and on the floor mattresses and hot bottles and air-cushions and bed-pans, and cradles for wounded limbs.

6 June
I am writing in bed although I was up part of the day, as I have a touch of fever. The typhus scare is practically over although some people are very ill indeed. Here is the history: the Narednik had it first and was promptly removed – then Mrs Stobart was taken ill – then Nurse Read, the operation sister – Dorothy Picton, Nurses Willis and Boothe and Miss Johnson, the manager of the laundry. The doctors said 'typhus', and all were removed to an isolation hospital. I felt ill but vowed that as long as I could I would keep on my two feet. I did not feel that I was in for a terrible illness and I did not want the isolation tent – so I just made myself scarce when temperatures were taken, and kept on – then I got too bad and had to give up, and by the time this happened the illness was beginning to mystify the doctors, as it was not continuing in the way that typhus should, and some of the patients were beginning actually to get well. I simply feel hot and 'soppy', and dissolve into tears at intervals during the day

and night. My prickly heat sticks on to the blankets (oh, for sheets!) and my hair is in wet lumps.

War is the devil's own. When I see these wounded here I have got a new obsession. I don't see you and Geoff and Chris hurt, but I see all the men that you and Geoff and Chris are going to hurt as these men are hurt – and that is the unbearable thing.

There is an article in the *English Review* on Nationality – which I feel in my bones is true. It is this madness of Nationality, this false patriotism, that makes wars. As long as men grab land and think it noble to die for their own bit there will be wars. As though a nation depended on its land! It depends on its spirit and its ideals. The Jews are a nation and they have no land.

This war will not bring peace – no war will bring peace – only love and mercy and terrific virtues such as loving one's enemy can bring a terrific thing like peace.

Do you know, these Serbians can do nothing but fight – their whole talk is of fighting – their fathers did nothing but fight before them – they are human beings wasted. As soon as they are well, they want to go and fight again.

9 June

I have not been able to write yesterday or the day before because I am only just getting better and had an immense amount of work. We have ten nurses down now with this unknown fever – everybody is doing everybody else's work. My two helpers have gone – one is ill and the other is nursing her. They seem to get worse and worse in that isolation tent – oh, thank God I had the sense to keep outside! With me the fever seems to have taken the prescribed time – ten days from first to last – but I have a very high temperature every night to which I seem to have grown accustomed, for I don't feel ill with it.

12 June

Eleven people are down with this deadly fever that has no name. [In the margin: We know now – Enteric].

Poor Dorothy Picton is very ill with complications. I have not seen her for ten days – they are all separated from us. Seven of the sick are nurses, three orderlies, and Mrs Stobart. Poor things, it came very quickly. This terribly hot weather is against them too – words can't express the heat of this camp at midday.

I have got over my attack, though I have my breakfast in bed and have to knock off work from twelve to four.

I am not suffering from anything at present but fleas at night. Fleas! You never saw anything like these fleas – they have snouts like walruses – and sulphur, Keating, and vermicelli are just pleasant little tonics to them.

Some men came over from Vrnachka Banya – RAMC – a barrister, some artisty people, very respectable. We had a tea-party for them (that is, four of us had, not the Unit). In course of conversation the most precious of the lot said, 'You know there is never a tea-party in Serbia that doesn't begin with lice and end with latrines'. The latrines here are perfect, and everybody has to be shown them. You see, we have a woman to do this – an Irish girl – and women are naturally fussy about these things. You should see her digging her trenches. It is a miracle, for we are over 200 people, and there are always baths and heaps of water, and the refuse and mess from two great kitchens to deal with.

I have learnt a fearful lot here. I am altered in heaps of ways. I think it has been the lack of discipline in camp life that has struck me more than its discipline – 'pinching' things, for instance – and one's powerlessness. When I first came I simply never got a bath, for I felt I could not fight for hot water. I used to put on my water to boil, and invariably somebody who watched me do it used to 'pinch' it when I was gone to get my india-rubber bath. Now I sit over my water, and if I have to leave it for a minute to get anything, I throw bricks at anyone who goes near it.

Tuesday
Yesterday I knocked under with this fever – typhoid – but mild, owing to inoculations. Don't worry about me …

Dr Elsie Inglis

Scottish Women's Hospital, Kragujevatz, Serbia

Serbian Military Hospital – Czar Lazar Hospital – Krushevatz, Serbia

Dr Elsie Inglis, a qualified surgeon, became honorary secretary of the Scottish Federation of Women's Suffrage Societies in 1909. When war was declared she was Commandant of an Edinburgh VAD detachment and went to Edinburgh Castle to offer her services to the Royal Army Medical Corps. These were refused with the words, 'My good lady, go home and sit still.' A fund-raising campaign was then started and she persuaded the Committee of the Scottish Federation of Women's Suffrage Societies to help organise units staffed by women who could be sent to countries desperate for medical aid. The Belgian and French Red Cross asked for help and the first Scottish Women's Hospital, led by Dr Alice Hutchison, worked in Calais for a few months, nursing patients when typhoid broke out in the Belgian army. By December 1914 Dr Inglis had established the Scottish Women's Hospital in Royaumont, France.

'Send us where we are most needed', was always Dr Elsie Inglis's insistent demand. The Serbian authorities also responded to her offer and in December 1914 the 2nd SWH unit sailed from Southampton. Their chief medical officer was Dr Eleanor Soltau. On their arrival in Salonika the Unit was sent north to Kragujevatz where they found appalling conditions in the hospital they were to take over. Men suffering from frostbite, dysentery and typhoid, the limbless, the dying and the already dead, lay crowded together. It was impossible for a man to move without disturbing his neighbour. A great many had been lying with their wounds undressed for at least a week. There were only a few doctors and nurses working night and day against all odds – there was very little medicine and major operations were performed without anaesthetics.

Conditions in the unventilated wards cultivated typhus fever, which added to the misery and confusion already prevailing in the hospital. The fever soon became an epidemic sweeping from one end of Serbia to the other.

On their arrival in Kragujevatz the women of the 2nd Unit took over 250 patients desperately in need of care. They soon had an efficient hospital running. The wards were emptied, cleaned and whitewashed and the patients given clean beds with bright red coverlets.

By the end of March the unit was in charge of three hospitals – one surgical, one typhus, and one for 'Relapsing Fever' and general diseases – with a total of 550 beds. Although the typhus epidemic was still severe, the suffering gradually eased as help was sent from almost every country in Europe and Serbia was 'fast becoming the cleanest country on earth'.

Then Dr Soltau became ill with diphtheria and Elsie Inglis, at the age of 51, arrived in May 1915 to take over as chief medical officer and general supervisor of all the Scottish Women's Hospitals in Serbia.

Over the following months she wrote letters to her family and also detailed reports to the SWH Committee in London.

SWH. Kragujevatz
May 30/15
We have had a busy time since we arrived. The Unit is nursing 550 beds, in three hospitals, having been sent out to nurse 300 beds. There is first the surgical hospital, called Reserve No. 3. It was a school, and is in two blocks with a long courtyard between. I think we have got it really quite well equipped, with a fine X-Ray room. The theatre, and the room opposite where the dressings are done, both very well arranged, and a great credit to Sister Bozket [sic] [Sister Boykett].

There are two other hospitals, the typhus one, No. 6 Reserve [under Drs Janet McVea, Janet Laird and Catherine Corbett, an Australian], and one for relapsing fever and general diseases, No. 7 Reserve, both barracks. We have put most of our strength in No. 6 and it is in good working order, but No. 7 has had only one doctor [Dr Elizabeth Brooke], and two day Sisters and one night, for over 200 beds. Still, it is wonderful what those three women have done. We have Austrian prisoners as orderlies everywhere, in the hospitals and in the houses. The conglomeration of languages is too funny for words – Serbian, German, French, English. Sometimes, you have to get an orderly to translate Serbian into German, and another to translate the German into French before you can get at what is wanted. Two words we have all learnt, 'dotra', which means 'good', and which these grateful people use at once if they feel a little better, or are pleased about anything, and the other is 'boli', pain.

The day before yesterday we got our orders for a new bit of work. They are forming a disinfecting centre at Mladanovatz, and Colonel Grustitch, who is the head of the Medical Service here, wants us to go up there at once, with our whole fever staff, under canvas. They are giving us the tents till ours come out. Typhus is decreasing so much that No. 6 is to be turned into a surgical hospital, and there will be only one infectious diseases hospital here. I am so pleased at being asked to do this, for it is part of a big and well thought out scheme. The surgical hospital is to remain here. Alice Hutchison goes to Posheravatz also for infectious diseases.

Nish, 4 June 1915
What brought me up to Nish was to see Sir Ralph Paget [British Commissioner for the British Relief Units in Serbia] about the new scheme, and also Dr Hutchison. Her Unit had been stopped here, because a bridge has come down in the floods north of Kragujevatz and south of Posheravatz. Dr Hutchison's equipment is, however, south of the bridge, and it has been suddenly decided by the Serbian authorities that she is to go to Valjevo at once, as the bridge cannot be mended for ten days. Of course she is delighted, as that means work at once; but it knocks the 'scheme', which was a very much bigger thing, on the head. The scheme was to block the whole infectious disease, which always appears in every army, up north, by these three big disinfecting camps, and to bring only surgical cases south to Kragujevatz. Now we again begin simply attacks on isolated centres like Valjevo, which from all accounts is bad enough, but unless we can make Mladanovatz very fine and effective, I am afraid whatever attacks the army will attack Serbia – as typhus did. I am writing quite frankly, as this letter is to be brought by hand.

You can think of us really being of use – all three hospitals at Kragujevatz have been full and very busy. In the surgical one last week we had twenty-three operations.

Kragujevatz, 10 June 1915
And now about our camp at Mladanovatz. After innumerable delays, finally Mrs Haverfield [Evelina Haverfield, the administrator], Dr Laird and I went off in Colonel Gentitch's car, with him and another Serbian officer, to Mladanotatz for the wildest motor drive I ever had in my life. We skidded at least fifty times in the course of the day, but we never upset. We bumped all the day, and at one time charged a string of boulders, which had been used to mend the road, and got over them; but it was the most glorious run as regards scenery. For a long way the road ran along the top of hills, and we had the most wonderful distant views of hills and valleys, and the lights and shadows were magnificent. I don't know when I enjoyed anything so much. And we did the business we set out to do, namely, chose our site on gently sloping ground, with a good water-supply, and an iron shed at the back where we can put stores.

Kragujevatz, 22 June 1915
The Valjevo camp is beautifully situated, lower down the valley than that at Mladanovatz, but on sloping ground with a good water-supply. It is, of course, thoroughly well arranged, and every detail well thought out, as you would expect from Dr Hutchison.

Wood is very precious here, so we have decided at Mladanovatz not to put down our wooden floors, but to use the planks for dividing up the magazine. The only tent in which we will put a wooden floor is the operating theatre, and there we shall make it in four pieces. There will be no heavy beds, and we shall empty the theatre once a week, take out the floor and scrub it, and spray the ground with formalin.

In the other tents we have cleared away the thick grass, beaten the ground hard, and dug a deep trench round to carry off the rain-water. The ground in the tents is sprayed with formalin every morning.

There were seventy patients in yesterday morning at Mladanovatz when I left, and they are coming in at the rate of fifteen to twenty a day – medical cases entirely. Some of them seem to be cases of pure fatigue. They arrive with a temperature of 103 or 104, they are put to bed, given milk and some light supper, and the next morning the temperature is normal. Then after a day or two they begin to rouse up. There are two bad pneumonias in, a case of rheumatic fever, and a man who might possibly be enteric.

When the move comes, and I suppose that will be when Constantinople falls, or the Russians gain a decisive victory, there will be a tremendous need for us!

The whole army is massed on the frontier, a quarter of a million men (I am offending the Censor, so you will be careful – won't you?). We see them streaming past at Mladanovatz, and they have only about 300 Serbian doctors altogether. One hundred and twenty-five of their doctors died during the typhus outbreak; so you will see how short-handed they must be.

P.S. Just home from the conference at Mrs Stobart's [qv]. General Soubititch, Head of the Red Cross, was there, and Capt. Javanovitch. There is no uncertainty about it at all. Col. Gentitch said definitely that no one is to leave, and all Units on the way to come at once. Capt. Javanovitch put it that this is the 'lull before the storm'. It is reported today that the German Emperor has invited the Prime Ministers of Bulgaria and Romania to visit him at his Headquarters. If they go against us there will be savage fighting here. Then there is a possibility that Germany may try to break through to help the Turks in the Dardanelles. In any case 'there is a storm brewing and we must have everything taut for the gale'. They did not mince matters at all, and I pass it all on to you, knowing that you will remember that the *Censor has not seen this letter.*

Kragujevatz, 1 July 1915
I only wish you could see both camps at Valjevo and Mladanovatz. They are both in perfectly lovely country and well placed. It was curious to go up on the hill the evening I was with Dr Hutchison, and look down on that peaceful valley, and the clean little white town, and think what a change had come there since the winter.

With Miss Holme arrived the two motors – the Welsh ambulance and the seven-seater. Will you tell the donors how very pleased we were to see them, and how much they have been admired, especially the Welsh ambulance, which we have been told is the finest ambulance in Serbia. I cannot say I hope they will soon be in use, but I can say this, if the need arises, which is expected, it is a great thing to have two such cars ready.

Everything depends so much on events over which we have no control, and there are so many possible contingencies that it is very difficult to say definitely what should be done, but this much is certain, that if anything does happen, this plucky little country will need help more than any other of our Allies, and we have definitely undertaken to help them.

One way and another I have been able to see a good deal of the country going from one of our Hospitals to another, and up to Belgrade, and so on. Most people find the travelling very tiring, but I must say I have enjoyed it all. I have had the most extraordinary luck – the Government have given me a free pass over all the railways. Once I got into a Sanitary train and was invited to breakfast by one of the doctors in charge. I generally find my travelling companions most interesting and ready to talk: twice I have travelled with Serbian officers, who have told me a lot about the country.

Kragujevatz, 10 July 1915
The typhus is over, there is no fighting for the moment, and the country is wonderfully healthy. Sir Ralph Paget is coming to Kragujevatz tomorrow – and has summoned a Conference of the Heads of British Units to consider the position. I shall finish this letter tomorrow after the Conference and tell you what takes place. My own feeling strongly is that we should wait here in readiness for emergencies which must come, and when they come there will be no country in more need than Serbia – with under 300 doctors and no nurses whatsoever. In the meantime it seems to me there is a good deal we can do here. As soon as our drugs arrive, and our tent-poles – which have stuck for some unknown reason in Salonique – Dr McGregor is going to open a dispensary for the civil population at Mladanovatz.

Then we are arranging for Dr Hollway and the new doctors, with some Sisters, to take over a Serbian hospital at Lazarovatz, and run it.

We are waiting to hear from Lazarovatz. And I think it ought to be a most interesting bit of work, and also a very fine experiment. I should like to see what could be made of a Serbian hospital, using their own workmen and their own things, and see how much more is really needed. And Dr Hollway likes the Serbians so much that it ought to work out well. In a small way, I have been trying the same in our Surgical Hospitals here – for the new theatre and the improved sanitary arrangements, etc. In the theatre, for instance, instead of taking the glass cupboard for instruments, I have had a first-rate wooden cupboard made by an ordinary carpenter, and painted white.

Getting the courtyard in order has been quite exciting work. The cesspool, they admit, has not been emptied for four years. I think it is more like ten. We have pumped and pumped and pumped, and then last night they tried to empty it with buckets. One of the carts broke down and upset the whole awful mess in the street. It was perfectly awful.

They sent down ten Austrians to fill in a dreadful pit of dirty water, but they sent no picks or shovels! There were exactly two shovels and one pick in Hospital, and when I went down, eight Austrians were lying under the trees smoking – two were leisurely throwing loose earth into the pit. When they got to the end, another man dragged himself to his feet and broke up some more ground with the pick while the two overworked shovellers smoked. I watched this for about ten minutes, and then I descended on them. I asked for the officer in charge; they said there wasn't one. Ten Austrian prisoners and nobody in charge. Eventually we found the Serbian non-commissioned officer asleep at the back of the bathroom. I stood over them for two hours, and I don't think those Austrians can have worked so hard since they came to Serbia. They worked in five-minute shifts three at a time, one breaking up earth and the other two shovelling. In two hours we had made the slope where the cart is to stand which is to carry away our dirty water, and thrown all the earth into the pit.

Then I went up to Col. Gentitch's office and said that if they wanted me to spend my time standing over Austrian orderlies I was quite willing to do it, but I thought it was a job for their officers. They were horrified. So all yesterday and today there has been feverish energy and the place is tidied out of knowledge. We have half (!) emptied the cesspool. We have built an incinerator for all the dressings (which before went into the pond!) and solid refuse from the kitchen. We made a 'tamp', namely, a slope in which a cart with two barrels will stand, and all dirty water will be emptied into them, and carted to the fields. We are to have two carts and a yoke of oxen. And we have filled in the awful pit or pond – and the Serbians have tidied up the grass, which is so like them, the dear things. While we struggle with the cesspool they make the grass nice.

The Conference is over. Sir Ralph and Lady Paget arrived here at seven o'clock for breakfast, and we had the Conference in our dining-room at 10.30, and half the people stayed to lunch, and everybody came back to tea and Miss Patrick's Scotch scones!

The resolution, which was unanimously passed, ran as follows:

'That in view of the possibilities of the situation this Conference decides that no British Unit at present in Serbia shall leave the country. The Conference shall meet again early in September.'

It appeared that, counting the two doctors and nineteen nurses just coming to us, we are only 270 strong.

Kragujevatz, 19 July 1915

The Serbs are a strikingly handsome race. Our patients are delightful. The other day Dr Chesney got up a gymkhana for them in the Hospital yard – a very simple affair – and they did enjoy it so. A good many of the things had to be done by the Austrian orderlies – for instance, a stretcher race, where I thought it distinctly safer to have a well man in the stretcher. But there were several events for the patients: an egg-and-spoon race, and a crutch race, and a needle-threading race – when the Sisters threaded the needles. I went into the wards in the middle to give some tobacco to the men who could not come out, and heard the laughter and cheers, and I could not help thinking, there we all were – Turks and British and Serbs and Austrians, all playing together as happy as possible. Perhaps if we played more together and knew one another better, such awful things as this war would not happen.

I wish you could have seen us last Sunday afternoon. That was one of the unexpected things that happen. We went up, some of us, quite unsuspecting, on a quiet, sunshiny afternoon to the Stobart Camp for service (by the way, we have one here every Sunday), and instead of a calm service we spent the afternoon hanging on to tent-ropes and rescuing patients from under collapsed tents. The wind suddenly got up, and in about two minutes a peaceful camp was a roaring chaos. Eventually, when it died down, there were seventeen tents down, and five centre poles broken. Almost everybody's hair came down. One patient with a crutch hurled himself out of the tent, and twisted himself and his crutch into a rope and sat down on it. In another place the patients were all found sitting in a row – on the fly – but I must say they saved the tent. Mrs Stobart took it awfully well, and as nobody is any the worse we can all laugh as much as we like. I was so stiff I could hardly move the next day. The achievement was the cooks'. When we eventually emerged with time to look round, we found the kitchen fire still alight, and the evening meal being cooked, though all the tents, kitchen stores, etc., were down. I am not sure that Mrs Stobart did not equal them, for she invited us all to stay to supper! But we didn't.

Skoplje, 10 August 1915

The Committee will be surprised at this address. Lady Paget [qv] wired to me last Sunday and again on Monday, asking me to come down and help them, as they had some bad surgical cases and no surgeon.

I shall go off tomorrow night – straight to Mladanovatz, and from there to Valjevo, where they are in great trouble – six cases of enteric – three doctors and three Sisters.

After Valjevo I shall go to Lazarovatz – which lies between Valjevo and Mladanovatz – and see them fairly started. Dr Hollway's account is very interesting. It is a village, and the 'Hospital' which consists of 200 beds, is in eight different houses – really miscalled 'gast houses'. It is a junction, and will be a splendid dressing-station some day.

Lady Paget's is a beautifully organised hospital – on a hill about a mile out of Skoplje. They have 350 beds, and could expand in an emergency to 1,000. Lady Paget is the 'soul' of the place. I have lent them three of our new nurses. It really is a place to be proud of – and so beautifully situated with glorious views of the hills. There is a first-rate laboratory, and they have their own carpenters' shop and mechanics and everything. Skoplje itself is very interesting – quite Turkish.

Mladanovatz, 13 September 1915

First about the opening of the Fountain here. This took place last Tuesday. Colonel Gentitch and Colonel Michalovitz came up from Kragujevatz for it. We came up in two cars – our seven-seater and an ambulance car belonging to the Government. We started at 6am. You remember I told you what an awful road it was, the first time Mrs Haverfield and I came here with the Colonel to choose the site. Positively this time I thought the road quite good! It was a much colder, greyer day than last time, but still very beautiful, and we all enjoyed it. We got here at a quarter to ten, having stopped for coffee at Topola.

It was a dedication ceremony, five Greek priests performed it. All the Bevis Camp (the 1st British Field Ambulance Corps) and all our people who could be spared, and Serbian officers representing the artillery, the cavalry, and the infantry, about twenty of them – and some engineer officers, friends of the architects, and the squad of men who did the actual building. The Fountain is between the camp and the village, on the same hill, looking right across to Kosmai, the mountain where they fought one of their big battles last year.

A table covered with a white cloth stood in front of the Fountain, and on it a silver crucifix, a bowl of water, a long brown candle, lighted, and stuck in a tumbler full of sand, and two bunches of basil, one fresh and one dried. The priests in their canonicals ranged themselves behind the table, and the Colonel who is in command here, and Colonel Gentitch, and the head of the Medical Department, stood facing them and all the rest of us, round about. Quite unconsciously we all got together on the right, the Bevis people and us, and the Serbian officers on the left, which was just as well when it came to the blessing and sprinkling with the Holy Water. It would have made an awful muddle if we had all been mixed up. The very first thing that happened was so impressive with them all standing together like that. The service was intoned, and at the first note, just as if it had been a word of command, each man swept off his cap, and crossed himself – just in a flash, like drill. They cross themselves the opposite way to Catholics, from right to left. The singing of the service was very beautiful; the priests passed the books from one to another, singing alone, and then together. A peasant, dressed in ordinary rough peasant clothes, swung the censer towards us and the others and the priests, and whenever it was swung towards any side the people there bowed. The service went on, and the crucifix was dipped in the bowl for some time. They blessed King Peter of Serbia, Nicholas, Tsar of Russia, and George, King of England. Then they turned round and blessed the Fountain, sprinkling the water on it with the bunch of fresh basil, first in front, and then all round to the back. After that, one of the priests made an address, of which, of course, we understood nothing except Lady Paget's name; but later on Colonel Michalovitz translated it into French, and it was a very pretty little speech, saying how grateful they were to the Scottish Women's Hospitals, and that they are a poor people, and cannot do big things, but they had done this little thing to show they were grateful and to keep the name of the Hospitals 'for ever' in the countryside, so that the peasants always would remember.

Colonel Michalovitz stood in the middle and said it all to me, and I felt, as a Suffragist who can speak, I ought to make a speech in reply! But in the first place I should have had to speak in French, and in the second I knew they weren't used to women speaking, so I just said I thanked them a thousand times, and they did not seem to expect anything more.

However, I have run ahead, for Colonel Michalovitz did not make his translation till later. After the Fountain had been blessed, and the address given, the priest came to the front of the table, holding the crucifix in his left hand and the basil in his right, and all the officers there went up one by one, beginning with Colonel Gentitch, and the priest sprinkled the water from the basil on their heads, and they kissed the crucifix, and some of them kissed his hand. Then he went round to where the squad of men stood, and sprinkled them, but just walking along in front of them, not individually.

That was the end of the service, and Colonel Michalovitz made his translation. The priests gave me the two bunches of basil, the fresh and the dried one, and these are some of the few things I shall certainly keep.

The second interesting thing is the work at Lazarovatz … As I told you, the Hospital at Lazarovatz is housed in various houses in the village, private houses, and inns. I don't know if the Censor will let this pass, but as I want the red blankets, I must tell you the number of beds! We are expected to be ready for 600 beds there.

They are having quite a rush of work, considering how healthy the country is. One day a division passed through and left 100 sick behind them. This more than filled every bed we had ready. So you can imagine our feelings the next evening when we suddenly heard that fifty more were coming down the line. It was really like war work, as one imagines it! We went and turned out a gast house, people who had been sitting there in the cafe helping to clear out the tables and chairs, the proprietors helping too, and showing us where extra wood was to be had, and so on. We swept the whole place out to the light of storm lanterns, made a roaring fire, got on some boiling water in the little kitchen place, and then down on us came the patients, beds, bedding, all together. Some of the men were really ill, and all of them were dead tired. We packed that house as no English Hospital would ever dare to pack! But we got a bed for each man. There was no question of bathing, of course! We just tore off their uniforms and their heavy muddy boots.

Kragujevatz, 26 September 1915
You probably know more of what is going on at home than we do here – but the last week has been full of rumours. What seems to be certain is that Bulgaria is mobilising – probably to attack Serbia; that Greece and Romania are also mobilising – object unknown; and that an Austrian – some say German – force is massing on the frontier, and that there is certain to be an attack on Belgrade.

I travelled up from Nish yesterday, and the whole line was blocked with trains full of soldiers and transport. We took twenty-one hours on the journey. Last week Austrian aeroplanes were 'announced', and the authorities evidently believed the report; for the Arsenal was emptied of workmen – and they don't stop work willingly just now. So – as a Serbian officer said to me yesterday – 'Serbia is exactly where she was a year ago.' It does seem hard lines on our little Ally. If only they could have sent a British Expeditionary Force up here this summer, it would have made absolutely all the difference – all the Balkan States would have declared on our side, Germany could not have got ammunition through to the Turks, and probably things would have been easier for Russia.

Well, as to how this affects us. Sir Ralph was talking about the various possibilities. As long as the Serbians fight we'll stick to them – retreat if necessary, burning all our stores. If they are overwhelmed we must escape – probably via Montenegro. Don't worry about us. We won't do anything rash or foolish; and if you will trust us to decide, as we must know most about the situation out here, we'll act rationally …

On 5 October 1915 the Austro-German army, which had been gathering strength for weeks along the river Danube, started an intensive artillery bombardment of Belgrade followed by a massive assault. Three days later Belgrade fell to the enemy.

At first the Scottish Women's Hospitals in the north of the country at Mladanovatz, Valjevo and Lazarovatz remained busy coping with the wounded, but as the situation deteriorated, and the Serbian army was relentlessly driven back, the women were ordered to retreat.

Dr Beatrice McGregor's Mladanovatz unit left their severely wounded in charge of a Serbian doctor and some Austrian orderlies and took their valuable equipment, medicines and some patients in ox-wagon ambulances to Kragujevac. They then opened a large dressing-station and a hospital where they had 600 beds. Over the next two weeks they nursed some 10,000 casualties, many of them severely wounded men.

Dr Alice Hutchison and the Valjevo unit had to encourage their walking patients to return to their homes and left many other wounded in the care of a small Serbian staff. They evacuated the remnants of their patients and equipment over the Sumadija hills, and across streams where bridges had been destroyed. They managed to reach Vrnjacka Banja where they opened a dressing-station and a hospital for the casualties who were pouring in and overwhelming the facilities of the existing hospitals in the town.

Dr Edith Hollway and her staff were not told to leave Lazarevac until gunfire was within hearing distance. They reached Krushevatz after a difficult journey and immediately set up a dressing-station in two large storehouses. Here they were joined by Dr Inglis and her staff.

On 12 October Bulgaria attacked Serbia, advanced over the entire Eastern Front, and two days later officially declared war on Serbia. From the north the Austro-German armies were advancing and in the south the Bulgarians swept towards Skoplje. When the Bulgarians marched into Skoplje on 22 October, Lady Paget and her staff had already unanimously decided to remain with their patients in their huge hospital; the First and Second Serbian Relief Fund units therefore became the first British aid workers to become prisoners of war.

As the enemy continued to advance rapidly on all fronts Serbian authorities became increasingly disorganised and chaos spread throughout the country. Roads and passes became choked with continuous streams of retreating humanity – hundreds of thousands of soldiers and civilian refugees, ox-wagons full of wounded, vehicles, equipment and animals – and there was only one escape route out of the country which lay across the bleak Montenegrin and Albanian mountains to Scutari and to the coast.

Sir Ralph Paget had been ordered by the Foreign Office in London to ensure the safe evacuation of the British relief units and all their valuable hospital equipment. His wife had already decided to remain with her hospital in Skoplje and when the other unit heads met him at Vrnjacka Banja he was told that they had no intention of deserting their hospitals either. He warned them that they would inevitably become prisoners of war and repeated the option of escape over the mountains. A few, with personal reasons to return home after a long tour of duty in Serbia, chose to leave.

Dr Inglis, Dr Hutchison, Dr Chesney, Dr Hollway, Mrs Haverfield and most of the SWH staff decided to remain.

Krushevatz, 5 November 1915

We are in the very centre of the storm, and it is anything but pleasant to be part of a beaten and retreating army.

Dr McGregor has trekked with her whole party from Kralievo (where she was sent from Kragujevatz to form another dressing-station), and I think intends to form a hospital at Novi-bazar. But we have missed one another every time, and I only know what Miss Pares told me. Getting no answers to our telegrams, and hearing nothing, and with there being no trains, I went up today to Kralievo in the Welsh Ambulance (which is now the Field Ambulance really), to the undisguised distress of the officers at Headquarters! Campfield drove, and we did not see the shadow of a German. Col. Antitch is left there with 700 wounded – three assistants and no nurses. The dressing-station moved two days ago to Rashka – he understood for Novi-bazar, to form a hospital. They have not a scrap of equipment, and cannot get it.

Just now one can think of nothing but these poor little people in this awful hole – with the country they have fought so hard for overrun from end to end. They can hardly speak to one without breaking down – even strong men among them. They look at one so eagerly, and say, 'When will your men be up?' When? The road to Kralievo today was crowded with refugees in their shaky bullock-carts full of all their household things. And there were groups of stragglers from the army. As we came back these men were being gathered up by officers. The whole of Serbia has been thrown back on this Western Morava valley, and now there is nothing left but a further retreat south, and then – surrender?

I have forgotten to tell you that we have a Hospital here in the gymnasium – 200 beds – very nice building, and all our equipment.

At first the Units worked in two parties: the one in the Girls' School, which was arranged on the lines of the Hospital at Kragujevatz, with the equipment brought from there; and the other at the Serbian Military Hospital – the Czar Lazar Hospital – where they were given charge of the annexe formed in the storehouses. The Hospital at the Girls' School had a short, if brilliant, career, for it was seized, with all its equipment, by the Germans two days after their entry. After the loss of the Girls' School both units worked at the Czar Lazar.

The German occupation of Krushevatz was heralded in proper form by bombardment. The Serbs blew up a railway bridge, which attracted their fire, and they threw three bombs and several shells into the town. We felt that we had had our baptism of fire.

Their entry next morning, 7 November, was almost in the form of an anticlimax. We turned into the principal street to find a German regiment lined up there. The best of the Serbs had left, white flags were hanging out of most of the occupied houses, and Krushevatz was taken.

The Czar Lazar Hospital was in a building designed for the barracks, and could have held comfortably 400 beds. In the grounds were two small buildings, intended as the hospital in connection with the barracks, two big stores, or magazines, as we always called them, and numerous outhouses. When we went up there, there were 900 patients, 300 of them in the magazine under Dr Hollway. During the greatest pressure the numbers rose to 1,200. Patients were placed in the corridors – at first one man to one bed, but later two beds together and three men in them. Then there were no more bedsteads; mattresses were placed on the floors. We filled up the outhouses. The magazine in full blast was a sight, once seen, never to be forgotten. The ground flat had an uneven earthen floor, not the place one would choose to nurse surgical patients. Dr Corbett and Dr Scott – the latter had come home from New Zealand 'to do her bit' – in charge. But upstairs in Dr Hollway's domain, the patients occupied the shelving which ran the whole length of the building in four rows. There were three tiers, the slightly wounded men in the highest tier. The time of day to see the magazine at its best – or rather worst – was in the gloaming, when two or three feeble oil lamps shed an uncertain light over the scene, and the tin bowls clattered and rattled as the evening ration of beans was given out, and the men swarmed up and down the poles of their shelves, chattering as Serbs will chatter. The Sisters called the place the 'Zoo', the only name to describe it.

We could not take away the men's uniforms either in the magazines or corridors, for the weather was bitterly cold, and there was already a shortage of fuel. This fact, taken with the overcrowding and the condition of the men – fatigued, depressed, and underfed – made the possibility of an outbreak of typhus a very real danger. At the request of the Director of the Hospital, Major Nicolitch, we opened a small building in the grounds as an infectious diseases hospital, and he appealed to the Austrians for the use of another building to relieve overcrowding. 'There is no other building', was the answer, though all the time the upper storey of the prefecture was empty (the lower one was used as a store for Red Cross equipment, which they had taken from us without receipts), and the fact was brought to their notice. But we soon realised that no help was to be expected from that quarter, and that we must help ourselves. So we improvised a bathroom in the corner of the magazine, took over all the bathing arrangements for the Hospital, set the two French disinfectors going, with the help of a Russian and one of ourselves, who was something of a mechanic, and last and most important of all, we took over the laundry, and the Hospital got clean linen. We worked round the Hospital, bathing and disinfecting every five days. In this connection we must always remember Sister Strange's name, who took over this very necessary, if uninteresting work, from the point of view of a fully trained nurse, and carried it through triumphantly. We had not a single case of typhus.

Only two cases of typhus appeared in our little infectious diseases hospital, and they were both from among the civilian population. We heard that there were a great many cases in the Austrian Army.

Later the Director made over to us the whole downstairs flat of the Hospital, with the room for dressings and the medical ward, as well as the little hospital for infectious cases, the magazine, the laundry, the sanitation. There was one bit of work which we were offered and refused to take – the care of women suffering from venereal disease. It was very difficult to refuse, with our modern vision of the solidarity of womanhood; but the Hospital was not opened for the safety of the women, but for the protection of the Army. To have taken over that work would have been to encourage vice, and that we could not do.

Perhaps the most important department was the sanitation. We had not an expert amongst us; but when Dr Hutchison's Unit passed through, her Sanitary Inspector, Miss Gordon, came up to inspect us, and was pleased with the result. When we arrived, that hospital compound was a truly terrible place – the sights and smells beyond description. We dug into the ground the rubbish, emptied the overflowing cesspools, built incinerators, and cleaned, and cleaned, and cleaned. That is a Briton's job all over the world, and our three untrained British orderlies took to it like ducks to water. It was not the pleasantest or easiest work in the world; but they did it, and did it magnificently. Miss W. especially developed wonderful powers of command – managed her men, fed them, clothed them, and left that hospital compound not, it is true, exactly like an English park, but at least clean.

The prisoners taken in the south were brought through Krushevatz on their way to the Concentration Camps in Hungary – one day as many as 3,000. We had seen these men all through the summer just beyond our camps at Mladanovatz and Valjevo with their heads held high, and conscious of the good work they had done for the Allies in driving back the Austrian 'punitive expedition'. They used to say to us with such childlike pride, 'We are the only ones who, so far, have beaten our enemy.' They came back to us broken and dispirited men, over-fatigued, and dirty, and underfed. They were turned into the Hospital grounds, given their scanty ration of beans with a little meat and half a loaf of bread for twenty-four hours. For some weeks they got only a quarter of a loaf – one loaf among four men. Their campfires flickered fitfully through the long, bitter cold nights. Every scrap of wood in the enclosure was torn up: the doors and windows from the buildings wrecked by the first bombardment; the little foot-bridge over the drains; the trees hacked down. One night the scene might have been the retreat from Moscow. The ground was white with snow, a fine blizzard was blowing, almost blotting out in the distance the crouching figures of the men as they sat in their ragged uniforms round the fires.

There was a shortage of food even while we were there. Remember what a hospital diet usually is, and then remember that we had to feed our patients on beans and a scanty allowance of meat – which was not always good – half a loaf of bread a day for each man, and some weak tea. One day the Director got 500 eggs, but they were seized at the Hospital gates by the Austrians. There was rice in the stores, and we had some sacks too, and we boiled it up with condensed milk and made 'sutlyage', which added something to the diet, but when sugar failed, as it did eventually, half the good of this addition failed also. Our Administrator, Mrs Haverfield, scoured the country for milk and eggs, and we bought what we could with the Scottish funds, but it was not enough.

These months at Krushevatz were a strange mixture of sorrow and happiness. Was the country really so very beautiful, or was it the contrast to all the misery that made it evident? There was a curious exhilaration in working for those grateful, patient men, and in helping the Director, so loyal to his country, and so conscientious in his work, to bring order out of chaos, and yet the unhappiness in the Serbian houses, and the physical wretchedness of those cold, hungry prisoners, lay always like a weight on our spirits. We got no news and we made it a point of honour not to believe a word of the German telegrams posted up in the town …

Mrs Mabel Stobart

First Serbian-English Field Hospital, Serbia

At the outbreak of war Mrs Stobart was already experienced and hardened to a tough and dangerous way of life. For four years at the beginning of the century she farmed under frugal conditions in a remote area of the Transvaal, and in 1912 she took a Unit of women doctors and nurses to help in the desperately understaffed hospitals in Bulgaria during the First Balkan War.

On 5 August 1914, the day after war was declared, Mrs Stobart, founded the Women's National Service League, 'with the aim of providing a body of women qualified to give useful service at home or abroad.' After her offers were repulsed by Sir Frederick Treves, chairman of the British Red Cross Society, she went to Brussels at the request of the Belgian Red Cross. Before she could set up a hospital the Germans occupied the city and she became a prisoner-of-war, condemned to be tried for high treason. She was released after a hearing in front of a lenient judge. She then took her unit to Antwerp but they had to evacuate the hospital there after two weeks. For the next five months her unit worked under the auspices of the French Red Cross at the Anglo-French Hospital, No. 2 in the Château Tourlaville, near Cherbourg.

In February 1915 Mrs Stobart was asked to organise and direct the Third Serbian Relief Fund Hospital Unit. She recruited forty-five women to the newly formed unit – seven surgeons and doctors, eighteen nurses, cooks, orderlies, chauffeurs, and interpreters. John Greenhalgh, her second husband, accompanied them as honorary treasurer. One of the orderlies was Mabel Dearmer [qv].

The unit reached Salonika in the middle of April. With their medical equipment, stores and tents, the women then went by train to Kragujevatz, where the Serbian army had its headquarters and a large ammunition arsenal. They chose a disused racecourse for the site of the hospital and by the following evening members of the unit had pitched tents for wards, staff quarters, offices, X-ray facilities, a dispensary and kitchens. The efficient organisation of the hospital ensured its mobility to pack up within a few hours.

The wounded men, at least half Austrian prisoners, arrived from the front line almost every day and they accepted women surgeons, doctors and nurses with cheerful confidence in their professional skills. The Unit also opened several wayside dispensaries within a radius of some thirty miles of Kragujevatz, to treat the civilian population, suffering from typhus, diphtheria, typhoid, smallpox, scarlet fever, tuberculosis and many other major and minor diseases.

There were increasing rumours that the Austrian army was massing on the Danube Front and Bulgarian troops were gathering on their frontier. At the end of September Mrs Stobart was asked to fulfill the promise she made to the military authorities when she first arrived – to accompany the Serbian army to the front with part of her unit as a flying field hospital. She was appointed to command the column of men and women and sixty Serbian soldiers who served as ambulance men and drivers of the thirty oxen and horse wagons used to transport all the hospital equipment. The staff and their personal baggage travelled in the six motor ambulances. The members of staff included Dr Payne and Dr Coxon; nurses Cockerill, Collins, Giles, Newhall and Kennedy; chauffeurs Little, Marshall, Colson, Holmstron, Jordan, and Miss Sharman; Mrs Dawn, the cook; orderlies Miss Benjamin and Miss Chapple; John Greenhalgh; and two interpreters. Mrs Stobart was given the rank of major but preferred to be known as 'Maika', Serbian for mother. The remainder of the unit, under Dr Mabel King-May, were left in charge of the hospital in Kragujewatz. Before she left for the front Mrs Stobart did not consult Sir Ralph Paget [the commissioner for the British relief units in Serbia] and he later reported her to the committee in London.

On 1 October 1915 Mrs Stobart and The First Serbian/English Field Hospital left Kragujevatz by train and arrived at Pirot near the Bulgarian frontier two days later. On 5 October the Austro/German army invaded Serbia and three days later Belgrade fell. On 12 October Bulgaria attacked from the east. Serbia was in a hopeless situation and over the next two weeks her army suffered increasing defeats and was forced to fall back from the fronts. On frequent occasions a mounted orderly from headquarters brought Mrs Stobart a white square envelope with orders for the column to move on to another destination before they had the opportunity to set up the field hospital. At these times her weary staff began to question Mrs Stobart's decision to remain with the army. They felt they would be of more use at a base hospital.

As all the roads became more and more congested progress was desperately slow and Mrs Stobart realised it would be difficult to keep the column together as the cars, horses and oxen went at different paces. Therefore to ensure that the horses and oxen travelled at the same pace the cars drove on for half an hour and then waited for the others to join them. She also knew that the only way to lead her column was to ride on horse-back. Every day and through many nights the fifty-three-year-old woman rode astride on her black horse at the head of the column, with Vooitch, a young Bosnian Serb, her faithful interpreter and bodyguard, riding close to her. Before arriving at the next destination an interpreter rode in advance to find food and water and Mrs Stobart also went ahead with Vooitch and a Sergeant to choose a site. When the column arrived, horses, oxen, wagons and motor ambulances were directed to a separate area; wood fires were immediately started, tents pitched, surgical boxes unpacked, and the kitchen set up. As soon as the doctors and nurses were ready in their white coats and aprons, a pole flying the Red Cross flag was placed in the ground near the hospital tent. Even in the worsening chaos the Serbian transport system was still working and most of the wounded were sent from the front by train to the main hospitals, but on 14 October when the column reached Palanka the first wounded arrived in pouring rain and wind from the battlefields. Over the next days and nights as the column continued to move the wounded followed for operations, treatment and food. The wet, cold soldiers, piled into rough, springless ox-wagons, were often dead on arrival after a long journey over terrible roads. The dead dressed in their torn and blood-stained uniforms were buried, in coffins, near the roadside. When possible a candle was put in their hands and plain wooden crosses, marked with the name and regiment, were placed on the grave.

By 17 October Mrs Stobart and her column realised that the Serbian army and the Serbian nation were in retreat – 'and we never advanced again', she wrote.

The next day (18 October) things seemed to be going badly. Piteous processions of refugees from villages bombarded and threatened by the Germans, were streaming southwards along the roads.

We again received wounded. During that evening and throughout the night we were kept busy; 102 badly wounded men arrived in batches from the battlefield close at hand.

By noon (Tuesday, the 19th) our wounded were all evacuated. This was fortunate, as at one o'clock came the order to move on at once. News from the front was bad; the Germans were pressing on, and were now close behind us. The guns sounded very near. We had not far to go, only to Uvidno, a two-hour trek. It was difficult to find a camp site; the whole country near the roadside was mud swamp from the continued rain. We pitched the hospital tent between the road and a wood, and three tents, one for the doctors, one for the men, and one for the women, were pitched in the shelter of the wood. The cars stayed on the road. There were not many wounded that afternoon – that was a bad sign. It meant that the enemy were giving no time for collecting them from the field; they were also firing on the ambulance parties, and only the least severely wounded came straggling in as best they could by themselves. We evacuated them when their wounds were dressed.

The news grew more and more serious. The Bulgars had taken Vranya, the Germans were at Valievo, and also at Michaelovatz. An unending stream of refugees passed along the road, and whole families of women and children, babies in arms, infants that could just toddle, boys and young girls, all sheltered at night near us in the wood, constructing as best they could rough arbours of branches for protection from rain and wind.

On Thursday, 21 October at 9am we received the order to go to Palanka, and to establish our dressing-station in the casino, opposite to the Hotel Serbia. Rooms for the staff were found in the Hotel Central. I slept in the car as usual.

Palanka, when we entered it, was already evacuated in readiness for the Germans. The houses were deserted, the shops shuttered, the mud, churned by thousands of oxen, horses, and wagons into gelatinous paste, was a foot deep. Heavy rain was falling. In the main street a continuous stream of fugitives – old men, women and children – were splashing through the mud, carrying their bundles of household treasures on their backs, and driving hurriedly before them their precious pigs and goats and little flocks of sheep.

The news from the front, which was, alas, behind us, continued to be bad. Work, therefore, for doctors and nurses was slack; there is never time, in a retreat, to collect all the wounded.

After a little time the mounted orderly came up with the white envelope: marching orders, and we moved on immediately.

We arrived at dusk, after much trouble with the cars owing to the mud, and took up quarters near some old stone quarries.

Wounded came again during the night and we evacuated fifty in our cars and in wagons to Ratcha. The wounds were terrible and some men were already dead when they arrived. The transport of the wounded was always an anxiety, lest the job should not be completed and the motors should not have returned before the next order to move should come.

I went to bed at 1am, and was up again at four. We made ready for departure and packed everything except the surgical dressings, and then more wounded came so they were tended. One man died at dawn and we buried him. At six o'clock the order came to go towards Ratcha, to a place only distant one and a half hours. We encamped in a field by the roadside and immediately wounded arrived.

On 24 October at 5.45 we again retreated, this time to a field beyond Ratcha. The roaring of the guns was now terrific and the scenes along the roads, which were crowded with refugees who were all mixed up with the retreating convoys of the army, were heartrending. But this day, for the first time since we left Pirot, the sun shone and we were at least physically warm for a few hours.

The direction of the place detailed for the next halt (25 October) was still southerly. It was 9pm when the order came. Immediately everything, tents, surgical boxes, kitchen materials, etc., were packed in readiness for departure, when suddenly, as we were about to start, a batch of fifty badly wounded soldiers arrived in ox-wagons from the battlefield to be dressed. We could hear that the Germans were now close behind us; their big guns were banging ominously as the wagons discharged their burdens on the ground and disappeared. At once I gave the order for the necessary surgical boxes to be unpacked.

The night was cold and dark, and by the light of hurricane lamps the doctors and the nurses set to work and cut away the torn and bloodstained garments and dressed the wounds of the gory, groaning, battered objects, who were placed upon the ground round impromptu bonfires which we made of hay, straw and wood to give warmth.

One man was already dead; I ordered a grave to be dug and then sent to another column for a priest. I stood beside the priest, a few yards behind the scrimmage round the bonfires, whilst he, in his gay embroidered robe, chanted, all out of tune in the old Slavonic language, the words of the Greek Church burial service. He held the prayer book in one hand and read by the light of a small piece of tallow-candle held in the other. The groans of the wounded and the thunder of the guns, coming ever nearer and nearer, made an effective accompaniment.

The Germans were coming on fast behind us. They had taken Palanka in the afternoon and there was no doubt that as we had received the order to move a couple of hours ago, we ought not now to be here; but we still had our fifty wounded to evacuate. We had been told in the morning that we were to send all the wounded to a hospital along the road leading to Kragujevatz, in a south-westerly direction. It was evidently intended that the retreat should follow that route. But now the orders were to move the Column to a place which was, as the map disclosed, along the road leading to Krushievatz in a southerly direction. I knew that the Germans had, since the morning's order, taken Palanka close behind us, and that if I now obeyed the morning's order and sent the wounded and the chauffeurs along the Kragujevatz road they would almost certainly be cut off by the enemy. I also knew that to disobey a military command is to incur grave responsibility; but I incurred it, in obedience to common sense; and as there was no time for hestitation, I decided at once that the wounded must come along the Krushievatz road with us. I was sure that there would be a hospital, sooner or later, along the road.

But how were we to move the patients? Three of our motors had gone with wounded earlier in the afternoon, along the Kragujevatz road, and had not yet returned. That left us with only three motors for the staff and for the wounded. The ox-wagons which had brought the patients from the field had disappeared and, owing to the nearness of the enemy, no other wagons would be available.

There was only one thing to be done if the whole hospital was not to be taken by the enemy. The staff who usually travelled in the motor ambulances must walk, until the three motors from the Kragujevatz road caught us up; the worst wounded must go in the motors, those who could crawl must crawl. At that moment empty artillery wagons were passing and they gladly took the residue of the wounded; and two soldiers were left to tell the three cars to follow on.

The road was abominable, with mud and holes, and narrow and broken bridges and in the dark, dangerous. We were continually, all through the night, obliged to lift the wounded out of the ambulances and carry them over the dangers, and hold our breath whilst the motors – those wonderful Ford cars, wonderfully handled – performed acrobatic feats inconceivable to orthodox chauffeurs at home. The three other motors caught us up after we had been trekking for two or three hours and the staff were again able to ride. This was, fortunately, just before we came to a bridge which was the scene of six motor miracles. I was riding, as always, in front of the Column and when I was half-way across the bridge I discovered just in time that the planks on either side, a few yards in front of me, had been broken off, presumably by the wheels of the heavy gun-wagons which had preceded us. There was no parapet and the bridge was so narrow that it seemed doubtful whether there was room for a car, even if it could steer straight enough, to avoid the precipice on either side. If the wheels skidded in the mud the car must overturn; and just beyond the bridge there was a mud-hole three or four feet deep; and there was no other road.

The wagons, being warned, passed safely, though some stuck in the mud-hole and had to be dug out. But the men then cut branches of trees and found some kukurus stalks. We stopped the mud-holes with the trees and laid the kukurus on the skiddy mud on the bridge, and the road was now mended for the motors. The wounded were lifted out and carried on stretchers over the bridge; the first chauffeur had a final good look at the place, then mounted the car and made a dash. It seemed impossible that the other five chauffeurs should all be equally skilful and equally lucky but soon we left that danger safely behind. There were plenty of others ahead of us, and continually, all through the night, the cars had to be pushed and lifted out of mud-holes. We reached Gradatz at 9.15 next morning.

Our encampment was in a field near a small stream with high hills on the other side of the road. At noon the Staff mounted-orderly rode up – instant departure.

I was not surprised, for the guns were making a deafening noise close at hand. We had already despatched our last wounded, so we packed and were away within half an hour. There was no time for lunch. Berzan, the other side of Batuchini, was our goal.

When we reached the village, shells were whizzing over our heads and falling clumsily rather close to us. We pitched camp in a field at the back of a disused café, specially designated in the orders as our site. The approach was down a narrow by-lane which was a bog of mud. Wounded arrived at once and kept us busy with the hospital and evacuation work, but when the cars finally came back about 11pm, we sat round the wood fire and enjoyed a supper of turkeys which had been spitted over the wood fire by our cheery cook.

30 October. We moved at 8.15. We were told to encamp on the other side of a bridge near Kriva Alpregan. The whole country was a swamp, but we found the bridge, and as there was no village we took shelter in a wood. Between the field and the wood was a deep and broad ditch of mud which we had to cross continually, but we were glad of the shelter of the trees.

On Sunday, 31 October, the order to leave for Voliovtza came at 10.30am. This time we were able to pitch our bivouac on dry ground, on short, sheep-eaten grass by the roadside, just outside Jagodina, and we received at once some wounded. We only had a dozen and they walked in. They told us that the severely wounded were being left upon the field; the enemy would give no time for collecting them, and they were, as usual, firing on the ambulance parties. Only those men, therefore, came for treatment who could move themselves.

On Tuesday, 2 November, the situation looked desperate. It had never looked so black. The Germans had taken Kragujevatz.

Then came a sudden influx of severely wounded – 96 that day up to 10.30pm.

After supper we received a message that we were to hold ourselves in readiness to depart at any moment and we accordingly packed our hospital tent. But the wounded continued to arrive. The doctors and nurses now attended them in the open by the light of hurricane lanterns. Then came a further order that we were not to move until the morning, so we put up the hospital tent again, for it was raining and shelter for the wounded must be provided.

The situation was growing more and more serious. We had retreated 40 miles in the last two days, evidently not without reason, as the Germans had entered Jagodina at noon on the day we had passed through at 2.30am. Remarkable indeed was the dignity and orderliness with which, from start to finish, the retreat of the Serbian Army was conducted. And the silence! Hour after hour, day and night after day and night, week after week, thousands upon thousands of soldiers, trudging wearily beside their slow-paced oxen, or with their regiments of infantry, or driving their gun-carriages or, as cavalry, riding their horses – in silence. No laughter, no singing, no talking; the silence of a funeral procession, which indeed it was.

The retreat in which we took part was the retreat, not only of the Serbian Army, but of the Serbian nation. This meant that thousands of women, children, and old men, driven from their homes by the advancing enemy, were in ever-increasing numbers, as we progressed southwards, adding to the difficulties of the safe retreat of the army, by mixing with the columns of artillery, cavalry, infantry, engineers, field hospitals, and swelling the procession.

Wagons filled with household treasures, beds, blankets, chairs, frying-pans, even geese, slung head downwards at the back of the cart or balancing themselves with curious dignity upon the uneven surfaces of indiscriminate luggage; a look of pained astonishment on their faces at their rude removal from their own comfortable pastures.

Or, more frequent and more painful still, wagons filled with little children; the oxen, weary and hungry, led by women, also weary, hungry, and footsore. I saw one woman dragging by the rope two tired oxen drawing a wagon in which were eight small children. I saw a tiny boy leading two tiny calves, which were drawing a tiny cart containing a tiny baby who was strapped to the cart. I saw a woman, evidently not wealthy enough to possess a cart and oxen of her own, carrying her two babies, one on her back and one in front; and in one of the crushes which frequently occurred, the baby on her back was knocked off by the horns of a passing ox. And in this and other ways hundreds of little Serbian children perished.

We arrived at Kupci at 3pm on Saturday 6 November. Amongst the refugees, who swarmed along the road, were thousands of Austrian prisoners. They were without guards.

Food for everyone was getting more and more difficult to procure, even for money; for prisoners without means it was almost unprocurable. They had to rely on scanty bread rations. Half a dozen of these prisoners straggled into our camp at Kupci and their eager gratitude when we gave them some food – which we could ill spare – was horrible to witness.

That evening I had a talk with the Commander and the PMO. They told me confidentially that the situation for the army was, at this point, critical. The road from Kupci to Blatzi led through a narrow defile and there was grave fear that the Germans, who were already at Krushievatz, might overtake us in the rear and enclose us on the northern entrance, and that the Bulgars might dash across from Nish, which was now in their hands, and cut us off on the southern exit. The Austrians also were on their way to Mitrovitza, and might wish to have a hand in drawing the net around us and in annihilating or capturing the Serbian Army. Hope of help from the Allies was now extremely faint and all efforts must be concentrated in the endeavour to save the army. I must, therefore, push the Column through the defile as speedily as the oxen and the congestion of convoys would permit.

We left Kupci at 5pm on 7 November. When we entered the gorge (Maidevo end) it was pitchy dark and the murky mountains, almost meeting overhead, shook their sides, echoing and re-echoing the thunder of the guns. On our right, the narrow road adjoined precipitously the river (Racina) which, below us, surged. The mountains descended vertically, from hidden heights, to the river's farther bank, and on our left they towered perpendicularly by the roadside.

It was raining. Progress was at snail's pace; there was no one in control of the way, and wagons belonging to army Columns or to refugees all intermingled, blocked every inch of the road, either in single file or two deep, according as the breadth of road allowed.

A stoppage in front caused increased congestion and confusion behind, as everybody then tried to pass everybody else, and the result was an entanglement of wagon-wheels and a general jumble, which was as big a nightmare as human brain could picture – with the cannons bellowing on every side.

If a wagon stuck in the mud, which was sometimes two feet deep, it held up the whole procession for miles. Then the drivers, urged by the impatience of those behind, lightened the load by pitching the contents of the wagon into the river. The example was contagious, and soon barrels of benzine, packing-cases (some containing food), tents, chairs, beds, were hurled indiscriminately over the precipice, and bobbed or floated or sank in the narrow swift-flowing waters. If a wheel came off, the wagon, with its contents, was hurled over the precipice. It was necessary to watch carefully, lest our own drivers should adopt this simple method of easing the burden of their oxen.

There was that night neither moon nor stars. Black clouds hung over the mountains which were dimly discernible, precipitous, close upon either side of us. The darkness was complete, and all night long the guns thundered ceaselessly against the mountain-sides. At any moment annihilation of our Columns was possible; the scene of what might happen in this narrow gorge if the enemies overtook us – from both ends – was easily imagined.

The crush of wagons in the gorge grew worse and worse as the night went on, till at 1am all movement stopped, and the block seemed permanent. Were the Bulgars closing in upon us in front? Or were the Albanians taking this easy opportunity of attacking Convoys?

There was barely room to pass, but I rode forward with Vooitch, scraping and bruising my legs against the wagon-wheels and hard, wooden pack-saddles, to try and discover the reason for the long halt. We found, as we had suspected, that a little way up the line some of the oxen had decided that it was now bedtime, and they were calmly lying across the road, and the complacent drivers, in the absence of officers, had acquiesced. The soldiers were seated around the promptly lighted fires. Vooitch and I were both wearing thick boots. We dismounted, and walked along the line of the Columns ahead of us, kicked the oxen out of their slumbers, called the men from their dreams, and provoked a move.

We then journeyed continuously, except for short compulsory halts, due to congestion of convoys, all through that night and the next day, till six o'clock in the evening – a twenty-five hour ride – till we reached Ravni, in an opening which ended the first, or Maidevo, half of the gorge. This opening was also the entrance to the second, or Yankova, portion of the defile.

The following night we tackled the second half (Yankova portion) of the defile. The first stretch of road was terrible for the cars, very soft and deep in mud and holes, but the soldiers all helped to push and carry, and the chauffeurs mastered all difficulties.

The situation is extremely black. The numbers of the infantry were rapidly diminishing; 1000 had been left dead and wounded on the field near Bagrdan. It had been impossible to move the wounded; the Germans had fired on the ambulance parties. Officers were now reduced in numbers by one-third. Now I heard for the first time that, if there was no hope of being joined by the Allies, the army must retreat across the Montenegrin mountains to the coast of Albania.

The column continued the retreat via Spantzi, Marzovatz, Podyevo, Banya, Dubnitz in increasingly appalling, bitterly cold weather conditions, with the rain and sleet turning to snow. They crossed the historic battlefield of Kosovo plain, where 'every few yards the corpses of horses and oxen and bodies of wounded and dying men kept the image of death foremost in mind' and arrived, cold and hungry, at Prishtina on 19 November. Finding food for themselves and hay for the horses became a greater problem every day and although the town was almost abandoned, no orders came to move on. Bulgarian guns thundered louder and nearer on one side, and the German guns on the other. Mrs Stobart's staff was exhausted and depressed by the constant moving and by the fact that there had only been a few wounded over the past two weeks. Although there was friction between Mrs Stobart and Dr Coxon and Dr Payne, the doctors, nurses, and orderlies were dedicated, disciplined and brave women who admired and respected Mrs Stobart as a leader and, on many occasions, made allowances for her strong-willed and autocratic behaviour. The part of the unit left at Kragujevatz, under Dr King-May, had been ordered by the Austrian military authorities to evacuate the hospital and they had arrived in Prishtina. It was suggested to Mrs Stobart that she should reunite the units and accompany all the other British units to Scutari and then to England. The Serbian army was no longer fighting and there was no need of a flying field hospital. She refused to do this, determined to lead the Serbian army's medical column to the end of their retreat. On 22 November Mrs Stobart received her orders to take the column to Petch, near the Montenegrin frontier. Montenegro was Serbia's only Balkan ally and the Serbian authorities realised that as there was no hope of any other Allied assistance the entire army must be on a full-scale retreat which would take them over the Montenegrin mountains to the coast of Albania.

The congestion occasioned by the retreating of all the various Convoys of an army 200,000 strong, with their innumerable oxen and horse wagons, plus the refugees, with or without wagons, along bad and narrow roads, was now the more dangerous – because four enemies – the Germans, the Austrians, the Bulgars and the Arnauts or Albanians (who made sporadic and murderous raids upon the Convoys for the sake of loot) – were all close upon our heels.

We travelled all through the day and all through the night and a second night must be spent without sleep. At twilight, on this evening, at the top of a steep descent, an officer in command at this point of the road ordered way to be made for us, and we started in the dark on a narrow road, which was worse that anything we had yet met, with deep holes and mud up to the axles. I could not believe that the cars could possibly get through, but Mr Little walked ahead with me, and said it might possibly be done. The cars made the descent safely and, finding that a road which was being reserved for Artillery was better than the road which we and all the other Columns must follow, we obtained leave for the cars to take that road and to meet us at Dreznik. And thankful I was that this was done, for the road on which we travelled would have been impossible even for our wonderful cars and chauffeurs.

Before dawn (on Wednesday 24th) came the moment when we had to take advantage of other Columns who might be dozing, and get into the line before them. There was no road, only a track through beech scrub and up a steep ascent. We continued all through that day in one ceaseless struggle with mud and ploughed fields. At 9pm the oxen could go no farther, and we outspanned for two hours in a wood by the side of the road, till 11pm. Then into the line again. We reached Dreznik at 4pm on Thursday 25 November. We had left Prishtina at seven on the morning of Monday the 22nd, and had thus travelled continuously, with only occasional short halts, during three days and nights.

At Dreznik we had a lovely dry camping ground, near a farm house, and we slept in a tent on beds for the first time and the last for many weeks. The night was cold but dry, and we had a real supper round the camp fire and arranged to start at daybreak the next morning when a snow blizzard began and continued all through the day.

The word 'road' is a euphemism for the river of mud into which we immediately plunged; indeed, all day long we met no road, but journeyed over ploughed fields, bogs, now covered with snow, rivers, mud banks, and stick-hills. My horse was continually over its knees in mud and was growing weaker every hour; but it was necessary to ride up and down the Column through the slough of mud to watch that when a wagon stuck or broke and had to be left, that the load was not thrown away, but was distributed amongst other wagons. Horses fell and their riders were thrown into the slush; wagons overturned; the road was one long pandemonium. At one bridge, over the River Drin, the scrimmage was even worse than usual. The bridge was so narrow that passage could only be effected in single file, and an officer near me estimated that 5,000 wagons were struggling at the entrance for places in the line. Everyone's nerves were overwrought, and suffering and discomfort were universal.

Monday 29 November the cold was horrible all day and the route was worse than ever; over hedges, ditches, rivers, bogs, ploughed fields and slippery ice all the way to Petch which we reached at 4pm. Our cars were on the other side of the town near a monastery, and that sounded very hopeful and peaceful. I found that the doctors and nurses and their cars were inside the monastery walls; the other cars, with the remainder of the staff, were outside, beside a stream. On the other side of the stream we placed the Column. It was pleasant to be welcomed by the staff after a separation of six days.

Dr King-May and the Unit from Kragujevatz were in the town on their way to England, so I went to see them and found that Doctor Curcin, who had at Kragujevatz been officially responsible for the welfare of foreign Units, was in charge of the party and that all arrangements had been made for their journey with ponies to the coast. It was now decided that the two doctors [Coxon and Payne] of our Serbian-English Field Hospital, two nurses and three chauffeurs should go home with them. I was pledged to the army and to the Column as long as my services were needed. We helped them to buy ponies and they left Petch on 1 December for Andreavitza and Podgoritza.

The cold that first night at Petch was intense, and in the morning we couldn't put on our boots till we had unfrozen them at the fires. In the morning (Tuesday 30 November) I went into the old Turkish town, picturesque with Mosques and narrow streets, to get orders on the telephone from the PMO. I was told to do whatever was done by the Fourth Field Hospital. He also said that the roads would be even worse now and I must cut our four-wheeled wagons in half and make them two-wheeled carts. He then said that he and Headquarters were very pleased with us, that we had done well in difficult circumstances, and he referred, with congratulations, to the fact that we had had no deserters, a trouble which had befallen other columns. He was glad that having come through so much we were still sticking to the work.

Thursday 2 December was a busy day; the first job was to cut the wagons in half; the back portion would be left behind and we should carry on with the front portion. Then came the sad business of sorting hospital material. Half must be left behind (we gave it to a hospital in Petch), also most of the equipment and the tents, except one bell tent to which we clung in case of desperate weather at night.

We guessed that it might be possible that even the two-wheeled carts would not be able to continue to Scutari, so we set to work to buy ponies, upon which to pack food and kit, in case the carts must be abandoned. Jordan, Colson and Vooitch cleverly managed to find a dozen ponies, in various stages of decay; these were subsequently our salvation. But they must be rough-shod, or they would be useless in the ice and snow, and there were no blacksmiths left in Petch. Nearly everyone had now gone, and the town was deserted except by the passing soldiers and fugitives. But this difficulty, too, was overcome by the triumvirate. It was also important to procure a store of food. We luckily found some of our precious mealie meal, also a little rice and a few beans and we carried these in sacks, and they ultimately saved us from starvation.

We were up at 3.30 the next morning, Friday 3 December, to pack the ponies and get ready to start at daybreak. We must now leave our much-loved and faithful cars behind; we gave them to the Prefect, with instructions that he must burn them if the enemy arrived. We should badly miss their sleeping accommodation, but for me it was one anxiety the less. Possessions are at the root of all anxiety.

At 6.30am our reduced Column, with its deformed carts, set out through the narrow streets of Petch, to be swallowed up in the great Mountains. Nothing was visible except the endless stream of two-wheeled carts, oxen, horses and soldiers, behind us and ahead of us. The road that day was not worse than usual, and we encamped at dark in a tiny but dry field behind a farmhouse in which Headquarters Staff were spending the night. That was the last time we saw or heard of them till we reached Scutari.

We departed soon after 1am 4 December and in a quarter of an hour we arrived at a block which, in the darkness, seemed to be composed of all the carts and oxen and soldiers of the universe. It was too dark to see what lay ahead, blocking progress, and no one knew anything except that movement was impossible. So we lit fires and sat around them till daylight at 6.30 when we had coffee, and moved with the multitude a few hundred yards. But we were at once again hopelessly blocked.

We took advantage of the halt to send the drivers for hay for the oxen and horses, and we outspanned for two hours. The snow was now melting under a hot sun and making a miry slush, which was not warming for the feet; but by the time we had procured hay it was daylight, and as we could then see that there was no road, there seemed to be no object in waiting, so we wriggled out of the chaos of other Columns and took a track of our own – an awful track over rocks and scrub and amazing mud, but in the right direction; and at night we bivouacked on the slopes of a wood overlooking plains and mountains which lay in the direction of Macedonia.

We could see the shrapnel-fire, and hear the mountain guns close to us all evening. In deep ravines in the track in front of us lay dead horses and oxen and broken carts. At daybreak a message came from an officer in charge of the way to say that we were to abandon wheels, and continue as best we could with any ponies we might have; how thankful we were that we had bought some; we could otherwise have carried no food or blankets. Our oxen were now reduced to thirty-two. They could carry nothing, but they must go with us and be saved if possible.

The abandonment of carts meant the abandonment of our beautiful hospital material and camp equipment; all our treasures must be left upon the ground. But I determined to save the instruments and to carry them with us at whatever trouble they might cost us; they were valuable and belonged to the Serbian equipment. But, to my horror, the man in charge of them had taken upon himself to loot the box, and had already begun distributing the knives and other useful implements amongst his friends. I was just in time to save them. I wrathfully made the man return the instruments. I then took them out of their box, which was heavy, and placed them in my own brown canvas rug bag, to be carried with my personal goods, instead of something else which I left behind. But they were stolen on the way.

At daybreak I called the men together. We must now, I said, be prepared to meet discomforts and difficulties; but though we were abandoning much, we must take with us good-will and a courageous spirit; these would be of more use to Serbia than the ointments and bandages which we were leaving behind. If any man wanted to turn homewards and risk being shot by the Germans, the Austrians, the Bulgars or the Arnauts, he had better go now and save us from the trouble of feeding him over the Mountains. Those who wanted to stay could put up their hands. And every hand went up with a shout of loyalty and determination to keep together to the end.

We had only been able to procure one pack saddle, and all the other loads, containing food and blankets, we tied to the horses' backs with string and cord which we had brought with us.

At 11.30am we turned our backs on the ruins of our Column – burnt and broken carts, beds, tents, personal clothes, surgical boxes and hospital equipment. Our bivouac looked as though burglars had been interrupted in looting operations, and in their flight had left the ground strewn with the spoils. Goodbye to our hospitable field-kitchen; goodbye to tents and beds and the last relics of comfort; goodbye to all hope of hospital work; and, worst of all, goodbye to all hope of rescue for Serbia.

Into the land of Montenegro, the land of the Black Mountains, which already threatened precipitously to bar our way, we must now force an entrance on foot. I went first, and led my horse, for though there were plenty of men to lead it, I guessed that I should better be able to sympathise with the difficulties of the road if I had to overcome them first myself; and I wished to choose the route. Our skeleton Column was followed by other skeleton Columns, and during all that day we tramped and splashed and slipped and scrambled over rocks and through scrub, in mud and over slopes of ice and snow – a route impossible for carts.

Roads had now ceased and even the tracks were only those which had been trampled by the multitudes in front of us; over passes 5,000 feet high; between mountains 8,000 feet high; through snow, ice, boulders, unbroken forest, mud-holes, bridgeless rivers.

It would be impossible to trek at night, and at dusk I noticed ahead of us a mountain slope covered with trees, which would give us partial shelter from the cold wind. Only another half-hour's scramble down a steep incline in a thick wood, and rest and fire and supper would reward us. The last hundred yards of descent were precipitous, and at the top, my horse and I slipped on the ice and rolled together to the bottom. We picked ourselves up and walked on.

We were now in a narrow valley, with steep mountains close upon either side of us. We scrambled a little way up the slope on our left and found that the whole mountain-side was becamped, and we secured a small level space for our fires with difficulty. We scraped away the snow and made a fire with wood, of which there was plenty, collected some clean snow for tea water, warmed some tinned food, and had supper. Except for the snow there was no water available during the next three days. No hay was procurable for the animals, and all we could give them to eat was dead beech leaves which we unburied from the snow.

We slept round the fire, and prevented ourselves from slipping down the mountain-side by logs of wood placed at our feet. The men, with their fires and the horses and the oxen, were close to us. And then I noticed that not only was our own hillside ablaze with camp fires, but that the lights amongst the trees upon the mountain opposite, from which we were only divided by 200 yards of valley, were also camp fires, and not, as I had fancied, stars.

It took us at first a long time to pack the ponies, but we were away by dawn (Monday 6December), climbing up the mountains, through the fir trees, over slippery ice, and rocks which were half-hidden in snow. There was no longer a defined way; the whole earth was now an untrodden track. Whichever way you looked, oxen, horses, and human beings were struggling and rolling and stumbling all day long in ice and snow.

As the physical difficulties of the route increased, the difficulty for all the Columns of securing bread for men and hay for oxen and horses increased also, with the result that the track became more and more thickly lined with the dead bodies of oxen, horses – and of men. Men by the hundred lay dead; dead from cold and hunger; and no one could stop to bury them. But worse still, men lay dying from cold and hunger and no one could stay to tend them.

Except from time to time, the congestion this day was not so great, because the mass of Columns was now spread out over the Mountains and the Commanders chose their own tracks; it meant that the responsibility for route now lay with me. Life is a sequence of choices during every moment of existence. Even if we choose not to choose, that is equally a choice.

Progress was slow, the ponies often fell and their loads had to be readjusted. My horse and I had many a stumble, but that served as useful warning to the others behind. As the day wore on, the way became steeper, and more and more slippery, both up and down the mountain-sides. In the afternoon, when we were half-way up a steep hill, which was covered with snow – a foot, and sometime two or three feet deep – we reached a space which was a solid block of oxen, men and horses, all jumbled together in chaotic confusion. Evidently there was only a narrow outlet into the thick forest of pines and beeches which covered the valley to which we must descend. To avoid the block some Columns were climbing higher up the mountain in order to make the descent at a further point. The majority were trying to join a track which entered the wood on the south side, and, like sheep through a gate, they were all tumbling over each other in the scramble for places in the narrow line. We had not heard close-range guns of late, and we were now surprised to hear again loud, continuous and near firing. We were soon told that a party of Arnauts, or Albanians, had entrapped, for loot, some Convoys which were close behind us, in a narrow gorge, and that they were now murdering the members of the Convoy.

We should have had to wait for hours, perhaps all night, before our turn came to get into the main line of entrance to the wood, therefore, as the further climb up the mountain must be avoided, an alternative route into the wood must be found.

But the wood was as bad as anything we had yet met – steep, slippery, with rocks and stones, tree trunks across the track and low branches overhead hitting you in the face. The wood was interminable, and it seemed as if we should never reach the valley bottom, but we must get out of it before night. Besides, we could not stop; we were in the narrow line of Columns.

It was now dark, and we must wait for stragglers who had got cut off in the wood. When these had collected, we went on another 2 or 3 miles up the river-bed of mud and rocks, which opened into a narrow road of mud, with a thick wood on either side. With thousands of others we bivouacked for the night, at eleven o'clock, sleeping on the ground, round a fire.

Next morning at daybreak we were about to sit round the fire for breakfast when an excited officer rushed up and shouted to us to get away at once, as the Arnauts were close behind us. As we moved off, daylight revealed dead men, unnoticed last night, lying close beside our camp, and as we plunged into the muddy road we saw that dead horses and oxen by the hundred were lying on the track.

We were up at five on Thursday 9 December. The loud firing near us all day, and news that a stiff battle was pending, put spurs into weary feet. The strain and effort of wading through mud, sometimes above the knees, during hour after hour of a twelve-hour day, made such a spur sometimes useful for safety. Along, and up, and down mountain-sides, and in woods, through mud lanes which never saw the sun, we scrambled till dusk. Then we outspanned on a grass slope at the edge of a wood of firs and beech trees.

On Friday 10 December we were up at dawn as usual and we trekked along a better road to Berani. We obtained twenty-five kilos of bread for the men and ourselves and secured some hay for the animals. We trekked till dark, and bivouacked partly in a paddock and partly in two rooms of a house belonging to an Arnaut and his wife.

On Saturday 11 December, the usual routine. Over mountains and through mud which had been churned into jelly by countless hoofs of oxen and horses. Towards the end of the day we were near Andreavitza; our road led near to, but not through the town, and we cherished hopes of oil and candles, meat and bread. We arrived at four (dusk) at the cross-roads, and placed the Column in a convenient field amongst trees on the eastern side of the bridge. But the only triumph in the town was a tiny bunch of tallow candles, and a promise from the Prefect of bread for tomorrow. Always bread tomorrow; never bread today.

Next morning, Sunday 12 December, we were late in starting, as we had to wait for the return of the men sent to fetch the bread from the military station in Andreavitza. As long as bread was procurable the men need not starve, as trek oxen could always be sacrificed, and I frequently had the melancholy task of deciding that the weariness of death was coming over such and such an ox; he had been lovely and pleasant in his life, and now in his death he must be divided. As for ourselves our supply of mealie meal and rice and beans still held out. We said goodbye to butter, jam, milk, sugar and biscuits long ago, but we were in luxury compared with many thousands.

But now, on this Sunday, to our surprise, we found ourselves upon a road which was more like a Corsican than a Montenegrin road. Steep, very steep, all day long, but with excellent surface and excellently graded.

Next day, Tuesday 14 December, the weather gave us a variety. Rain and hail and sleet and bitter cold all day. We had found hay for the animals last night, but none for the morning's feed, and we were still 54 kilometres – a two days' journey – distant from Podgoritza. No wonder that animals were lying dead in hundreds. Bread, too, became more and more difficult to get. Was it a wonder that men also were lying dead and dying in hundreds by the roadside.?

After trekking for three hours we heard that there was hay to be bought some way up a mountain on our left. So we halted at a cottage while the men climbed the hill to fetch the hay.

We had lost two more ponies today; left on the road too weak to rise, and it was doubtful whether my horse could go much farther. But the men found a fine strong pony on the mountains when they went for hay, and this was a great help.

We were too late to get bread that evening, but we were told to come again in the morning. That looked hopeful; but when next morning, Wednesday 15 December, we arrived at the military station, the officer said that no bread had come, and that he had just received a telegram saying that all bread, when it came, was to be sent to the soldiers at the front – an effective silencer.

Our route lay in narrow valleys between steep mountains of grey rock; bare of vegetation, bare of life, bare of everything but inhospitable jagged peaks. The rocks were grey, the sky was grey, and yet suddenly, at a sharp turn of the grey track, a grey precipice pointed grimly all the way down, 3,000 feet, to a tiny ribbon of the most brilliant green water that ever flowed in fairyland.

There was that day another moment of stolen joy, when, before beginning the descent towards the plain in which lay Podgoritza, the grey prison walls slid open and revealed vast stretches of open country, distant mountains, valleys, and, in the middle of a grey mist of mountain ranges, glinting in the midday sun – the Lake of Scutari.

Thursday 16 December, the last day in the mountains of Montenegro consummated the impressions that had been stamped upon our minds of the gaunt, desolate nature of this country. Rain fell all day as we trekked through valleys which were only wide enough for the narrow road, and for that bright green ribbon river which, below us, ran between mountains of bare precipitous rock. On all sides grey prison walls, and mist and rain, shutting out earth and heaven; only the track visible, and on the track dead oxen, inside out; hungry men slashing with knives the still warm carcases, and marching off with hunks of bleeding flesh in their bloody hands; dead horses; dying horses who understood, and forbore to harass you with the appealing eye; and dead men at every turn – men dead from hunger, cold, fatigue, and sorrow. With the dead men the pathos lay, not in their deadness but in the thought that these simple, ignorant, peasant soldiers had, in these desolate mountains, laid down their lives away from military glory and renown, for an idea which must, for many have been blurred and indistinct, almost subconscious. The idea that the soul of Serbia must be free to work out its own salvation. Home, family, even country, count for nothing if the soul of Serbia is not free.

At two o'clock that day we could scarcely believe our eyes. In front of us was a break in the imprisoning rocks, and we saw an open plain, and on the far side of the plain a town – Podgoritza.

We were soon in Podgoritza. Leaving the Column in a side-street, Vooitch and I went first to the military station to ask for bread and hay. The Captain in command was extremely genial and kind. But he said that no bread was available till tomorrow.

He tried to persuade me to go to Scutari by boat across the lake, and to leave the soldiers to come by themselves, with the ponies and the remaining oxen, by road – only ten oxen were now left. The road was, he said, execrable and we couldn't make the journey in less than three days. But as long as there was one man and one ox left, I couldn't desert the Column. There seemed no reason, however, why the British staff should not take advantage of the offer; they could meet me at the other end of the lake and save themselves from days of discomfort. But the suggestion was met with scorn. Having gone through so much together they loyally insisted on sharing with their chief the fate of the Column.

Next morning, Friday 17 December, we did not leave till noon as we had to wait for the bread, and for the shoeing of some ponies. Fifty-four loaves came, and these had to last us and our sixty men till we reached the next military station. We only had four loaves for ourselves.

The first few miles of the road were passable over an uncultivated plain, but as the Mountains of Montenegro closed behind us, the Mountains of Albania opened threateningly before us. The grass plain became a swamp, and soon we were playing the same old game, wading and splashing through mud and water, no road traceable. After we had crossed a river, with a bridge broken off at both ends, our route lay across an expanse of basaltic rock which looked impassable for horses and oxen. By that time it was dark, and it seemed wise to wait till daylight to attack the new enemy, so we bivouacked in a tiny grass enclosure, near an old ruined chapel.

On Saturday 18 December we saw at once that it was goodbye to our hopes of a better road between Podgoritza and Scutari. Our route this day was, if possible, worse than anything we had yet encountered, dead oxen, dead horses, dead men, every few yards. Sometimes thick scrub, with spiky thorn bushes and with slippery foothold, was interlarded with the mud and boulders; then came basaltic rocks, superimposed in fantastic fashion, and mountainous boulders with beech scrub, and berberis, and juniper between; but always, whatever else there might or might not be, there was mud, two and sometimes three feet deep. Today this was of a rich red colour.

In one wood there were many dead men. In a patch of grass near one poor fellow, who was lying where he had fallen in the snow, green buds of young snowdrops were bravely peeping through the dead leaves as though to adorn his grave. Beside him was his tin mug from which he had been drinking his last drink of melted snow.

We picked bunches of snowdrops in that wood whilst waiting, during moments of congestion of oxen, men, and horses, which was now worse than ever. In another wood a long halt had to be made whilst Convoys ahead of us took precedence at the narrow exit. One Convoy, which said it had been waiting there for two days, had with it hundreds of oxen, and was on the point of pushing past us, but at the critical moment a friendly officer came to the rescue, claiming that our horses should have precedence of oxen, and he shouted and insisted and bluffed and pushed both our Column and his own, which was even smaller than ours, into the line. He came with us and we bivouacked together for the night in a tiny walled paddock, a couple of miles (over rocks and mud) above the end of the Lake of Scutari and outside the hut of an Albanian.

The latter at first refused us the hospitality even of his field, but he eventually yielded to the money bribe. The captain and his lieutenant supped with us. We gave them hashed and warmed tinned Serbian meats, of which we still had a few, with white beans, and a second course of boiled rice, which was one of our mainstays. We were a quaint-looking group as we sat round the fire all smothered to the waist in thick red mud. We were obliged to let it dry upon us as there was no water to wash it off. We had no change of clothes; we had left the last relics of such superfluities behind, when the carts were burned.

We could see, from the convergence of Columns from all directions, that we should have trouble tomorrow in getting into the line of the narrow track along which we must travel. So we were up at 4.30am on Sunday 19 December, and as the result of combined tactics, our two Columns eventually pushed into the narrow track of mud and rock.

Some distance below us was the north end of the Lake of Scutari – at the other end – Scutari, our goal.

After standing blocked during four hours in the mud, we advanced four yards. There was evidently some extra bad place causing the crush ahead of us; the horses had had no food, either last night or this morning, except for the nibblings of the nearly bare paddock and the delay might prevent us from reaching hay today. A slow move, a yard at a time, brought us eventually to a wood and we understood the cause of the delay. Owing to the size and number of the trees, there was only one narrow track, and progress was only possible in single file; the descent to the level of the lake was steep and slippery, over a jumble of huge boulders, half-covered with melting snow, and ice, fallen tree trunks, deep mud-holes, and dead bodies. In one hole we had to trample over the bodies of three horses, one on top of the other, the top one not yet dead. Bodies of men who were dead were lifted to the side of the track; the oxen and horses had to be left where they fell.

After some hours of horrors in this wood, we eventually emerged on to a narrow lane which was a sea of gelatinous and slippery mud; two steps forward and one back.

We must continue till we reached the military station or some place where hay could be found.

Our Captain of last night had gone ahead, and in the evening, when it was dark and there were symptoms of fatigue amongst the staff, and rain was falling, as it had fallen, in heavy showers all day, he appeared on the road and said that he had found some kukurus, both for his and for our animals, and a good camping-place for us near him. In return we gave him some of his favourite rice for supper, and porridge of mealie meal before we started in the morning.

We were early on the move on Monday 20 December, and hoped to reach the military station within an hour or two. The route began with its usual ferocity of mud, and the continuous effort, during hour after hour, of dragging the feet out at every step was wearisome. Rain fell in torrents all day.

We reached the military station at Ritzik at 11am. The office was in an old monastery, and we waited for our turn to be served with bread in an upper room. There our hosts were two Albanian (Franciscan) monks. The ponies and oxen had to wait in the pelting rain. There was, after all, no bread, but mealies were given instead, both for the men and ourselves. We were disappointed but made no comment, and as we were leaving, the officer in charge gave me two large corn loaves of his own.

The weather grew worse all day, and at dusk a heavy thunderstorm, with drenching rain, made shelter desirable. We were already wet to the skin and the night was now pitch dark, though there should have been a moon, and as we moved away from the slight shelter of some haystacks into the road, the heavens shook, and thunder, lightning, wind and hailstones hurled themselves in unrestrained fury on us and progress on the invisible road, which was full of mud-holes, was difficult. After we had been walking for an hour, a flash of lightning suddenly revealed that the road had disappeared and that we were on the edge of a broad expanse of lake. Another lightning flash showed us that there was no way round the water, unless we climbed steep hedges, impossible for the pack ponies. But it could not be Scutari Lake; it must be flood, and there was nothing to be done but to plunge into the water.

It was my job to go first; so I jumped on my pony and told the others to wait and see what happened. There was nothing to guide me as to the depth of the water, and I couldn't see a yard ahead, except when the lightning flashed; but the worst that could happen would be a ducking. I plunged. The water was up to the saddle girths and there were holes and boulders every few yards; but we all crossed safely. We were now doubly wet, from rain above and from water below, but this was a useful encouragement to everyone to continue in spite of fatigue.

At this point we decided that we would be bold, and push on to Scutari, as no earlier military station seemed likely. A hot drink might save some of them from catching cold, but we couldn't light fires or stop in the pouring rain, and we had no brandy or whisky, so I concentrated thoughts on obtaining some refreshment.

The miracle always happens, if you will it to happen and look out for it. We were trudging along silently, no sign of life anywhere. All the other Columns had mysteriously disappeared, and we had the dark road to ourselves, when I noticed a house, 100 yards back from the road on our right. I told Vooitch to go up to it and knock, and to ask the inhabitants to give us something hot to drink. He went and knocked, and the door was promptly but charily opened. I rode quickly up, and went in before they could shut the door, and I saw that the house had been a wine and spirit shop. Round the walls were shelves on which stood bottles. A fire was lighted in the middle of the floor, and three or four men were seated round it on the floor, smoking and drinking. The owner said he had no wine and no rakiya in the place. He had closed his shop and had sent away his wares. But he couldn't get away from the fact that the men round the fire were drinking cognac. He would give us what he had, but he was nervous lest we should let it be known to others that his shop was open. We reassured him on this point, and within a few minutes we were all inside that room drinking cognac out of tiny glasses, and every man and woman of the Column had his or her share. We then divided amongst us all the two cornbread loaves given us in the morning, and we all felt much refreshed.

And at 10pm we reached Scutari – Military Headquarters. It seemed too good to be true. We had reached our goal, and the human portion of the Column was intact. Nunc dimittis …

Lady Paget

First Serbian Relief Fund Unit at the Bulgarian Military Hospital, Skoplje, Serbia

Leila Paget, wife of Sir Ralph Paget, commissioner for the British relief units in Serbia, was the administrator for the First Serbian Relief Fund Unit, which arrived in Skoplje in November 1914. Skoplje was the main military and administrative centre for the south of the country and Lady Paget established a 600-bed hospital, with laundries, workshops, and outbuildings for stores in a collection of old buildings on a hill outside the town. During the bitter winter of 1915 Lady Paget and her staff suffered in the basic conditions of the hospital as they nursed typhoid, typhus and dysentery in addition to severely wounded men. In March sixteen members of the staff, including Lady Paget, collapsed with typhus. They were very ill for a few weeks but recovered, and although tired and weak, they returned to their work in the hospital.

On 12 October 1915 the Bulgarian army attacked Serbia and within a few days were marching towards Skoplje. After a meeting with General Popovic, the city governor, who told her the situation was desperate, Lady Paget decided to go to Salonika and ask the British and French army commanders for military aid. She was told that there was nothing the allies could do to help Serbia and she returned to Skoplje miserable at the hopelessness of the Serbian plight. Sir Ralph Paget, obviously afraid for his wife's safety, and responsible to the Foreign Office in London for the British relief units in Serbia, pleaded with her to evacuate the hospital while there was still an opportunity. After differences of opinion with some of her staff who wished to leave, Lady Paget finally persuaded them that they would be greatly needed, not only to nurse the wounded but also to care for refugees, and they all decided to remain with her. At midday on 22 October shells fell on the town. Lady Paget wrote: 'Our motor ambulances went out to meet the advancing Bulgarians and announced that the British Hospital had remained in Skoplje and asked for permission to pick up the wounded, both Serbian and Bulgarian off the field and bring them up to the hospital.' That evening the members of the British relief unit were prisoners of war.

I knew that until we had won the confidence of the Bulgarians and convinced them that we were acting in good faith, we should have no security for ourselves or power to help the Serbians. My policy was never to take any step, with regard to staff, patients, or refugees, without first consulting the wishes of the Bulgarians and gaining their consent.

It was necessary to safeguard myself and the unit by getting a written permission, signed and sealed by the Military Commandant, for anything I proposed to do. The organisation and administration of the Bulgarians, at this time, were of necessity unsettled and chaotic. The country was, of course, under martial law, and as the battle-front advanced, officials in the rear advanced also and their places were taken by others. During the first month of Bulgarian occupation we were under four different military Commandants. The result of this unsettlement was that the different departments worked without connection, and the same department without continuity. A distribution centre which, by consent of one department, we opened in the morning, would probably be invaded and summarily closed down during the afternoon by the underlings of another department, and this precipitate interference caused intense misery and suffering, hundreds of people being left without food. It therefore became necessary to have an order signed by the highest Bulgarian official in the town, so definitely authorising any relief or other work we undertook that no department would dare to interfere with it; and this I accordingly took care to obtain from a very early stage.

The Bulgarians entered Skoplje on Friday 22 October, and by the beginning of the following week the sufferings of the town from famine had already begun. The Serbian army had sent away the main part of the food supplies, driving the flocks and herds before them as they went, burning their crops and destroying all the railways behind them. When the Bulgarians arrived they found but little food or fuel, and for the time being no means of bringing even the most essential supplies from elsewhere. What little was left they at once commandeered for the use of the army, sending as much as they could transport by bullock-wagons to the troops in the field. The civil population, therefore, which was increasing daily as the refugees poured in from the surrounding country, was without bread or the means of subsistence.

In our hospital stores we had 2 or 300 sacks of flour, as well as a quantity of rice, while of clothing we had an almost endless supply. As these were practically the only stores available in the town, I suggested to the Bulgarians that we should distribute relief to the destitute until they were able to bring up their own supplies. At that time they believed that the reconstruction of the railways would be a matter of only two to three weeks at most, nevertheless they realised that in the meantime they would be quite unable to cope with a situation which every day was getting more out of hand; they therefore assured me that they would be very grateful if we would assist them until they were able to undertake their own responsibilities, and on Wednesday 27 October, we opened our first centre for distribution in the town.

Though the Bulgarians had given us practically unlimited freedom, and the independent use of our stores, there were many among them who viewed these privileges granted us with annoyance, and though the head officials had the sense to realise that it was to their own interest that the population of Skoplje should be clothed and fed, the discontented minority bitterly resented any help being given to the Serbians. At the instigation of the malcontents, the house where the distribution took place was raided the Monday after it was opened by an officer and three soldiers, who had orders for the immediate suspension of the distribution. I appealed to the Governor, an official who by a sudden shift of events was for a few days in control. But the moment was not auspicious. The Bulgarians had had a severe set-back in the hills, a short distance away, and were feeling their tenure very precarious. The Governor was extremely angry and agitated, and flatly refused to authorise any continuance of the distribution. The situation, therefore, was dangerous in an extreme degree. Skoplje might be retaken, and there was a risk that, the atmosphere being so electric, hunger and riot might end in massacre.

By great good fortune next day I met several Bulgarian officials of high rank as they were passing through Skoplje, on their way to the front, and I seized the opportunity to put the whole matter before them in all the gravity of its bearing. It seemed that certain biased informers accused me of favouring the Serbians and giving only to them, while I turned Bulgarians away. This charge was surged against me on several different occasions, and invariably resulted in a sudden order for the stoppage of relief; but it was never at any time true. I explained to them that the policy we followed, which I believed to be the only fair and reasonable one under such conditions, was to give to all who were absolutely destitute and without resources, regardless of nationality. I pointed out that those who lived in the town had either work or relatives to support them, whereas the refugees were utterly without means of subsistence. Since, therefore, the genuinely destitute were the refugees, it stood to reason that by far the greater part were Serbians; but never at any time did we turn away starving Bulgarians or Macedonians when investigation showed their cases to be deserving of help.

The Bulgarians, when they understood, entirely appreciated the principle upon which we worked, and we were given permission to continue on our own lines, while, as a guarantee of greater freedom from interference in the future, the Governor, to whom I strongly objected, was removed to another sphere of action.

Owing to the rapid increase in the number of refugees, and also to the confined space at our disposal for distribution in the town, the last few times the crowd had become somewhat unmanageable, struggling and pushing to get in, with the result that a few were injured. In order to obviate these difficulties in future we decided to put the matter on a different footing. We divided the crowds into refugees and townspeople and started two separate centres, that for the townspeople being as before in the town, while that for the refugees we moved to the hospital. Henceforth, rations for two days were distributed on alternate days to both groups simultaneously to prevent any one being served twice. The hospital was most convenient for the refugee centre, having two large rooms intercommunicating (in the block nearest the town and close to the store-rooms) with doors at opposite ends – an ideal arrangement for dealing with large crowds. Moreover, our small staff had no longer to transport the stores into the town, and it was a very great advantage to me to be able to keep the whole business more effectively under my own control.

On Wednesday 3 November, we began work on the new lines, and on the 5th the number of persons relieved had risen to 800. On the following day I received a petition from the Mayor of Skoplje asking me to take over a further list of 300 Macedonians, who were daily clamouring for food at the Opstchina, or Town Hall, and whom the Bulgarians found themselves at the moment powerless to help. I agreed to do this so long as our stores lasted, or until the Bulgarians could get their own supplies up; and only a few days later, on the 10th, we also had to assist the Croatian Roman Catholic population. Their Bishop, Nikola Glasnovitch, had come to me in extremity; he said they were a poor community with no friendly influence to help them, and if we did not succour them they would have to face starvation.

From now onwards the suffering of the people grew daily in intensity, and for the next three months Skoplje was in the grip of famine. The winter set in unusually early; the earth soon became icebound and for weeks the snow lay deep. In addition to the refugees who were daily pouring into the town, there were thousands of Bulgarians constantly passing through, foraging far and wide for food and fuel. The life of the hospital, on the administrative side, became one endless struggle to obtain the barest necessaries for its upkeep, while the medical staff were deprived of all the first essentials for work. The wards were packed with heavy cases, and the theatres were working from ten to fifteen hours a day, for seven days in the week. At that time it was no uncommon thing, when one returned at midnight or later from the quest for food or fuel in the town, to see the lights from the theatre, where they were still working at high pressure, shining out over the snow. At this time there was no bright illumination in the wards to shine out at night; after the sun had set the sisters had to content themselves with a single candle in a ward of forty to fifty beds, carrying it round from bed to bed to do the heavy, painful dressings, while the rest of the ward was swallowed up in darkness. The temperature of the wards in which the sick and wounded lay was as cold as that of an ice-house; and the bedrooms of the staff through the coldest and darkest days of winter, except for a solitary candle, had neither light nor warmth.

For weeks, even months, it was only by dint of the utmost exertion that we could extract from the exhausted town sufficient wood and petrol just to keep fires going in the kitchens and sterilisers in the theatres. Sometimes days came when even that failed; then the staff ate cold food and the theatres closed down. Those were strange times, and in the common struggle for mere existence it did not occur very much to any one to consider who were friends and who were enemies. At the military and municipal Headquarters, we forced our way into the stores along with a jostling throng of Bulgarians and Macedonians, all clamouring for supplies, and on the whole we were quite as successful as they.

Our staff had to be in the town all day, haggling and extorting. It was only natural that each department should keep a jealous watch over the remnant of its stores and fight to retain them, for no one knew if any more would be forthcoming on the morrow. The Commandant or Mayor in the first place, after a certain show of reluctance, would write an order for the amount required. When this was presented at one of the stores the frenzied intendant who guarded the treasure would shower imprecations on our head and vow, probably with complete truth, that there was not so much to be found in the whole town; then he would write the order down to a tenth part. This done, the next problem was to arrange for transport, as our own ambulances were unavailable owing to the impossibility of procuring petrol. Sometimes only two ox-carts were available, and the journey might have to be repeated four times over; sometimes there was none, and the work had to be done by clattering, mangy ponies; and when even these failed it meant that the whole business had to be started over again next morning, from the Commandant downward, as an order stamped one day was never valid the next. By that time the chances were that the store on which the draft was made out was empty, and that meant yet another fresh start. Luckily the day when permit, ox-carts and stores all coincided, and the hospital fires and lights all brightened up for a bit.

That the shortage was real and extreme was beyond a doubt. Not only did we have to tear down for fuel large wooden sheds which had been constructed during the summer, but when the pinch became most severe the Bulgarians and Austrians had to follow suit, even pulling down houses, while the Commandant himself like us could not use his car for lack of petrol.

The money problem had early on become acute. After encouraging announcements made by the Bulgarians during the first week of their occupation, to the effect that until a settlement could be effected Serbian money would remain current at its full value, a proclamation was suddenly issued stating that the dinar was worth only 65 centimes, instead of 100 as normally, and that the banka (a note worth 10 francs) had no value at all. As the supply of Serbian silver coinage was extremely limited, and as there was no Bulgarian money to be had, the town was practically without means of purchase, and though a vague promise was made as to the early arrival of a Bulgarian bank, it was many weeks before this actually occurred.

As our stock of rice and flour could not long withstand the drain that was being made on it, I saw that the only way to carry on was to raise a loan from the Bulgarian Red Cross and to obtain the right of purchase of flour in the town. All foodstuffs had at once been commandeered for the army, and the army itself was placed on very low rations; the permission, therefore, was not very easily obtained, although the authorities assured us that they would do all they could to help us to carry out our scheme.

Permission to buy flour, we learned from experience, was not of any use by itself; it was necessary also for the merchant to have a permit to sell to us, otherwise he incurred the pain of imprisonment, the order being that none but the military could purchase. When this was obtained we were told that there was no flour available nearer than 12 kilometres from the town, and as no means of transport could be provided the whole transaction became abortive. I made strong representations to the authorities as to the impossibility of working unless the entire system of petty obstruction were abolished. Finally we got the business pushed through, including grinding rights in the mill, which had threatened to be yet another spoke in our wheel.

Our own supply of flour for distribution had meanwhile given out, and in order to keep the refugees alive we had to deal with small private holders in the town. Secrecy in these transactions had to be guaranteed to the vendors before they would part with their flour, because they feared that if it became known their whole stock would be commandeered. To avoid rousing suspicion they would only part with a few sacks at a time, and it had to be collected by us after dark from one of the hidden underground storerooms with which the Turkish town abounds.

Just as the new scheme was started, with purchase rights and grinding rights all in order and first consignments of flour delivered, the informers once more endeavoured to impede our work. This time their method of interference was different; instead of the closure being applied directly to us, a manifesto was issued placing the hospital out of bounds, and ordering any refugees who attempted to leave the town to be shot at sight. The following day, the last day on which the distribution was to be allowed at the hospital, it was dark and icy with deep snow on the ground, and the wretched refugees wailed and wept as they went away with their last dole.

I decided to have it out with the Commandant. I suggested he should put sentries on guard in the room where the distribution was taking place, so as to satisfy himself that nothing improper was happening. In the end he agreed to all our proposals, and henceforward we distributed relief under the watchful eyes of two sentries. When the work grew more than we could cope with, we made them help, and when the day came round for the giving out of money due for rents, they voluntarily assisted the children in the kindest and friendliest way to hide it about their persons so that it should not be lost or stolen on the way home.

From now onwards the cold became intense and snow lay deep for weeks. Doubtless this was what saved us from disease, for it was only the frost that prevented the earth and air from becoming pestilent. Scores of unburied carcasses of horses, mules, oxen and buffaloes lay in sight of the hospital where they had fallen weeks before. The skins had been taken by the Turks for shoe-leather, and the bodies lay there bloated and purple in the snow, while roving bands of pariah-dogs and flights of carrion-crows tore them to pieces. It was difficult to go more than a few hundred yards in any direction without finding a ditch choked with putrefying carcasses which had been tipped there to get them off the road. There was no one to bury them so they remained; and after a time one's senses became too blunted to notice the foulness. It was not only the beasts that had to wait over-long for burial; the corpses of soldiers did not count for much more when there were so few to look after the living. The first few days after the battle the death-rate was very high, and as the bodies overflowed the mortuary they were laid out in the artillery sheds, near to the Chancery. Daily returns were sent to the Opstchina of the number of deaths during the twenty-four hours, and it was the duty of the civil authorities there to provide priests and coffins to carry them away. There was no time for us to visit the mortuary while the wards were in such dire need of help, and it was not until the hideous smell of corruption warned the Chancery of danger that we discovered that the Opstchina was taking no steps to remove the dead, and that the mortuary was choked to the entrance with rotting bodies.

But though the cold kept down pestilence it caused unspeakable misery. Hundreds of those who had fled to Prishtina and Mitrovitza tried to return on foot to Skoplje, but few arrived at their journey's end. The vast majority either died of starvation or were frozen in the snow, and most who succeeded in getting through arrived with frost-bitten feet and open wounds caused by lice. Many were raving mad from hunger; they had had no bread for nineteen days, nor food of any kind for five. When they left Prishtina, eggs were selling at five dinars each, and bread for nine or twenty-three dinars the loaf, according as it was black or white.

It was not only the poor who now came to us for food, but Serbian ladies, wives of officers and officials, well dressed and living in their own houses, stood out in the snow for hours with the rest, waiting for half a kilo of flour or rice. Their Serbian money, of which some had a considerable amount, was useless to them, and they were as near starving as the peasants and beggars. The number of the poor dependent on us was ever increasing. By 16 December we had 3,117 in one day; two days later 3,371; and after that for a while the number was over 4,000.

The method I adopted for distribution of relief was as follows. Each adult member of a family received a half kilo per head, small children a quarter kilo per head. When there was any sickness in the family we gave them a little money for firewood and other necessities. Clothing we gave out according to the need. Sometimes women accompanied by several little children would arrive from Prizrend or Prishtina, having come all the way on foot [over 60 miles through snow and mud]; they would invariably be in rags and nearly always barefooted. These we would clothe from head to foot, as well as the little children of all ages who would turn up alone, having lost both their parents and having also returned on foot, over the snowclad hills, depending entirely on the kindness of the Bulgarians and the passers-by for scraps of food to keep them alive. Some of these children, one might say the majority, were usually adopted by women who had lost one or more of their own. Those few who arrived alone, little motherless babes, often such tiny mites, looked so forlorn and miserable with their white, pinched faces and tragic eyes. We placed them either in the Orphans' Home in Skoplje, or if they had a relative left in Serbia we would send them in charge of some responsible person to see that, failing to find this relative, they were placed with some other family willing to take them in the village from which they came, we paying their maintenance for six months.

Some Serbians, residents from Skoplje, returned to find their household goods had been looted, so that they had no beds, mattresses, linen, etc. To these we gave all the above, except beds, but with mattresses they slept most comfortably on the floor. Sick male refugees were at once admitted into the hospital and kept until they had regained their health and strength.

A very large number of Serbian soldier prisoners came up to the hospital on the distribution days, and to them we gave from two to five levas each, as well as socks, shirts, mufflers, and other warm garments. Their condition was pitiful in the extreme, and if they were ill they also were put to bed. The Bulgarians were very good, and never once objected to our making use of the Bulgarian Military Hospital for Serbian civilians.

We opened a dispensary in the town for the benefit of the civilian population, who would otherwise have been without medical aid. Two American doctors from our unit undertook to prescribe at the dispensary to those who were slightly ailing in the morning, and the afternoon was reserved for house to house visiting; they also attended confinements. Our hospital provided most of the drugs and dressings for the dispensary, but the Bulgarians were very generous and gave us as much as they could spare of the two latter. In this way no Serbian was without medical help, and if any were very seriously ill we either brought them up to the hospital or arranged for a nurse to attend them at their homes. They received drugs and everything free.

Young mothers-to-be came and begged for a small piece of flannel in which to wrap their babies when they were born, having no clothes for them and no money with which to purchase material for making clothes; other young mothers, with tiny babes of only a week old in their arms, would come three times a week and wait for hours in the snow for their allowance of flour, which was probably all they had to live on; or for baby clothes, of which they had none, their babies being wrapped in old shawls lent to them by neighbours. When we had to tell the refugees we had no more food for them they did not complain; they received the news in silence, but a look of utter despair crept into their faces, and tears poured down their cheeks. They came and kissed our hands or our dresses, murmuring heartfelt gratitude for what we had already done for them, and departed.

Towards the end of November there arrived on foot from Prizrend 105 Serbian school-boys and two professors. They had trudged through the snow for days, and arrived in Skoplje shoeless, destitute, and covered with lice. The professor in charge of them had at once applied to the Commandant for help, and was given two rooms in the town in which to lodge the boys, and for the rest was advised to come to us.

Knowing from experience of the previous winter how great a danger such centres of dirt and over-crowding would be to the town, we discussed the matter, and at once made arrangements to have the boys brought up to the hospital, bathed, and their clothes sterilised. The method decided upon was as follows. Half the boys were to be brought up one day, bathed, and their clothes sterilised, while one of the rooms in the town was disinfected; then, when ready, they were to be put back into the clean room while the second half of them came up for similar treatment. But, unfortunately, owing to the disconnection between the various Bulgarian official departments, the scheme miscarried; for while the first batch of boys were up at the hospital being cleaned their rooms were taken from them, in order to provide quarters for newly arrived troops. We therefore found ourselves suddenly, late at night, with over 100 boys to be fed and lodged in the hospital, where every nook and cranny was already filled, and where even the outbuildings and stables bristled with troops and horses.

Of course it was a great convenience to the Bulgarians that we should take the boys off their hands; and since it enabled us to see they were well fed, clothed, and cared for, we were more than glad to keep them, even at the cost of serious difficulties to our domestic arrangements. We stowed them away in corridors and tents, and in spite of the wet and cold they throve and were happy …

Lady Howard de Walden

Convalescent Hospital No. 6, Alexandria, Egypt

At the outbreak of war Tommy Scott-Ellis, 8th Lord Howard de Walden, went to Egypt as second-in-command of the Westminster Dragoons. Shortly after the birth of their third child his twenty-five-year-old wife, Margherita, who was a trained opera singer, left the three children at Chirk Castle, the family's country seat in north Wales, and followed him to Egypt.

When her husband went to Gallipoli with the 29th Division, Margherita and her friend Mary Herbert, wife of Aubrey Herbert, answered the appeal for hospitals and nurses in Egypt and found a building, Maison Karam, outside Alexandria, that would be suitable for a hospital. She returned to England and engaged a Matron and eleven private, fully qualified nurses. She then 'ordered hundreds of jolly-coloured striped pyjamas. Jams and chocolate, stores, and medical stores, instruments, blankets, sheets, etc., and foodstuffs and much more besides.' Towards the end of July 1915, four days before she was due to return to Egypt, Margherita Howard de Walden was asked to report to General Sir Alfred Keogh, Director General of Army Medical Services at the War Office. He refused to give her permission to start a hospital, telling her everything was well in hand and that he did not 'require or wish for any private enterprise in Egypt', and she was also intimidated by the matron-in-chief who joined General Keogh in his office. When she burst into tears the General gave her permission to 'go out and see her friends', but he ordered that she must not take the nurses and stores. However, the following day Margherita Howard de Walden, Mary Herbert, the Matron, eleven nurses, stores and equipment left for Egypt.

After an uneventful journey during which we got to know our nurses a little, we arrived, and the ship anchored off Port Said. The Captain came and told us that he had just received strict instructions not to allow us to land. This was indeed a shock! General Keogh had cabled to General Sir John Maxwell, then in charge of Egypt saying, 'Forbid these women land. Please uphold authority.' So he had no choice but to inform the captain of the P & O. We felt very low, and equally very determined. We calmed the nurses and hung over the rails, watching the last of the passengers disembarking.

At that moment, an open launch came alongside and a woman dressed in black stood up and called out, saying, *'Je suis l'emisaire du White Slave Traffic de la part de Sir Ronald Graham. Ou sont Lady 'Ovard de Valden et ces autre dames?'*

We rushed down the gangway, we jumped into this splendid life-saving boat. We thanked the good lady profusely and she laughed and told us that Ronald [Sir Ronald Graham, Advisor to the Ministry of the Interior] had been blessed with this brilliant idea on our behalf.

We got into a hotel and chose our own rooms in strategic positions so that nurses would not go out without our hearing them. There was a balcony running along the front of this place and they stayed on it well into the night, thrilled with the new sounds and smells and the dark faces looking up at them.

Egyptians and 'all sorts' waved to them and once or twice we butted in saying enough was enough. Eventually they quieted down and went to bed. Some were older but several were very young and rather attractive, and they had not been abroad before.

We got the whole company and the packing cases somehow or other to Alexandria and the address Sybil [Lady Sybil Graham, wife of Sir Ronald Graham] gave us. Here Sybil met us and explained that Maison Karam belonged to a rich Syrian merchant. It was out at Ramleigh, and a twenty minute tram ride from Alexandria. And he was willing to let us have it for a small rent.

It was a huge house, covered in stucco work. One approached through big wrought-iron gates. There was a fountain and a large laid out garden and a drive up to this pink and white palace. Wide steps and a very big front door.

Inside the hall was of marble and there were marble pillars, and a wide marble staircase and gallery. The rooms off this hall on the ground floor were either covered in murals of camels and sheiks or had small mirrors inserted into a tangle of stucco work on walls and ceilings. A truly remarkable place.

It took days and days to eject the whole of the Karam tribe: for it is the custom for poor relations and their families and retainers, and the retainer's families and poor relations, ad infinitum, to find shelter with their powerful and rich relatives. They hid in cellars and underground rooms and back rooms upstairs. There must have been literally a hundred of them tucked away about the place!

The next thing was the drainage system. This was quite simple for there was one big pipe which at night took all dirty water and sewage out into the landscape – and every morning the clean water came to the house by the same pipe. Thank goodness one had taken an interest when the bathrooms were being put in at Chirk and Brownsea [Brownsea Island, Dorset, her childhood home].

So while I dealt with the new drainage system and supervised a sad gang of Armenian refugees, and chose a suitable site for a cesspit and arranged where to store coal and other such matters, Mary worked at getting us accepted. The authorities could not allow us even to set up a hospital, so a compromise was come to and we became Convalescent Hospital No. 6.

In fact this was a wise decision. Casualties went first to the authorised hospitals and after being operated on they were sent to us, leaving free beds for the next batch of men.

There was difficulty and opposition in getting a doctor and finally they appointed us a young one temporarily up from a southern district.

While Matron supervised and the nurses unpacked those cases, and stored the stuff away, I was busy persuading Messrs Thomas Cook and Sons to find or make us beds and get mattresses made in the bazaars.

Someone helpfully engaged servants and within a few days, and before we had the beds, and before we were fully unpacked, with broken tins of jam still sticking things up in the hall, the troops started to come in. We had over a hundred lying on mattresses on the floor in the big rooms and around the gallery.

The nurses were magnificent, and so were Mrs Alcard [Mary Herbert's cook] and Annie Tyler [Margherita's maid]. With no Arabic to help them they managed to produce light diets all round and our patients were nursed and comforted. The nurses showed ingenuity and true discipline and their morale was first-rate. They knew their work all right and when not sure how to cope or what was best to be done in some unusual situation came and asked one of us, and we in turn sometimes asked for their opinions. The names of our nurses were – Sisters Broom and Sims, both very reliable, Lamble was full of fun, and Millidge and Pryde, Burton, Gibb, Marr, Houston and Dickson were all quite excellent, as was Whittuck, to whom so many patients lost their hearts.

It was at times awkward being so young. I used to talk of 'our' hospital, but Mary said, 'No, it must be yours.' This was generous of her because I could not have even got started without her. But there has to be a head and the staff accepted me, thank goodness. When we did not know the answers, we invented what actions we thought would best fit the case.

The big landings at Suvla on the Gallipoli Peninsula were on 6, 7 and 8 August 1915, and shortly after that these tragic hospital ships began to return. Casualties absolutely poured in. They unloaded them on to the quays where vans and lorries picked them up. In the meantime some had an hour or several hours lying unattended with the blazing sun tearing their nerves. So many wounds had developed gangrene on the voyage over, with a shortage of nurses and frequently no one at all to change the dressings.

Here Mary's mother-in-law Lady Carnarvon worked. She collected other women and sunshades and organised cups of hot tea to cool and refresh these unhappy men. She was tiny, and white-haired with a quiet manner: the heart of a lion and indomitable determination and very persevering. Everyone knew her and respected her.

I had to go to Hospital No. 21 to discuss with them what type of patients not to send us. I asked not to have anything infectious, and also no operations yet to be done, since we had not always a doctor.

It so happened, however, that a young soldier with a bullet in his chest had been sent on to us, presumably by mistake. One could see where it was, about half-an-inch under the skin, and he had a high fever. The nurses said something must be done and at once; but unfortunately, that week we had no doctor at all. I suggested that one of them should extract it, but all were adamant on that point, and none would contravene nurses' etiquette and training. So Sisters Whittuck and Burton, I think it was, persuaded me to do it under their instructions. I was told which sterilised scalpel to use and how to make the incision, and to make it long enough and deep enough, and then was given forceps with which to hold back the skin. They helped with squeezing the bullet out, and cleaning the wound, and then handed me threaded and sterilised surgical needles and told me how to sew it up and tie the gut.

And that poor boy never said a word. But the fever went down and he soon healed and was fit again.

The hospitals would send us jaundice cases, until I utterly proved that it was contagious. One man in a ward and the others got it, surely that is proof! Also an occasional dysentery case was sent by mistake, and would infect others.

Our days and evenings were full, as there was no secretary and every man's papers had to be made out in triplicate. The catering had to be done. (All stores and food we bought from Greeks in the bazaars, and hard business-men they were.) Costs were worked out and accounts were kept. We wrote rules, and continually one or other of us went round to see if things were all right and to remedy any situation which had been overlooked.

Each morning one gave Mrs Alcard the list for the day which would look probably something like this: 70 full diets – 60 light diets – 70 slops only, and there were ourselves and the nurses to cater for as well.

A bad moment was when, for no reason that I ever discovered, all the servants left. They just did not turn up in the morning. Not even our fat laundresses.

Everyone was alerted, and those good nurses all helped, and between us, dishes and dishes of rice puddings and Irish stew were produced. All did what came to hand. I, because I could not ask anyone else to do so, washed out and disinfected the dysentery lavatories and wash-rooms. But presently we became organised and had some spare time.

The rules were simple and effective and were on the whole carried out. As the men arrived their uniforms or hospital blue clothes were exchanged for striped pyjamas, and their uniforms stored in labelled sacks in the cellar. In this way one hoped to prevent them, when well enough, from wandering out of the grounds and trying to get into Alexandria.

Some did so, of course, and one would be rung up by the Military Police who soon began to recognise these brightly striped pyjamas and brought men back out to us again! Egyptians used to sell them bad spirits through the railings and this too had to be watched.

There was an Irishman on whom a strict eye was kept, but he fell downstairs being properly drunk one day, and it was discovered that he kept under his mattress red ink in a ginger-beer bottle! This he drank, and it worked!

We built an open-air hut big enough for all mobile cases to eat in, and then again with some Armenian refugees and no architect other than oneself as a sort of foreman, a room to hold a lot more beds, and used an old asphalt tennis-court as the floor of it.

I eventually got a projector from England and some films, and in this hut we held cinema shows, which the men could watch comfortably from their beds.

Now we were able to take 200 patients in easily.

And then we could get no doctor any more.

The Mayor of Alexandria weighed 33 stone and was a dear man, and respected by all. He it was who had replaced our staff with servants he knew, and said to them that the day any of them left me or were dismissed he would see they got a hiding they would not forget. Under the circumstances this, though strong, was necessary; anyway they stayed! And he said he had been a doctor in his youth and would come every other day to No. 6. and do what was necessary. And he did so, panting and puffing up the stairs. And so we carried on.

Our convalescents sat in the sun, on the steps or wandered around with and some without crutches. They sat around the hall to keep cool or on their beds and most of them were co-operative and friendly.

We had enormous Maoris, Australians and New Zealanders, Welsh and Scottish and English, Irish, Zionist mule corps and the Navy.

The senior of the walking patients took the other 'nearly fit' men for a daily walk: and every Tuesday a military band was sent to play for them.

Very soon the Westminister Dragoons, now also in Gallipoli got to hear of our hospital, and touchingly wore labels saying: 'If wounded, please send me to No. 6.'

The head of the Red Cross in Egypt [Dr Ruffer] was very efficient and helpful. He offered to pay, as he did to other hospitals, so much a head per day. And it was through him too that we acquired a small open car and 'Hassan' as driver.

Mary was splendid at seeing people, and did most of the talking and the persuading. My forte was more on the practical and organising side. We made a very good team.

When Rupert Brooke and Patrick Shaw Stewart came through with the Naval Division we had all foregathered in Cairo – Aubrey and Mary Herbert, Sybil and Ronald [Graham], Mervyn Herbert and Hugh Thomas, and one or two others.

I had not known Rupert and Patrick before, but was made one of the party and we rode on donkeys by moonlight through the silent deserted winding streets and around the tombs of the Mamelukes. It was both eerie and romantic and then we had scrambled eggs and coffee at Shepherds Hotel.

How clever Patrick was, and how utterly charming Rupert Brooke. He had a transparency and simple beauty. He was quiet and yet easy, and loved life, and beauty and health, and his poetry has not been equalled.

They sailed the next day and did not return.

His Highness Prince Hussein, Sultan of Egypt, was a delightful old fellow. Slight and medium height. His hair brushed up at the back and plastered round his head, and a tarboosh on the top with a long black tassel. I can only think of him in a stiff collar and black frock-coat. He was affable and pro-English and intelligent. The cruel British had in fact dragged him from a peaceful intellectual life in Paris to take the place of the Khedive Abbas Hilmi, whom they dismissed to Turkey.

He took to us and invited us to dine at his huge banquets, and I had to sing afterwards.

The enormous hall in the Kasa el din Palace with a very high ornamented ceiling held a vast amount of guests. All in Western dinner dress with a Turkish fez on the top, and behind very high up Muskrabia windows, sat his invisible but charming Sultana, hidden but able to watch.

We were given four or five different wines and liqueurs more or less at the same time. Then I would be led to the centre of the room to do my stuff.

The day came when I just had to go home again and see if all was well with the family. Letters were satisfactory but I wanted to see for myself; it was a long time now since they went to Scotland and I to Egypt.

The day before sailing I had a strong feeling most unexpectedly, that I did not want to go. I cancelled the passage and got another for the following week. That ship was sunk with all hands. Another rather soon afterwards was also mined, but many were saved. Dr Ruffer of the Red Cross was on board and the funnel blew off and fell on him, killing him.

We had in the meantime undertaken to feed on light diet some 5 or 600 men in a sandy camp close to where we were and who were having a lot of dysentery. The dusty sandy place did them no good and they could not eat the normal toughish rations doled out to them.

We had also turned the old Residency in Alexandria, by request, into an officers' convalescent hospital, called No. 11, for about thirty beds. And this time we were allotted the daily services of a doctor. Two of our nurses, Sisters Broome and Sims, were put in charge and Chrissie, the wife of Tommy's old friend Winkle Cave, was OC in the kitchen, and proved an excellent cook, with native help under her.

When in London I contacted my old enemy, General Keogh at the War Office. This time he was full of affability and when the Matron-in-Chief happened to come in and gave me a baleful look, he said, 'No, no! Not this time – Lady Howard is doing very well.'

So then I dared ask General Keogh that he remove not only the 600 dysentery cases on our neighbouring camp, but all the 20,000 such cases then mouldering in Egypt. I told him the circumstances, and how urgent this really was. 'Perhaps,' said he, 'you are not aware that I am the greatest expert on dysentery; and there is nothing I do not know about it or that you can tell me!' I went a bit pink, but answered, 'Well no, I did not know that, but in that case you will of course take them out of Egypt and put them on the West Coast somewhere, now that you know about it?'

On that we parted and to my amazement and everybody's delight he took the whole 20,000 away in a very short time, so my impertinence was justified.

The next thing I found myself embroiled with was that nurses from all the hospitals in their time off had nowhere to go. They stood about talking to their soldier friends on the streets, and a few went to 'Groppi' for tea. It did not look well and there were complaints. But what else could they do? So I found a bank that was high and had a wide gallery inside, and they very obligingly said I might board in their gallery and use it as a nurses' club. Sibyl helped enormously by getting together an important committee and I took the chair. There were about twenty, Generals and officials and important residents. I explained my good idea and they seemed to agree until I came to: 'And not only will it be somewhere to go and to meet each other, there will be a separate reading-room and tea, and also light meals will be served, to which they can invite their officer friends.'

Then the Matron-in-Chief for Egypt, in her smart grey uniform, fitting a little tightly over her somewhat portly figure spoke up and said, 'Not after six o'clock.' She evidently felt strongly about men friends not being allowed into a nurses' club after that hour. I left it to the others for a while, whilst thinking, and then with my very best smile I leant forward and said very distinctly, 'Do tell, Matron, is it your own personal experience that men are more dangerous after six o'clock?'

Well everyone coughed, and pulled out handkerchiefs, and she was quelled and gave in quite graciously …

Sister E. Campbell

Hospital ships *Galeka* and *Caledonia*, Dardanelles

Miss Campbell, an Australian nursing Sister, left Melbourne on 18 May 1915, with seventy-five other nurses, and arrived at Suez on 15 June. She was one of thirty-five who continued on by train to Alexandria. They were then sent to the 15th General Hospital, where Miss Campbell had charge of four wards of twelve beds each. After two weeks she went to another ward of sixty-three patients. The nurses slept at the Hotel de France and had their meals at the Hotel Regina. On 13 July Miss Campbell was told she was going on transport duty and sailed the next day on board the hospital ship Galeka.

16 July

Arrived at Mudros Bay at 1pm. Beautiful entrance. Many battleships and cruisers, *Lord Nelson* and *King George* amongst them. The twin ship to the *Lusitania* – the *Mauritania* – also *Aquitania* – biggest boats afloat. Four hospital ships, counting our own in harbour. We passed a German boat commandeered by Australia for stores, which had collided with something. She had a huge hole in her side through which the water was entering. The steel girders were twisted and she had a big list. She sent out a signal to us in the night (SOS) but we could not locate her and she managed to get into harbour. This was the first boat to take troops to the Dardanelles and she was just on the point of action. The crew witnessed the landing and shells were dropping all round and on to her decks. Before all the troops had landed, the wounded were being brought back to the boat.

One hospital ship left port on Sunday morn – 17 July – full of wounded. A French camp is on the beach just opposite to our ship and we can see them drilling. This morning we heard the firing of guns from a neighbouring man of war. This afternoon four Australian MOs went ashore to join their units – Bowman, Campbell, Slade, Beath. The Colonel went ashore this morning – Colonel Mayo Robson, who is an eminent British surgeon.

We have no news of the war, only that a big engagement is expected in a couple of days when we will probably go on to another boat. We are very comfortable on this boat, meals are very good and the weather is good. We have started to sleep up on deck.

22 July

Went ashore in the sailing boat to a Greek town called Talekna. When we got back found that wounded had been brought on board. The deck was fitted up with beds. Altogether 100 came on and more expected in the morning.

Saturday 24 July
Came on board RMS *Ionian* at 4pm. We were brought over in a barge from *Galeka*. It belongs to the Allan Line and usually runs between London and Montreal. It has been bringing troops backwards and forwards and is now waiting orders. The *Galeka* went out on Sunday morning, 25th, laden with wounded from Dardenelles going back to Alexandria.

Friday 30 July
Troops coming in on their way to the Front in ships and troops coming from the Front (wounded) all day long. Minesweepers mostly bring them from the Peninsular and put them on to hospital ships and Transports.

Captain from *Asearnig* paid us a visit in afternoon – had afternoon tea and music. Played bridge in the evening in Captain's cabin. Saw what was thought to be gun-firing on the Peninsular from bridge.

Tuesday 3 August
Got word that wounded were coming on board; 150 came. We all got to work and had them fixed up very soon. Some very ill. 8 Sisters are staying on this boat and 8 going on to the *Caledonia* (Miss Payne, Bennill, Ludlum, Chapman, Macdonald, Grigor, Blackie and self). 8 MOs came on board with 30 orderlies. Day very hot.

4 August
Helped with patients on *Ionian* all day. Went over to *Caledonia* at 7pm. Had dinner and got our cabins (state deck ones). 6 MOs and 35 orderlies on board.

5 August
Worked all day getting wards ready for patients. Expected 800 but none came. Prof. Farquahson is Ship's Surgeon. Captain Cook SMO.

6 August
Mac and I go on night duty tonight. We got 30 cases on board from Mudros at 11am. Helped with them. Had lunch then went to bed for couple of hours. News came for us to go to Cape Helles – to sail at 6am, escorted by the *Doris*. They say a big action is going on now. Sailed at 6 for Imbros. Arrived at daylight. Up all night. Many hospital ships passed us during night. Heard firing and saw flashes from guns on Aschi Baba.

Saturday 7 August
Worked to get place ready for wounded which arrived in pm. 1380 of them mostly stretcher cases and very bad. Some brought on dead. Had 20 deaths during voyage. Saw aeroplanes very close to us. One French one. Also submarines and TBDs [Torpedo Boat Destroyers]. Heard firing all day. Could see smoke distinctly … The *Aquitania* anchored near us – largest ship afloat. She was laden with troops going on to the Peninsular. We spent all the afternoon and night dressing wounds. We left at 8pm. Men in every corner of ship. Wards frightfully hot. A good many Australians amongst men. MOs operated nearly all night.

Sunday 8 August
Arrived at Mudros again in am. Stayed all day for no purpose. Very hot. Men very ill. Sailed in the evening. Worked hard all night. Beautiful sight going out from Mudros at 6pm. *Ionian* went at same time, waving to us from bridge.

Monday 9 August
In bed all day. Working at night.

Tuesday 10 August
Arrived at Alex at 1pm. Unloaded three quarters of men to various hospitals. Was on duty for rest of men who got off at 9am on Wednesday.

Thursday 12 August
Mr Johnson took Mac and me in Araybier out for day.

Saturday 14 August
Troops and Officers came on board at 6am for Mudros. 1,400 on board at 2.30. General Sextron sent word just as boat was leaving that all the Sisters were to get off boat. We packed up and off on to pier. Troops cheered as the boat went off. Captain spoke thro' megaphone to say Goodbye and sorry we were leaving. We went in a motor launch out to the hospital ship *Devanah*. Luggage came by ambulance. Lady Carnarvon went on first to *Devanah* to say we were going on board. MO met us.

Sunday 15 August
Expect to sail at 6pm. Communion Service at 7.30 for those who died on voyage. Word came that troopship had been sunk on way from Alex to Mudros. 1,100 troops on board. *Soudan* rescued 400 of them. It was torpedoed. No other particulars. Very comfortable on this boat – she is a P & O and very cool cabins. Heard that nearly 1,000 perished on *Royal Edward*. Slept nearly all day.

Monday 16 August
Passed Rhodes Island to have Memorial Service for those on board *Royal Edward* as we pass over the spot where she went down. Had service at 9pm. Ship stopped at the spot where disaster occurred and the Burial Service was read. Very impressive. Dead March was played. We saw a great deal of wreckage as we passed the region. Boats upturned, etc.

Back to *Caledonia*.

Wednesday
Went up to Imbros. Took on 1,000 wounded and sick.

Friday
Arrived back at Mudros. Stayed till Sunday night. On night duty all the time.

Sunday 22 August
Left Mudros for Gibraltar where we arrived at 3pm on Friday [27 August]. Beautiful

moonlight nights but very hot in 2nd class cabins. Patients feeling the heat terribly. Only 1 death to Gibraltar.

Saturday 28 August
7.30 discharged 30 patients to Hospital at Gib. RAMC men came to wharf with hand stretchers on wheels and the worst cases went off. Went to bed. Boat left at 3pm on Saturday. Champagne supper – 5 of us.

Monday 30 August
Life-belt drill 9am. Heard SOS signal in am to say that a boat was chased by submarine about 300 miles south of England. Everyone has life belts handy. We went out of our course for safety. Kept a long way from coast, away from submarine track. Ship in total darkness – even our lanterns we had to screen and keep below the bulwarks, all switches turned off. Had candles in cabins. 2 French cruisers escorted us after 8am till 2pm when British TBD and cruiser took their place. Former able to go 35 knots, circled round and back several times. Fine sight.

Tuesday 31 August
Got up at 2pm. All patients moved from decks down stairs.

Wednesday
Arrived at Devonport 8pm. Stayed on board all night. Very busy with patients. Breakfast at 7 – ambulances came then. We left the boat at 1pm for London …

Sister Kathleen Mann

Hospital Ships – HMT *Ulysses*, HMT *Marathon* and *Devanha*, Dardanelles

Sister Mann served at the 2nd Eastern General Hospital from August 1914 until July 1915 when she was given twenty-four hours notice to join the hospital ship Salta *to nurse casualties from the Gallipoli campaign. They sailed from Southampton on 25 July and enjoyed a relaxed voyage calling at Malta, Alexandria and Lemnos. A few days later Sister Mann and her unit transferred to the* Ulysses*, a blue funnel liner, and arrived at Imbros on 19 August. She kept a diary of her active service written almost every day over the following months.*

19 August
We expect wounded as soon as we arrive. We have only a minimum of stores including three wash bowls, 100 shirts, 600 towels and no extras, so we had to plan a bit over linen and stores. With a little tact we drew from the chief steward some ships' linen, pudding basins and pie dishes for operation bowls. The mattresses were laid out on all

decks, the lower troop deck first, all mess tables being removed. We had later to learn what the joy of nursing bad cases on the floor, on tiny mattresses, would be.

20 August
Wounded started to arrive at midday, and continued until one o'clock that night. I remained up for the last batch, but felt dead beat that night. I had only arranged for two night nurses, so was obliged to remain and do duty on lower deck.

Most of the cases were acute forms of dysentry and mild, some running high temperatures, some typhoid cases, and gun shot wounds. On the boat deck in a Hospital of 44 beds we decided to put all our acute dysentries and others on the same deck. Above the Hospital was an Isolation Ward. I had two sisters on duty for the Hospital and deck. I little knew then what the work would be there, two was not sufficient. One developed dysentry badly, I had to take her off and keep her in bed, and we also had to land another elderly lady I had on, who crocked up soon after leaving Imbros, so were short for that journey.

22 August
Many small operations have been done, and to my great disgust an appendix has turned up; the ship is too full of sepsis, I feel sad to think it is being done.

23 August
We lost a patient this morning, after he had had two operations, poor boy, it was sad, only 24hrs, and he had been through so much (gas gangrene); it was horribly sudden. I witnessed a burial at sea for the first time that day. It was held on the end deck after lunch, the body being placed on a slanting board, covered with a union jack. The burial service was read by the Captain, there being no Padre; others attending were the OC Troops and some of the medical staff. It was most impressive and quite reverently done.

24 August
One loses count of the days as had no time on the *Ulysses* to write or remember days and dates. I cannot remember the date of our arrival on Lemnos, but remained there about 48hrs, thinking to land some of our men, but did not do so. At sea again. What a splendid sight the great ship must be stealing along in the moonlight, with no lights. At sundown all port holes are closed and darkened, no lights allowed on deck, it being too risky; we have over 1,000 on board.

The work of those ten days we shall not easily forget, to organise and arrange food etc., for such numbers, one never seemed to get ahead of the meals. At night before retiring Sister King and myself generally went up for some fresh air. The Captain sometimes invited us to visit him. He had a jolly cabin. In spite of work all my staff seemed to enjoy themselves, the officers being quite attentive. I think some of my people have an officer on each ship, am wondering (if we continue this work) how many they will finish up with.

26 August
It took all day to disembark [at Alexandria], the ship stands too high for a gangway, so a slow process, there seems some muddle. I felt sorry for the bad cases, they waited all day, the last left about 10pm.

Next day all slacked feeling awfully tired. I had my camp bed on the deck, and enjoyed a good laze. In the evening we promised to go on shore with the 4th Officer, but ended by going with the Captain for a lovely drive through Alex, by moonlight, returning about 9.15pm.

Next day we landed to do some shopping. Lady Carnarvon visited us, regarding some Red X supplies; she gave us quite a number of things. Later in the day we received orders to go on to the *Guildford Castle*, a hospital ship lying close by, as the *Ulysses* was to leave for Australia, and we were to return to Lemnos to wait for orders. Great sorrow at leaving the *Ulysses*; we have been so happy on her.

30 August
Made a tour of the *Guildford Castle*. She is well fitted, with very fine store rooms below, quite a model floating Hospital. The Matron is a charming little person, so lively and awfully kind.

The staff are fixed up in two officers wards. I had a cabin, it is nice being alone. We are returning minus three of our staff. Am sad at leaving Sister Swain in Hospital, she was a nice little patient, and Sister Gould was taken off before leaving. Hope to pick up both on our return. The ship seems a great roller, all rather sick and being tired does not improve matters.

2 September
Were landed on to the *Marathon* at 5pm after waiting about all day [at Lemnos].

3 September
No medical stores have arrived on board, but patients are doing so. There seem to be many stretcher cases. No hope of stores today, usual muddle. Took 540 cases on, amongst them some bad cases, chiefly medical, dysentries, and some surgical cases.

Some sign of stores and a few Red X things turning up, but no time now in which to sort them. All have been landed into my office. Had a visit from Admiral Wemyss (Admiral of the Fleet), a rather important person, and no one at hand to receive him. He was very annoyed but since finding the OC and Captain, is in a better temper. Two French Red X ladies were with the Admiral. They came to see how work was managed on a transport, so went round with the Captain. Their dress was a work of art consisting of long white surge cloaks, Army caps, with light straw bonnets over same, short sleeves, white dresses and long white cotton gloves, Red X fancy aprons, white stockings and sandals. Such a quaint rig out.

We have a less number of dysentry cases with this Convoy but some seem very ill. Rather more surgical cases. This time the Hospital is in use for the Surgicals.

5 September
Left Lemnos at sunset, a safer time as the islands round are rather danger spots for enemy

submarines, and we travelled quickly. Before leaving all patients were ordered to have their life-belts handy, they were placed under their pillows, and all lights extinguished. We are taking a different route. Some journeys we take three days, others two and a half, some routes being safer than others, but the danger zone for transports is near the islands. It is rather a creepy feeling one has at times, not knowing what may happen.

7 September
Reached Alex at dawn, no mishaps. Came into berth without delay, and disembarked before lunch. Also got some clearing up done. The stretcher-bearers were splendid and disembarkation well managed. Slacked on deck all the afternoon feeling tired and depressed, having received the sad news of little Swain's death (one of our staff). It has made a big blank in our midst. All liked her so much.

10 and 11 September
Still on the *Marathon* awaiting orders. Went on shore in morning and returned to hear that we are to remain on the ship to take some convalescent patients to England …

There was little nursing to do during the voyage home but in spite of heavy seas and submarine threats, Sister Mann and her Unit enjoyed a relaxed ten days on board the Marathon *and reached Plymouth on 23 September. After two weeks leave she was appointed Matron-in-Chief on the hospital ship* Devanha *and sailed from Southampton on 8 October for the Dardanelles. The passengers included members of the Scottish Women's Hospital en route for Serbia.*

21 October
Left Mudros at noon. Passed Imbros at 3.30pm. We are bound for the beaches. The sea is lovely blue today and sun hot when out of the wind.

Reached Suvla Bay about 4.30pm and anchored but not taking on wounded at once as two other ships are on the beaches filling up. We can see the large shells bursting and hear the roar of the guns. There is a search light from a battleship playing across the hill, on a spot where the Turks have tried to cut through after dark.

22 October
We were wakened by guns this morning. Regular firing about 6.30am. There is a cold wind blowing, but sun trying to come out.

Sister Dodd has packed a lovely sack for the Tommies on shore. She brought out many treasures including biscuits, sweets, books, socks, mufflers and tins of compressed things.

Our first lot of men came off at 11am. A lot of bad medicals, also some gunshot wounds. Patients look tired and done up. Several lots taken on, but only half full so far.

23 October
Finished embarking at 7.30pm. Very busy evening. Finished work at twelve o'clock. Very thankful for bed then. The Captain sent me down a glass of port wine, which I had on retiring. Several operations have been done, but staff cheerful and keen. Had two deaths.

24 October
Left the beach at 6am. Three burials at 9am. An officer was operated on (Major Lowery). Amputation of left leg (gas gangrene). No chance. He died the same evening. Very busy but all running smoothly and all happy. Food a little worry, but bound to be with such numbers.

The firing last night was continuous. Started at sunset and did not cease, with occasional heavy reports from the big guns. We watched some of the shells bursting and through glasses can see some trenches. On the beach there is an enormous quantity of stores. There is also the clearing hospital.

Reached Lemnos about 11am. Remained until 5pm and then went off to Alex.

25th
Two more deaths today. All going well but the medicals make the nursing rather impossible. One cannot do all one wants to for them.

26th
Reached Alex 11am. Busy day disembarking. All patients are sorry to leave. They seem to have been happy. May be here for a week, for some repairs and also must get coal.

2 Nov
Have orders to leave at 5pm today. Four new nurses are due on but have not turned up. Had to land to make enquiries. They arrived finally at 5pm. Pilot was on board. Did not leave harbour until 7pm bound for Lemnos. Have several passengers. Two Lt Cols RAMC and Padre.

3 Nov
Fixed up some rules for orderlies nursing typhoid patients, as on the last voyage we had so many and they do not seem to understand the care of them.

4 Nov
Arrived at Lemnos 2pm. Colder and a strong breeze. Too rough to report at the *Aragon*. We are ready again for patients. Have rigged up some special gowns for the orderlies when attending to typhoid patients.

5 Nov
We had one of the ship's boats and rowed off to land. Had a jolly walk, explored some way inland. We landed on a temporary pier by the French hospital and walked to the top of the hill where we could look down on a pretty bay. Walking was difficult – so many stones and sand. The thistles were bad. We passed a French camp on our return and a great number of mules. We also visited the Greek church. The houses are very primitive. The inhabitants live upstairs and the cattle occupy the lower flat. Another climb brought us through another small village and we finally reached our boat. I helped to row back, as the orderlies are not good at it.

6 Nov

Left Mudros at 6am. Our journey was to Anzac which we reached at 10am. The first load of patients arrived at 11am. A great many walking cases. Our second lighter came out at 4pm, making our total 350. We shall fill up tomorrow. We have some acute surgicals. One died on admission.

Sunday 7 Nov

A lighter came out, but not yet filled up. Several operations done today. Some will hardly pull through, such nasty head wounds. Have 98 empty beds left. All very tired but fairly ship-shape in wards.

8 Nov

Another lighter came out at 11am. Firing has been continuous all night. Our monitors firing frequently. From my port hole this morning I could watch a monitor fire and see the shell land. The Turks machine guns seem very busy. They say it is to prevent us attacking them that they keep up a continuous fire. A whole line of transports came up this morning. An aeroplane was over us yesterday at which the Turks opened fire – also today, but she was too high up and the shots fell short each time.

On the beach is a small trawler. The Turks have got the range of her with some high explosive shells. She must be riddled.

Left Anzac at 1pm. Reached Mudros at 5pm. Saw several troop ships leave. There are a number of hospital ships in the harbour. We are leaving our Indian wounded at Mudros.

Have two officers who are badly wounded. One quite a young boy was shot through the neck and is very ill. Another with a bullet in his abdomen has had some removed on shore. A very long middle line incision with drainage tubes in.

9 Nov

Yesterday we lost both officers. We signalled to the *Aragon* for a priest as the young Lieutenant was a Catholic and we have not an RC Padre on board. We were overjoyed to receive Mr Cavendish again and he arrived in time, before the boy died, and remained with him to the last.

All Indians have gone off on a lighter, also all eye cases and now have orders to leave for Malta.

10 Nov

A nasty day, ship on the roll, several of the staff feeling sick. I, for one, am feeling miserable. The lower deck is most unpleasant.

12 Nov

Came into Quay in the Grand Harbour [Malta]. Started disembarking at 9.30am. All walking cases have gone off first. All finished at 2.30pm. We were sent out to a buoy to coal. Had a visit from the Governor, Lord Methuen, this morning, who went over the ship. I was introducted and invited to lunch. All my staff have an invitation to tea tomorrow at the Palace but we rather hope to be away.

Sunday 15 Nov
On our way back again to Mudros. The wards are getting straight. Unpacked stores today. I discovered we had a batch of baby rabbits on board so took them up on the deck for an airing …

17 Nov
At Mudros. No further orders.

20 Nov
Left Mudros at 5.20pm. This journey is to Cape Helles.

21st
Sea very rough, so moved in to embark. The first lighter out before lunch, mostly surgicals. All very cold on admittance and so glad to get on board.

We are so near the shore that we can see the dug outs and camps. Also the road, with the traffic winding its way along. But oh the wind, it goes right through one. The *River Clyde* is on the shore, also what looks like another transport and several boats seem to be on the beach. There are many cruisers about.

22nd
Patients coming on at intervals. Have been ordered to go out from beach, as an attack is expected.

23rd.
Left Cape Helles.

25th
A ripping day, quite warm, all extra clothing is being discarded. It is nice to be warm again, after the intense cold of the Peninsular. All patients seem to be improving with the exception of a few.

26 Nov
Arrived Alex and finished disembarkation at 5.30pm. Have several very bad cases, one a pneumonia who is very ill. Lady Carnarvon came on board early and sent us some clothing of which we were short.

29th
We are to take patients back with us to Mudros for the *Mauritania*. Leo (the Senior Medical Officer) taken off the ship and a new OC put on. All very depressed. We shall miss him.

30th
Leo left at 8am. All very sad. New SMO, a regular, intends to remain on if he can manage it. Left finally at 12.30. Very rough outside harbour. We rolled a lot. Wards have not been properly prepared. Everything seems wrong. There has been such a horrid upset over Leo.

1 Dec

We had an awful day yesterday. The sea bad. Most of the patients, as well as staff ill. All fairly cheerful today. Some Sergts amongst patients inclined to grouse, but in the Army that is NCOs' privilege. (The Army was only meant for certain people.)

2 Dec

Mudros reached at 12.30. We have no orders to disembark as yet. Many grumbles as to food and many other little difficulties today. Oh dear our new OC is going to be a bit difficult. I like not Army ways or people.

3 Dec

Disembarked at 10am and came out into stream. Had orders to leave again at 2pm for Cape Helles which we reached at 5. All seems quiet and we are not very near the shore. We have had a rush to get ready. SMO most trying. Informs me that 'He is IT' on this ship.

8 Dec

We returned to Mudros after embarking rapidly and on to Alex. It has been a horrible week. We hope to pick up Leo again. A spirit of discontent and decidedly insolent tone has arisen amongst RAMC, due to changes. Our OC has done no work. He was on shore most of one day. All admissions done by Orderly Medical Officer for the day. All fairly quiet at Cape Helles.

9th, 10th, 11th

Colonel Sexton was on board this morning so explained the present impossible situation to him, regarding Captain Turner [the Senior Medical Officer]. The Captain took me on shore yesterday. We motored out to Staffa and saw Leo and visited the Brewshers for lunch.

12th

Captain Guillimore came on. Told him how unsettled we all were under our new rule, and also that the man was not safe. He gave me a note to take back to Col. Sexton.

13th

We have Sir Warren Lowe on board. He had a talk to me about it and I think will help matters for us. He is so nice.

Our SMO is in bed today. Is to have an operation at 6.15pm. So his time for this trip will be spent in bed and I suppose Captain Archer will take up his position. It can only be for this journey. It has been a horrible experience.

What a day and what a muddle. Captain Archer OC admitted the first load of patients. Others sent to wards by NCOs. All medical officers fed up with the state of affairs.

An aeroplane was above us today and it was most exciting to watch. The Turks firing at her she quite suddenly disappeared into the clouds and came out again. A shell dropped into the sea about 50 yards from the ship at lunch time. I had just come out on the deck so saw it. We moved off at once, it being too risky to remain.

Colonel Lowe is operating on a head case. There are three more operations to be done, but Sister Carter never grouses. She is as bright and full of work at the end of a day as at the beginning. There is another nursing orderly off to do duty on the OC, leaving a ward without an orderly but one is not consulted. They must just manage.

We have orders to go up to Anzac so shall fill up from there in the morning.

16th

One lighter out at lunch time. Some bad gun shot wounds and bomb wounds. Firing has been continuous. We hear that Anzac is to be evacuated. The Australians are awfully sad. The ones on board very depressed. They hate giving in. Suvla has partly evacuated. Stores have been leaving the shore today. A lot of signalling after dark and the large guns are firing. We think the Turks must have received fresh supplies of ammunition by the way they are using it. We hear that our OC is to be put off at Mudros as he has DT. Pleasant to be commanded by a DT Man. I am thankful we have the Colonel on board. Had a second lighter out at 6pm. I think we are now full.

17 Dec

Great excitement last night but all very depressed on board. Suvla evacuation going on and Anzac. At dusk three transports crept up and stationed themselves near us and men began to leave the beaches quietly. There were no lights to be seen. The ships in total darkness but for the moonlight, which was rather bright, but in the last quarter. Stores have been coming off all day. The patients tell us that large guns are being blown up and all stores destroyed. Large quantities of petrol and paraffin have been taken off to fire the first line trenches, the hospitals blown up. Volunteers have been called for to remain and 300 have offered. In first lines 200 and 100 for the beach. Last night horses and mules were removed.

Three men came on who were wounded whilst getting on to transports. It is such a horrid feeling one has, not knowing if the last men will get off safely or not. The Australians are most depressed. It has been such a blow to them, after all their hardships on the Peninisular.

We had an uncanny sight, what with the evacuation and our SMO shouting and fighting with his orderlies in the corridor and on the deck. Some of the Sisters were alarmed, not knowing before of his condition.

18 Dec

About 12pm there was a flare of light on land. I got up and went on deck to see a huge fire on shore by the pier. Stores were being burnt. It was impossible to remove them. We thought it had been purposely done, but heard today that an Indian was suspected and one had been shot for signalling to the Turks. The fire was an enormous one and gave the Turks our positions and pier which before they had been unable to get the range of. It is depressing as one wonders how ever the last men will get away. The RAMCs on shore seem to have done good work and the Captain on the lighter waved us goodbye as he left the last load, saying they would meet us at Southampton in a week's time. Such cheerfulness. The remaining men have had a great time as regards food etc., being given a free hand to help themselves, so have feasted on tinned chicken, turkey, jellies, etc.

19th
Reached Mudros and went alongside the *Iona*, a transport, to disembark our patients on to her. It took the whole day to get 119 cot cases removed with others. No method. All muddle. The walking cases left at 6.30pm and finished at 8.30pm. Wards very dirty and untidy. I am fed up and weary of the whole thing. Feeling one has completely failed, although have tried to keep things going.

As the *Iona* is not equipped for wounded we are keeping our worst cases. No chance of our OC going off as we are to return to Cape Helles.

20th
Anzac and Suvla have completely evacuated with three casualties. We hear that Cape Helles is not to evacuate but things look rather black I fancy. There seem to have been numbers of troops returning in the night. As nine other hospital ships are in harbour I cannot understand why we have been sent back with no chance of clearing up or having our wards straight and no change of linen for this journey.

Our OC has been placed under arrest with six orderlies on duty as guard so suppose we are bound to return to Alex this time.

Arrived at Cape Helles. A gale of a wind and sea very rough.

22nd
Sea too rough to embark patients today. A terrific bombardment this evening on shore. We do not know which side is attacking.

We started to fill up about 10.30. A very large barge came out with stretcher cases. Also lighter full of walking cases. Had three loads, mostly wounded. Only 81 beds left empty.

23rd
Two lighters out so have filled up. Left Helles at 12pm, reaching Mudros at 4.30pm. Nine other hospital ships in the harbour including the *Aquitania*. No orders as yet.

24th
Orders to proceed to Alex where I hope we land Captain Turner.

Have some very sad cases on board. Last night we lost a young boy with sepsis. Some very bad wounds and high temperatures. I so wish we had some Xmas gifts for our men but have nothing. They have cheered up and are so bright.

25 Dec, Xmas Day
Was up at 6.15am. We were so late last night doing up some stockings for the boys of 19 and under. We found many odds and ends in the Red X store and filled about 40 stockings not omitting our Padre and the Ship's Captain. Sister Dodd hung a stocking through her porthole which was quickly filled. The Head Waiter was busy last night arranging bunting in the Saloon which gives a very festive air. All are sad at having nothing for the men. The Padre held a Celebration at 6.45am in D Ward and another in the smoke room at 7.40am. Then some carols and short service in the Wards throughout the day. On the whole I think the men quite enjoyed it. The Chief

Steward rose to the occasion and provided a nice dinner. A roast beef and plum pud. The orderlies had a nice dinner midday. We went down to wish them a Happy Xmas before they started and the Padre made a short speech. He is always ready for any emergency.

30th.
Landed after lunch today and visited a dentist. Met Leo and had tea with him. Passed Colonel Lowe who tells me that he is returning to the ship. Also Colonel Sexton arrived on board with new SMO, Major Dunn. Hope things settle down again.

31 Dec
A glorious day. Left Alex about 7am. We fear it means the evacuation of Cape Helles that we have been sent off so soon again. Wards are ready once more for use. Have seen very little of new SMO.

The Padre has arranged for a short intercession service tonight at 11.30pm …

1916
France

Miss V.C.C. Collum

SS *Sussex*, English Channel

At the outbreak of the war Miss V.C.C. Collum was working as a freelance journalist and in the press department of the London office of the National Union of Women's Suffrage Societies where she helped Dr Elsie Inglis [qv] set up the Scottish Women's Hospitals. She joined the staff at the hospital in Royaumont in February 1915 and received her initial training in the X-ray department, later becoming a highly skilled radiographer. Just over a year later she was on the steamer Sussex *after leave in England. There were 386 passengers, including 270 women and children, on board. The captain and the fifty crew members were Frenchmen.*

Never was the sea in the Channel more blue than on the afternoon of 24 March when the *Sussex* left Folkestone harbour for Dieppe. I felt in high spirits. My month's leave had been just long enough to clear away all the feeling of staleness that had crept over me after twelve months' work at the Hospital, and to give me an appetite for more. A year is a long time in war. In a year the members of a corps, a ship's company, or the staff of a hospital, get to know one another very intimately, especially if, as in our case, the unit is somewhat isolated. In a year our Hospital had become a living thing, and our Head Surgeon [Miss Frances Ivens, qv], a Chief who commanded something that is more than loyalty and respect, yet which an Englishman hesitates to describe as devotion. So I was right glad to be going back to a life I loved, to a Chief I delighted to work with, to comrades proven in long months of alternating stress and monotony and to a little group of friends. Then there was also the prospect of bearing a share in the terrific work of the expected spring offensive.

We steamed out punctually at 1.30 to the rousing cheers of British troops soon to follow us to France. In less than an hour we had a reminder that the enemy also keeps his watch by sea. We passed thousands of floating bags of jettisoned cargo – 'A sinister reminder of possibilities,' I said to my neighbour, a stout elderly man.

I turned to the sea again, and watched – for a periscope. It grew cold, and I was beginning to think of going back to my sheltered chair to roll myself up in my rug, when in a moment the whole earth and heaven seemed to explode in one head-splitting roar. In the thousandth part of a second my mind told me: 'Torpedo – forward

– on my right', and then the sensation of falling, with my limbs spread-eagled, through blind space.

When I came to myself again I was groping amid a tangle of broken wires, with an agonising pain in my back and the fiercest headache I have ever known. My hair was down and plastered to my chin with blood that seemed to be coming from my mouth. There was more blood on my coat sleeve. I was conscious that I was bleeding freely internally with every movement. My first definite thought was: 'If only it is all a ghastly nightmare!' But I remembered. My next thought was a passionately strong desire not to die by drowning – then I crawled free of the wires that were coiled all about me and stood up. In one unsteady glance I took in a number of things. Near me a horrible piece of something, and a dead woman. (Afterwards I wondered why I was so sure she was dead and never stooped to make sure.) Below me, on the quarter-deck and second-class promenade deck, numbers of people moving to and fro, many with lifebelts on. I never heard a sound from them, but it did not strike me as odd then. Now I know I was deafened. So I had been blown up on to the top deck, to the other end of the ship. I swayed to and fro, and looked for a stairway, but could find none, and began to be aware that I had only a few moments before consciousness left me. Something must be done if I was not to drown. I forced my will to concentrate on it, and came to the side, where I found three men looking down on a lowered boat. I also saw a life belt on the ground. I picked it up, and not having the strength to put it on, I tried to ask the men to tie it for me. Then I found I could not speak. So I held it up, and one, an American, understood, and hastily tied it. Then I saw one of them catch hold of a loose davit rope and swarm down it to the boat. There was my one chance, I decided. My arms were all right, but would my legs work? I took hold, and made a mighty effort to cross my knees round the rope: I succeeded. Then I slid down till I was just above the water. I waited till the roll of the ship brought me near enough to the boat to catch, with my right hand, another rope that I saw hanging plumb above it, while I hung on with my left. It came within reach: I caught it, let go with my left, and lowered myself into the boat. Then I wanted to sink down in her bottom and forget everything, but I dared not, for men were pouring into her. I saw a man's knee hooked over the side of the boat where I sat. I could not see his body, but it was in the water, between us and the side of the *Sussex*. As in a dream I held on to his knee with my left hand with all the grip I had left, and with my right held on to the seat on which I sat. I could do nothing to help him in, but on the other hand, so long as I remained conscious, his knee-hold should not be allowed to slip. No one took any notice of either of us. Gradually I began to hear again. The men in the boat were shouting that there was no more room, that the boat was full. One last man tumbled in and then the people in the boat pushed away, and men on the *Sussex* helped. Others continually threw gratings and planks overboard.

Our boat was dangerously overcrowded. Already she was half swamped. I wondered when she would upset. A man on either side seized gratings and towed them alongside. One made a herculean effort and pulled the man whose knee I had been holding into our boat, and nearly upset her. No one said a word. He was an elderly man, and his fat face was white and piteous. His hands never ceased trembling. He had had a terrible fright. Some one suggested getting out the oars, and others said it was impossible, as they were underneath us all. However, it was managed, and several men stood up and changed places. Again we nearly upset. I joined with the others in commanding these wild folk to sit still. Three oars were produced. One was given to a young and sickly-looking Frenchman opposite me. He did not know how to use it. Everyone shouted to get away from the steamer. The water had now reached my knees, and I began to notice how cold it was. I saw three other women in the boat. They sat together, white and silent, in the stern, nor ever moved. They were French women. Someone noticed that the water was increasing, and there was a wild hullabaloo of alarm. A Belgian – the man who had pulled into the boat the man whose knee I held – called for hats with which to bale, setting the example with his own. But we were so tightly packed that no one could get at the water, whereupon the Belgian climbed overboard on to one of the gratings I have already mentioned, and a young Belgian soldier followed his example on the other side. They held on to our gunwale with their fingers.

Sometimes the people in the boat baled furiously, sometimes they stopped and stared stupidly about them. Some shouted to 'Ramez! Ramez!' Others equally excited yelled 'Mais non! Videz l'eau! Videz l'eau!' I apologised to my immediate neighbours for that I had no hat to lend, and for that I was too hurt to stoop, but I put my hands on the erring oar the young Frenchman was feebly moving across my knees, and did my best to guide his efforts. As often as not he put it flat on the water, and sometimes he merely desisted altogether, and gazed vacantly in front of him. The Belgian asked for a handkerchief, and groping in the water at the bottom of the boat, found a hole and caulked it as best he could. Thereafter the balers kept the water from increasing, but did little to reduce it.

Looking around I saw our steamer riding quite happily on the water with her bows clean gone. Afterwards I learned that the torpedo had cut off her fore-part, to within an inch or two of where I had been standing, and that it had sunk. I saw another full boat being rowed away from the ship, and an overturned one with two people sitting on her keel. I saw a man seated on a grating. All were convinced that help would be forthcoming speedily. And still the *Sussex* floated. Four times I remarked – by way of a ballon d'essai – that it seemed as if she were not going to sink, and always there was an outcry to row, and get away from her. The Belgian and the Belgian soldier evidently thought as I did. They proposed that we should return before we were swamped ourselves. Once again an hysterical outburst. One man jumped to his feet and shrieked, and asked us if it were to hell that we intended returning? I began to be afraid that he and those who thought as he did would throw us others into the sea, but commonsense told me that to remain all night in that overcrowded half-swamped boat would be to court death.

We saw at last that the other boat was returning. This was our chance. Example is a wonderful thing in dealing with mob hysteria. Tentatively the two Belgians and I proposed that we should go as close to the steamer as prudence permitted, and ask the Captain if she were going to sink. If his answer were favourable, those who desired should go on board, and any who liked could go off again in the boat. If his answer were unfavourable, we would stand off again. The maniac still shrieked his protests, but the rest of the boat was with us. But no one seemed to know how to turn the boat. As soon as we told one to backwater, the other two did likewise. It seemed hopeless.

Finally, we let the other two oars pull, and I myself tried to induce my vis-a-vis to 'ramez au sens contraire,' which was the nearest approach I could get to 'backwater' in French! He was too dazed to understand, so I simply set my teeth and pulled against him, and in about fifteen minutes the boat gradually came round in a wide circle. How I longed to be whole again so that I could take his oar right away and cox that mad boat! With my injured back and inside I could only just compass what I did. The pain kept me from collapsing, and the exertion from freezing. Even now a mutinous mood came over the boat every few moments, and they wavered and prepared to flee the ship again. It was like a political meeting. The boat followed the wishes of those who shouted loudest. So we who wished to return shouted monotonously, 'Retournez au bateau'. When the oars ceased dipping, I called out as encouragingly as I could – subconsciously following, I believe, the example of newspaper sergeants I had read of in French accounts of battles – 'Courage, mes amis! Ramez! Ramez! Courage, mes enfants!' No one thought it odd. The dazed ears heard and the nerveless arms worked again. Finally, the Belgian dragged me aside that some one might have another tussle with the rising water. It looked as though we were to be swamped, after all, within ten yards of the *Sussex*'s gaping bows, for our crew, in their excitement, had forgotten to bale for some minutes. As we floated in under her sides I made a final appeal, which a young Belgian put into more forcible French, for everybody to keep calm and not upset the boat at the last.

The women now spoke for the first time – and it was to appeal to the excited boat's load to let me be taken off first, since I was injured. I found I could not stand, so sat in the middle of the seat trying to trim the boat while the men scrambled out. I was left alone at last; and the water that came over the gunwale poured over my legs to my waist, some of it soaking through my thick great-coat and chilling me to the bone. The boat was floating away. Someone shouted to me to get up. I got to my hands and knees on the seat and tried to crawl along the side, but the change of position nearly caused me to faint with pain. Then the Belgian managed to get hold of the boat and hold her, and some sailors leaned out of the hatchway in the *Sussex*'s side and grasped me by the arms and pulled me up and in as though I had been a sack. There were many far worse hurt than I, and they left me propped against a wall. The Belgian again came to the rescue, and half dragged me to the top of the second saloon stairway. I got down by levering myself on my hands on the rails, while he supported me under the arms. Once in the saloon, he and the young Belgian soldier took off my loosely fixed lifebelt and laid me on a couch. One forced a glass of whisky down my throat, which burned and gave me back renewed consciousness, while the other ran for brandy. I was terribly cold, and the good Belgian took off my boots and puttees and stockings and chafed my feet till one was warm. The other had no sensation for over twelve hours, and five days later, when it was radiographed, proved to be sprained and fractured. He placed a pillow over them then, and proceeded to chafe my hands, first taking off my bedraggled fur gloves which I still wore. He sat and held my hands for at least a quarter of an hour till they were warm. Then he disappeared to help 'the other women'. Meanwhile the young Belgian soldier came and gave me a glass of brandy, giving me no choice, but insisting on my drinking it, and spilling a good deal on my bloody chin and coat collar in his zeal. Soon I felt quite warm again.

Presently the electric lights were turned up, to my great astonishment. The Belgian surprised me still further by taking away my boots and stockings 'to dry before the kitchen fire'. I did not yet realise what we owed to the strong watertight bulkheads of that well-constructed little vessel.

After that, long hours of waiting. A woman shrieked incessantly up on deck. A man with a wounded head came and sat patiently in a corner. A girl, complaining of a pain in her chest, came down the stairs and lay down on a corner couch. She never moved nor spoke again. By midnight she was dead. None of us guessed, none of us knew. She died bravely and silently, quite alone. Another woman showed signs of approaching hysteria. A young Belgian officer, who had been attending her, suddenly ceased his gallantry, and standing sternly before her, said brusquely, 'After all, if the very worst comes, you can only die. What is it to die?' The words acted on her like a douche of cold water. She became herself again and never murmured. We others, perhaps, benefited too. It is nerve-racking work lying helpless in a damaged vessel, wondering whether the rescue ship or another enemy submarine will appear first on the scene. And no ship came. At intervals the Belgian boy soldiers came down to reassure us: 'The wireless had been repaired. Forty vessels were searching for us. There was a light to starboard. We were drifting towards Boulogne …' But no ship came. The light to starboard faded. Another appeared, and faded too. Then we heard the regular boom of a cannon or a rocket. We all knew that something must have blocked our wireless, but no one said so. The Belgian came down to sleep, fixing his lifebelt first. With him came a good French woman, who was very kind to me and washed the blood from my face and rinsed out my bleeding mouth. She was very hungry, and all I could do to help her was to hold her jewels while she went on deck to search for her hand baggage, and, later, to give her some soaked food out of my pocket. There was no food left anywhere. She said some brave words, too, about death coming to all, only coming once, and being soon over. How much one person's courage can help others at such a time! Then she tied on a lifebelt and went to sleep beside me. The ship was rolling now, and the seas slapped noisily against her somewhere, jarring her all through her frame. But the Captain had said she would not sink for eighteen hours, and we all believed his word implicitly. Still, it was an ugly noise, and seemed to betoken her helplessness.

And then at last the news of rescue! A French fishing boat was coming! 'Women and children first,' the young Belgians cried. My Belgian succourer roused himself and fetched my stockings and boots. My right boot would not go on. My putties he could not manage, and so he tied them round me. He was always cool and practical and matter-of-fact. 'I have been in the Belgian Congo,' he explained, 'and in shipwrecks before. I know what to do, and I am not alarmed. You can trust entirely to me.' And I did. There was a great bump as the fishing-boat came alongside, and a rush upstairs. Once more I was left alone, for my Belgian friend had gone up to see about getting me helped on board. He came back to say that the crush was so great that he would wait till it was over and then take me. It seemed a long time, but he came back at last, only to find he could not lift me. Then he went away calling for an 'homme de bonne volonte' to help. A young Chinese responded, and together they staggered up the heaving stairway with me. When they reached the ship's rail it was to hear that the boat had gone! A British torpedo-boat was coming, we were told, and so the fisherman had gone off with as many as she could safely carry to Boulogne. With her went my hope of reaching my own hospital in France. I was sure the destroyer would take her load to England.

Once more I was on the point of collapse, and very seasick to boot. The Belgian supported me as if I had been a little child, and I tried to convince myself that I was not in dreadful pain. Perhaps half an hour passed, and then the destroyer came. This time one of the French sailors helped him to carry me, and I was placed on my back, across the ship's rail, and when the roll brought her near enough to the destroyer, British sailors grasped my arms and pulled me over. For one sickening second my legs dangled between the two ships, but the sailors hauled me in just before the impact came. They carried me to the chart-house and laid me on the couch, and before long the Belgian joined me, and, utterly exhausted, lay down on the floor. From that moment I felt entirely safe.

It took a long time to transfer all the remaining passengers from the *Sussex*, for the sea was becoming restless, and the two ships hammered and thumped at each other's sides to such purpose that the rescuing destroyer had to go into dock for repairs when her labours were over and she had landed us all safely. The injured were at once attended to, and I had not been more than half an hour on board before the surgeon came to visit me. Having sent the Belgian below, he did all he could for me, and then, assured that I was by no means in extremis, he hurried back to attend to three others who were. The mate of the destroyer came and made me comfortable, and sent me tea, and a young gunner to keep me from falling off the couch when we should move, and reappeared at intervals to see how I was getting on. He gave me chocolate, which I ate quite greedily, having had nothing for over twelve hours. Unfortunately, as soon as the destroyer began its homeward race, I was very sea-sick.

Somewhere near 4am the kind mate came to tell me we were coming in to port. I was carried by sailors out on to the deck and placed on a stretcher, and then a RAMC surgeon with orderlies took charge of me and carried me aboard the hospital ship …

Miss Dorothy Higgins

Anglo-Belgian Hospital, Rouen, France

Dorothy Higgins, a British Red Cross VAD, was twenty-three when she arrived at the Anglo-Belgian Hospital in Rouen, northern France, in April 1915. She was a trained radiographer and radiotherapist. In pencilled letters written to her parents in Alford, Lincolnshire, she often mentioned her friend 'Tim' and her assistant 'Nick' (Miss Nicolson), fellow VADs, and admitted that she was 'awfully homesick sometimes'.

At the beginning of April 1916 she wrote that the hospital, which specialised in physiotherapy and orthopaedic cases, would soon be moving to a new large complex in Bonsecours, a suburb of Rouen.

9 April 1916
My patients and treatment grow apace. Bonsecours is getting on splendidly and we hope to be up there by the end of May. It is quite a city: such a wonderful looking place and all built by the Belgian Army engineers. It will be ripping up there as we are so fearfully cramped for room down here. I shall be very sad to leave our quay where I've seen so many interesting disembarquations.

21 April 1916
We are crazy on gardening and getting things ready for Bonsecours. The hut we shall sleep in is already up.

Tim and I went up on Tuesday last and dug the quarter circle bed and planted it with a few things. Thursday we took a lusty comrade and the three of us set to work on the long bed or border. We pegged it out with string and with great labour succeeded – completing a piece about as large as a dog's grave!! It doesn't sound much but we are inordinately proud of it. By complete I mean sods cut off and the ground properly dug and trenched to a depth of two feet. We cut the sods off quite a long way and put them aside. Then there was a lot of twitch to get out so it all took time. But it is so ripping having a garden to look after and play with. Tim and I are fearfully keen.

We have been appointed hospital gardeners and mean to do our very best to make it look smart and jolly.

Will you please pack a packing case or hamper with the plants (I'm sending you a list) and address it to Mrs Macdonald, College of Ambulance, Vere Street, Oxford Street, and put on it 'For Miss Higgins, Hôpital Anglo-Belge, Rouen. To be called for'. And a girl who is returning this next week will call there for it.

It is a regular city, this new hospital. Water, electric light, gas, telephone and tram all of its own. The tram line of the town goes round below the bluff on which the huts are built and they have made a branch line coming right into the hospital.

Plant list. Please put names inside packets:
Golden rod, catananche, centaurea montana (blue), Iceland poppy, helianthus, pansies and violas, cerastum, lychnis, meconopsis cambrica, phlox, geum, mallow (white), sidalcea, achillea ptarmica, sweet rocket, digitalis, doronicum, erigeron, eryngium, gaillardia, gypsophila (one of my little plants), alyssum saxatile, anchusa, antirrhinum, arabis pl. fil, thrift, Michaelmas daisies, delphinium, calystegia, campanula persicaefolia and C. pyramidalis.

Seeds:
Tropaeolum (the red kind of the Lake District), nemesia, myosotis, mixed sweet peas.

Ryders PP Catalogue:
Please send seeds and Ryder's catalogue as soon as possible.

30 April 1916
I have had a very hard week: I am now treating or superintending the treatment of 100 men a day and we have got two nurses isolated in a French hospice with 'hun-rash' measles: two have been on leave: one left in the middle of the week as she had

a tendency to tuberculosis and Rouen with its moist steamy atmosphere and airlessness is one of the worst possible places for such people. Another one a common little Canadian suburban mixture got married to a Belgian lawyer, and has left, rather in disgrace and so we have been working on about half the usual personnel. I have been doing half an hour's dispensing and preparing for the day's work every morning from 7.30–8. Back again at my electrical work from 8.15–12 and again from 1–4.30 or 5 except two days a week when I have free time from 2–6 and work from 6–8.30 with a break for dinner. Then with our short-handedness I've been doing half an hour or an hours duty in the wards from 8–9 or so, to relieve other tired folk so you may see I haven't had much spare time. What I have I've used to tear up in a tram to Bonsecours and grub with pick and spade making a long border by our sleeping huts.

16 May 1916
The plants you sent are top hole: they look as if they'd lived in our bed all their lives. We have now got 6 beds. One is all herbaceous perennials with a rose tree or two and a lavender bush and such-like oddments in it. There are a few patches of seeds coming up. The next bed has fewer perennials and more seeds in it – four nice clumps of sweet peas. The next two beds by the *lingerie* are all annuals seeded for stock to pick and the inside ones near the *lingerie* are seeds and perennials again.

There are two military gardeners belonging to the engineers building the hospital and they have been digging for us: they are such nice kind men but our conversation is somewhat limited as they hardly understand any French nor we much Flemish. I think they are astonished that we have got our garden so nice all by ourselves.

All against our hut on the garden side we've planted climbing nasturtiums and morning glory and mignonette to bush at the foot of the climbers.

It will be much nicer when we are up there as it takes half an hour to get up there and sometimes more, and when one only has 3 hours of free time it takes up such an age getting there and back.

27 June 1916
Our garden is looking awfully nice now. We have had some warmer weather with a few showers and the things are galloping up. The anchusa though small is a sea of blue and has a small shoot by its side which looks as if it might have flowers later on. The geum has flowered for ever so long. Then we have pansy edging all round.

Various people among the staff contributed a dozen or dozens of pansies which certainly make a delightful edging to our kind of cottage garden. Then there is a lovely patch of Canterbury bells, white and purple. There are very healthy Michaelmas daisies coming on, and lavender and rose bushes and your Iceland poppies are a glorious splash of orange. Then in the other bed there are sweet williams coming out and rocket, and phloxes growing tall and stout; a lupin nearly over, a hollyhock and campanula pyramidalis and sweet peas galore and lots of other annuals; gypsophila, nasturtiums, godetia, coreopsis and Shirley poppies.

My wrist is all right now and so is the hay fever, at least much better. I have got some new French stuff which is quite good.

I'm frantically busy and heaps of patients and new apparatus.

3 August 1916, Bonsecours
I find the garden perfectly lovely. Gypsophila, clarkia, nasturtiums, Shirley poppies, Iceland poppies, phlox and roses form the chief of our gay show. The sweetpeas will soon be out: everything has grown splendidly while I've been away

The plants I brought out suffered a little from the fact that they were wrapped in cabbage leaves which had rotted. The aubretia cuttings were quite dead. Could you send me the names of the sweet williams as I want to write for some seeds.

The work has increased even while I have been away. Fifty new patients during the fortnight that I was on leave and only about 10 left.

14 August 1916, Bonsecours
The weather here is very hot but today has been cooler with showers of rain, for which I have been very grateful as the garden wanted it badly. I am busy digging a new bed for the rose trees. It is two yards square, only a little job one would think, but the ground is like iron as it is virgin soil.

On Sunday I had a day off and as I was alone I set off on a walking tour. I left at 9.15 and walked by the long road to Pont de L'Arche, a fine old town higher up the Seine. I arrived there about 2.15 and ate a hearty lunch. Then I set off back again by the short road and got back to the hospital at 7.30 having covered 45 kilometres which is roughly about 27 miles!! Not bad was it! The staff wouldn't believe me at first. I got a bit footsore towards the end as the roads were covered with gritty dust which would get into my shoes, but I enjoyed myself no end and drank gallons of cider on the road in various small cafés.

The garden is lovely. I wish you could see it. I cut quite a lot of sweet peas on Saturday and the Shirley poppies are a sight, so is my campanula pyramidalis which is at least 7 feet high. I have a lovely double primrose-coloured hollyhock too.

20 August 1916
I would rather be at home with you and Father: nothing could be nicer. However I shall instead be feeding weak muscles and wounded nerves and bones and such like to the tune of 300 with their daily dose of electricity in its many forms.

3 September 1916
I have treated 484 patients in the month of August and given over 7,000 treatments – and for the hot air baths which are given by an orderly under my direction we treated nearly 300 patients and gave over 4,000 treatments. I didn't have the hot air baths before, they are in the same room as the electrical things and under Dr Stouffs direction but with a different nurse. Now they are put into my hands which has given me a lot more work.

17 September 1916
We have had some new beds made. One lies between our hut door and the mess. We have filled it with daffodil bulbs and oversown it with alyssum and a deep border of forgetmenot. The seeds are pouring up. The annuals are mostly over save a few climbing nasturtium and morning glories, annual coreopsis and annual lark-

spur. The latter we planted late and are quite a sight only just coming into flower and a good 3 feet high. The things I brought out did splendidly except the pink cuttings. Get Fuller to cut some more and not wrap them in rhubarb leaves: they rotted and made the cuttings rot too. I only want white pinks, we've heaps of pink ones. Also I would like 2 dozen Madonna lily bulbs, 50 chionodoxa, 50 camassia, 2 dozen grape hyacinths, one dozen fritillaria (spotted), and 50 snowdrops mixed single and double – also my gumboots.

14 October 1916
Most of the bulbs are in the ground. We have had 5 days running without rain here, almost a miracle. So we have been digging and forking and planting bulbs for all we are worth. I think we have worked every day for a fortnight in the garden. The campanula pyramidalis is still in flower. We have got 2 baby frames made of packing cases sawed diagonally in half and with lids put on them (glass of course). We put manure and soil in them and are raising seeds and cuttings for next year. The pinks haven't rooted yet but they look quite happy.

15 November 1916
I have been planting rose trees with Tim in the bed I dug on Sunday. It makes the garden look awfully swishy! Then we planted some belated bulbs. It is sickening how we've been delayed with our bulbs owing to the ground having been soaked. Yesterday the frost came and today it is awfully cold too.

My work grows apace: we are going to do X-ray treatments as well as X-ray photos now: it will be intensely interesting but very delicate work. There is always something new cropping up: new discoveries are being made every day and it behoves us to experiment with as many as we can.

30 November 1916
It is bitterly cold and raw and bites into the marrow of one's bones. Fortunately we have a big stove in the Mess and some little ones in our sleeping huts but in spite of them we scuttle quickly into our beds at night and throw on our garments in the morning very hastily.

The garden is feeling very miserable: things have a tendency to damp off in this beastly cold weather.

12 December 1916
Can you raise a big Turkey for Christmas? I have promised to be responsible for one. There are about 24 of us so it will have to be a hefty fellow. It must go to this address: Miss Moberg, 45 Princes Square, Hyde Park, London W. I hope this is not an awful nuisance for you and that you will be able to get it off in time, if not there will be 24 very hungry disappointed people on Christmas Day.

13 December 1916
We are full of preparations for Christmas. We shall try and make things as jolly as possible for the men. It is not so easy to plan for 1,000 odd as for 270 as it was last year.

We are doing a little show of our own on Boxing Day. Tim and I and four other nurses are doing two little plays in our Mess for the others and the doctors. One of them is 'Between the Soup and the Savoury', that hardy perennial. I am again doing the cook's part.

The weather is absolutely beastly. Today is a thick raw fog, bitingly cold.

27 December 1916
It was very sad that the turkey misfired. Miss Moberg turned up without it. She was very sad at not having received it, but these things will happen – especially in wartime. Luckily a benevolent Government provided us with one …

Miss V.C.C. Collum

Scottish Women's Hospital, Royaumont Abbey, France

After her rescue from the torpedoed SS Sussex, *Miss Collum was taken from the hospital ship to a small civilian hospital and then by ambulance train to a hospital in London. Here she was treated for spine injuries, internal bruising, a strained back and thigh muscles, and a broken foot. She was not allowed to return to Royaumont for three months, and arrived back to take up her duties in the X-Ray Department, just before the 1916 Somme offensive. Miss Frances Ivens was the chief medical officer. The other doctors at the time were Miss Ruth Nicholson, who was second-in-command and the principal surgeon after Miss Ivens; Dr Elizabeth Courtauld; Dr Agnes Savill; Dr Augusta Berry; Dr Elsie Jean Dalyell; and Dr Edith Martland. There was accommodation for 400 wounded in the hospital.*

1 July 1916! This is one of the half-dozen dates that will be branded for ever on the memories of every man and woman throughout France and Greater Britain.

We waited, full of tense, suppressed excitement. Our hospital had been evacuated almost to the last man. Our new emergency ward of 80 beds had been created in what had once been as big as an English parish church: our theatre and our receiving rooms had been supplied with a huge reserve of bandages and swabs, of lint and gauze and wool; our new X-rays installation had been fitted up to the last connection; our ambulances were waiting, ready to start at a moment's notice, in the garage yard. The incessant thunder and boom of the great guns had never been silent for days. This day, at dawn, the thunder had swelled to an orgy of terrific sound that made the whole earth shiver; then, a few hours later, had ceased, and we could hear once more the isolated reports of individual cannon. Those of us who had been at the hospital through the attacks of June 1915, and the more serious push in Artois, beginning on 25 September 1915, went early to bed. If the call came in the night, we could always be summoned – meanwhile we slept when we could.

2 July dawned. The morning hours dragged on, placid in the hot sunshine of high summer. Our ambulances were called out to await the first train of wounded at our clearing station. It was at noonday dinner that the telephone message came through that they were arriving shortly with bad cases.

The long blast of a whistle from the entrance hall. This was the porter announcing the arrival of the first convoy from Creil, sixteen stretcher cases. No sooner had the men been lifted out and carried to the various receiving rooms than the cars went back to the gare régulatrice for more. Trains were arriving from the Somme in one long stream. The drivers never ceased journeying backwards and forwards all that afternoon and all that night, and the three women and the man who drove our four ambulances carried over 100 cases during the first forty-eight hours of that nightless week.

They slept a little by turns, so that during the first twenty days of the great push there were always some of our cars at the clearing station, night or day, and the cases distributed to our hospital never had to wait there longer than was necessary.

Very soon, the first cases were brought, already washed and prepared for operation to the X-ray rooms. At first we worked the new installation only; then, as the men were brought up more quickly than we could deal with them, our Radiologist passed from one room to the other, making the examination herself, and leaving me to finish the photograph. Still we found we were not keeping up with the supply of fresh cases, and then she handed the smaller room, with the Butt installation, over to me, and herself worked the new Gaife installation, so that each case, as the stretcher was brought in and placed on the table, was examined at once, and we were able to deal with two at a time. The other assistant remained in the dark room, developing the plates.

Very soon the surgeon-in-chief was hard at work, with the anaesthetist and an assistant, in the operating theatre, each ward surgeon bringing up her own cases and assisting with them. It grew dark, and still the wounded came in. By ten o'clock we had a long line of stretchers lying in the corridor outside the X-ray rooms and the theatre. At one end wounded men waiting to be examined by us; at the other, those who had already been examined and who were waiting their turn for operation.

The two storekeepers, and the kitchen orderlies, who had gone off duty, organised themselves into a stretcher squad, and kept the X-ray couches and the operating table supplied. Down another corridor the other assistant radiographer had ranged her developed plates to dry – dozens of them. Some time after midnight our doctor had to retire to bed. She was not a strong woman, and she had to be ready for the new day's work at 8am. At four o'clock the other assistant, having developed sixty-three photographs since two o'clock in the afternoon, followed her. We knew the surgeons now had more cases ready for them than they could possibly operate on during the night. One or two of the ward surgeons dropped off, aware that they would have to begin work early in the morning. But the theatre went on, and the other surgeons who were waiting their turn to get their most urgent cases done, filled up the time by getting on with the list to be examined under the X-rays.

I went to bed when the theatre was closed for cleaning at 7am. The surgeons went to bed too, with the theatre Sister and her staff of two women orderlies, leaving the rest of the cleaning to be done by the night-duty orderlies from some of the less busy wards.

At eleven o'clock I went back to the X-ray room to find that the doctor and the other assistant had been hard at work since 8am, and that the surgeon-in-chief had already made great headway with her ward visits, while all the ward surgeons were busy with dressings. I went to the dark room.

Cases continued to come in all day, but as everyone was a stretcher case, and each car could only carry four, while the clearing station was 12 kilometres distant, the hospital was able to absorb them as they came in, so that there was little if any delay in attending to the poor fellows.

I worked through that day without pause after my four hours of real night sleep, and knocked off at about 11pm, leaving the other assistant single-handed to finish the night work. I had not been asleep an hour when there was a rap on the door, and an orderly called to me to come down at once, as a new convoy had come in and some of the cases needed immediate operation. I was wanted to develop the plates while the other assistant went on with the examinations. I do not think I have ever felt so sleepy and tired as I did when I got downstairs. We worked as in a dream. My legs and hands did not seem to belong to me, and I heard my own voice far away as if it came from somebody else. It had become impossible to work quickly, and I found it necessary to make great efforts to remember little things and to do them correctly. We got to bed again before the dawn.

The wounds were terrible. The men were mostly from the famous Colonial Division, or from such crack corps as the Chasseurs Alpins. They had broken the German line – but how they had suffered! Former cases treated in our hospital had been single wounds: many of these men were wounded – dangerously – in two, three, four, and five places. Gas gangrene was already at work in 90 per cent of the cases. Hence the urgent need for immediate operation, often for immediate amputation. The surgeons did not stop to search for shrapnel and pieces of metal: their one aim was to open up and clean out the wounds, or to cut off the mortifying limb before the dread gangrene had tracked its way into the vital parts of the body. The stench of it was very bad. Most of the poor fellows were too far gone to say much, but one and all bore their agony and the foulness of their terrible wounds with a bravery that must make every hospital worker know human beings to be, in some sort, divine. Those who cried out and moaned had passed beyond full consciousness and their own control.

There was one boy – a lad of twenty-one – hopelessly injured, though the surgeons never admit the hopelessness of any man's case till death has proved it. He was hurt in so many places that it was difficult and slow work moving him into suitable positions for his radiographic examination. He helped us all he could, and when it was over, and his stretcher was being lifted off the table, he apologised in the neatest of phrases for giving us all so much trouble when we must be very tired. He died a few hours later.

Each shift worked for twelve hours on end. But the surgeons could devise no system of shifts. Even when they got four or five hours in bed by a stroke of luck, they were constantly being called up to serious cases and to emergency operations. With such a high percentage of gas gangrene in the wounds, and with the men in such a state of exhaustion after hard fighting, cases were liable to take a turn for the worse at any moment, and further incisions, and often amputation, had to be resorted to in order to save the men's lives. By this time a second operating theatre had been improvised in the annexe of a small ward, and the junior surgeons dealt with the smaller operations here to relieve the pressure on the regular theatre.

The wards were an unforgettable sight. Light dressings and gallows splints were the order of the day. Morning dressings were no sooner over than evening dressings had to begin. Stretchers were constantly coming and going from the receiving room, the theatre, the X-ray rooms. It must have been heart-breaking to nurses accustomed to the clockwork round and the neat rows of counterpaned beds in civil hospitals at home. To the girls who were serving as ward orderlies – and during this period of stress often had to play the part of staff nurses – it must have been a long drawn-out period of dreadful strain and physical fatigue. The day staffs would work on till nearly midnight to help the night staffs; and the night staffs, instead of going off duty at 9am, would work on in the wards till dinner-time to help the day people. In the same way the kitchen staff, the laboratory orderly, the storekeepers, and Vestiare clerk, would wait up every night till long after midnight, working as a volunteer stretcher squad to carry the stretchers backwards and forwards between the wards and the operating theatre. When they went to bed, the cases were carried by the theatre Sister and her assistants; and if they were busy swabbing up a too slippery floor, the surgeons would carry them themselves. The ward orderlies were generally far too busy attending to bad cases in the wards to be able to spare time to carry their cases up to the theatre.

Several of the poor fellows died; the only wonder was that they had lasted so long, wounded as they had been, after an exhausting struggle and then sent on that long journey by ambulance and train from the Somme railheads to our clearing station. Many of them came from the Division Marrocain – not that first famous Division which protected the rear of the French Army in its retreat from Belgium – it had been annihilated – but the Division which cleared out the German first-line trenches in the Somme advance – cleared them, treading on the skirts of the wonderful French barrage, with long keen knives, that the picked French infantry might follow and hold them and use them as an attacking trench for their assault on the second and third lines.

These poor black fellows from Senegal, and the Arabs from Tunis and Algeria, were very severely wounded: men with less iron constitutions must have died where they fell of such wounds. Yet the agony of their wounds was as nothing to the terror of their minds when they realised that a visit to the operating theatre often meant the loss of a mangled and gangrenous limb. They spoke only a few words of pigeon French, and the horrible legend spread among them that the first visit to the theatre meant incisions – mere senseless slashes of the surgeon's knife, to their unsophisticated intelligences; the second, amputation. And the third, the slitting of their throats. It was days before their terror subsided, and weeks before their suspicious fear of the white women with sharp knives and wicked-looking forceps gave place to the dog-like devotion and gratitude that characterised their attitude to surgeons, nurses, and orderlies eventually.

One broad-nosed, woolly-headed giant, black as ebony, awakened from the anaesthetic (which drugged these coloured men much less deeply than their white comrades) on the operating table; he looked round in abject fear, though the instruments were all in the tray and the orderly had almost finished bandaging him; then his eyes lighted on the chief surgeon (divested of her gloves and gauze mask), who, as it happened, had dressed him in the ward and evidently gained his confidence. A black arm shot out towards her as she made towards the door, and clutched her hand, which he grasped and laid against his cheek, closing his eyes contentedly once more as he murmured, 'Moi connais toi'. Another, whose arm had just been amputated, and who, inconveniently coming round as he was being borne on the stretcher back to his ward, suddenly leapt from it and made as if to bolt. The head surgeon came out of the theatre, when he immediately calmed down, and, letting her take his remaining arm, walked docilely – and quite capably – upstairs and back to his bed.

Of actual physical suffering from their injuries they had no fear. Never have I seen such pluck as was shown by these native soldiers of France on our X-ray table. They never let a sound escape them, and they made every effort to do as they were bid when asked to move injured limbs or to assume difficult and painful positions. Once or twice I have known them ask if the rays were going to burn them – not in fear, but merely in order to know what they had to face. One little fellow of twenty-one, with a face like a child's golliwog, had enough shrapnel in him to kill three white men. His arm – both bones shattered beyond repair, and so full of metal that it would have been impossible to put a sixpenny-bit on any clear part of the X-ray photograph of it and not have covered a piece of shell – was amputated; but his thigh, from knee to buttock equally full of bits of metal, was left, since the buttock itself had been literally torn away.

One, badly wounded, and maimed for ever, would piteously ask: 'Why? Why?' His country was at peace, his village had not declared war, and his tribe had scarcely heard the name of France's enemy. Then why had they to fight and die with the French? None of them, I believe, understand that they belonged to an empire, and that their lives were being sacrificed for the security of their own homes no less than for those of their French comrades. They were fighting for the French, and they were proud of their prowess in the great war, and – most of them – they accepted death or maiming as part of the inevitable price of a great battle.

The Arabs were very different patients: highly strung, nervous, complaining of their sufferings, they nevertheless bore them bravely enough when they became almost more than human nature could support. Their mental pain must have been acute when the strange foreign women, rather than allow them to die in possession of their shattered limbs, took them off, and thereby closed for ever the gates of Paradise against them should they succumb after all. If they recovered, the loss of a limb troubled them little; but when they came face to face with death, it must have been bitter for the orthodox to face eternal banishment from Paradise as well. There was one little Tunisian who lost his arm, a mere lad: he was proud beyond belief of his two years of campaigning, and his devotion and gratitude to the foreign women who had looked after him was touching.

It is the courage of the French soldier that I remember most poignantly. There was one who was brought to my table with both shoulders horribly injured, and the wound in one already gangrenous. It was exquisite torture for him to be moved, lying, as he was, on his wounds: yet it would have hurt him impossibly to turn him over on to his face. I examined him under the rays, and found the clavicle on the right side broken, and five large pieces of shrapnel lodged in his shoulder. Then I found three pieces on the other side. I sent a message to his ward surgeon to ask what she wished done, and she asked that the larger pieces might be localised and both shoulders photographed. The poor fellow had to be shifted for each photograph. Then, after a rough calculation, it appeared that the pieces lay nearer the surface of his back than of his chest, but he could not be turned over for more accurate measurements to be made. So his ward surgeon, with our own radiologist, who left another case to come and see him, both came and looked at his injuries through the fluorescent screen, saw for themselves in what difficult positions the pieces of shell had lodged, and decided that the only means of getting the necessary information as to precise depth and situation was to have stereoscopic photographs. I was left to carry out their instructions. Before that man was taken away he had had two direct ray photographs taken, stereos of both shoulders (i.e., two photographs of each shoulder), and two or three localisations, and he had been lying there an hour on the hard table, suffering dreadfully. Yet he never uttered a word of protest or complaint, and murmured something cheery when we parted. A long wait, and then he was carried to the theatre to have the gangrenous wounds cleaned up. To endure all that after hours of tense waiting for the attack, more strenuous hours of fighting, and the noisy hell of a modern bombardment; then those two shattering wounds, and the long wait, under fire, for succour; and after that the painful journey to the dressing-station, and then the long journey by ambulance train and motor …

Miss Olive Dent

Race Course Hospital, Rouen, France

On 1 July 1916, the first day of the Battle of the Somme, the hospital was prepared for the wounded but no one had realised that the number of casualties would be so high.

We knew what to expect. For days and nights past we had heard the guns ceaselessly cannonading. So when the batman woke us at six one morning with the message that everyone was to go on duty as quickly as possible, we were not surprised.

We washed, dressed, and breakfasted hurriedly. It was a glorious morning with great glowing shafts of streaming sunlight warmly irradiating the camp. The tent walls had as usual been rolled back, thus making of the wards a roof and a floor.

In every walk there were wounded soldiers, a bus-load of the more slightly wounded cases at one marquee, motor ambulances with stretcher after stretcher of more seriously injured burdens bringing up the rear, men being carried pick-a-back by orderlies, others being brought on the 'four-handed seat', others trudging along with the aid of a walking-stick.

Tunics had been torn to free wounded arms, breeches had been ripped for access to injured legs, boots had been discarded in favour of huge carpet slippers or bandages, heads were swathed, jaws tied up, bandages stained with dirt and blood.

Almost every boy was clay-caked, the hair full of yellow clayey dust, the face thinly crusted with it, the moustache partly embedded in it.

The first batch of patients we treated stands out in any memory. They were fed, bathed, put into clean pyjamas, had their wounds dressed, were each given Blighty tickets and cigarettes, and lay with faces expressive of the personification of blissful contentment.

On and on we worked, forgetful of time and remembering our own meal only as we became exhausted. Trestle beds with a paliasse, or donkey's breakfast, as the boys call them, had been laid down in the wards. The church tent, the store tent, and the YMCA hut had been requisitioned, and some Indian marquees sprang up infinitely more quickly than the proverbial mushroom. These took the slight cases of which, fortunately, there was a very large proportion.

Everyone 'mucked in' in that magnificent whole-hearted way British people have when they are 'up against' anything. Rank and officialdom were forgotten, chiefly by those who held the one and were held responsible for the other. Everyone turned with enthusiasm to the task they had in hand. Whatever our hand found to do on that memorable day and the four following days, we did with all our might. Our colonel and medical major, kept waiting a few minutes in the middle of the night for a convoy they were to receive, put off their coats and helped cut bread and butter for the coming patients.

A dentist, finished his dental work, did nursing-orderly duty far through the night. The Padre ladled out soup and tea, at which he said he was an expert through long practice in soup kitchens and at Sunday School teas. He ran about unceasingly, too, giving patients drinks, quite a big item in the case of newly wounded men and with the weather very hot. He also acted as additional barber and went round with safety razor preparing for our further attention, surrounding surfaces of wounds on shin, cheek, jaw and head.

Laughter, tears, immense satisfaction and pleasure, immeasurable pain and disappointment were commingled that day. One lived very many times in a torrent of emotion, agonised by a flood of pity, racked by an intensity of sympathy, tortured by an exquisite, mental pain, almost overwhelmed by the passion to help to fight for those lives. So the day wore on and night came. Without – a night of glorious July summer, with palest saffron, flamingo and purple lights, and one gem-like star, a night of ineffable beauty and peace, and within – a vision of Hell, cruel flesh-agony, hideous writhings, broken moanings, a boy-child sitting up in bed gibbering and pulling off his head bandages, a young Colonial coughing up his last life-blood, a big, so lately strong man with ashen face and blue lips, lying quite still but for a little fluttering breathing …

Miss Mildred Rees

No. 4 Ambulance Flotilla, Barge 192, The Somme, France

Staff Nurse Mildred Rees was born and trained in New Zealand and arrived in England in February 1910. In August 1914 she had just completed her maternity training at Dundee Hospital and was immediately accepted by Millicent, Duchess of Sutherland as one of eight trained nurses who spent six weeks in Belgium in the Millicent, Duchess of Sutherland's Ambulance Unit [qv]. After she returned to England Mildred Rees applied to join the Queen Alexandra's Imperial Military Nursing Service Reserve (QAIMNSR). She spent ten months at No. 3 Stationary Hospital in Rouen and two months at No. 9 General Hospital in Rouen. After four weeks recuperating in London from 'influenza disability' she returned to France in April 1916 and nursed for a month at No. 10 Stationary Hospital at St Omer, followed by five months with No. 4 Ambulance Flotilla on the River Somme. She was then aged forty-seven.

[20 July 1916]
It is just about twenty days since the big advance began so during that time, at least by tomorrow night, we shall have carried exactly 300 patients in this one barge alone – all of them serious cases, in fact we get those that are not able to go in the trains. We have them on (board) from 24 to 36 hours, occasionally 48 hours, but as a rule only one night, for which Sister and I are very thankful, as we always share the night, Sister staying on until 2am, then I get up. Generally we are too busy to rest in the day.

As soon as we get them comfortably to bed we then proceed to cut off their dirty khaki, and as they are splattered with blood and mud you can imagine the state it is in. They, poor things, are out on the ground 12 to 40 hours before they are brought to the first Field Dressing Station, so you can think how exhausted they are. The marvel to me is that they recover and live, and they do in a most wonderful way, even when they are most frightfully wounded. As soon as we get their dirty clothes off we wash them and dress them and feed them, and they then sleep in a marvellous way, notwithstanding their terrible wounds. They love the barge and it does them (the trip) the world of good. I only wish it was longer. Last time we brought down some Australian officers, and I am afraid this time many, many men, as they have had an awfully bad time taking a village, but have done splendidly. So far there have been no New Zealanders in this part of the battle for which I am thankful.

I am writing this (3am) while looking after the men. We loaded up at 3pm yesterday. This is, so far, the least severe we have had since the first. Actually no amputations, only 5 compound fractures of arms and legs, 4 abdominals, and only 6 chest wounds, although many of the men are wounded in 5 or 6 places. Still they are not in the dangerous state the others were in. The last two trips we had a death each time. We are drawn in beside a lock, and as straight as the crow flies we are about 10 miles from the firing line, and the guns are going all the time – just one continuous thundering noise the big guns make at a distance. We are also near the railway line and the trains go night and day with troops or war material. Close beside us are barges with stores and things for the trenches, and roads, which are worked by German prisoners with French guards; in fact these days the whole river is most interesting. At one place we pass a large cavalry encampment and if this happens in the morning, all the men are grooming their horses, which are just dears, and so beautifully groomed.

Miss Lesley Smith

No. 129 General Hospital, Near Camiers, France

Lesley Smith, having attended Red Cross first aid classes after she left school, went to the Royal Sussex Hospital in Brighton as a VAD. She was called up by the War Office to serve in France and left London in November 1915. She travelled to Boulogne with fifty other VADs, one of whom, Miss Gratton, immediately became a friend. They were both sent to a general hospital near Camiers. This large hospital, under canvas, had '1,500 patients, several hundred orderlies and 15–20 medical officers'. In July 1916 after a few months nursing a constant stream of casualties, Lesley Smith went on night duty to 'B' Ward, one of three wards containing serious cases.

A, B, and C were the only huts in the hospital, and on nights they were all under one Sister with a VAD in each. A was mostly amputations with a very few abdominals. Most of the abdominal cases were taken from the CCS in barges to Abbeville or Amiens to prevent all unnecessary movement. B ward was heads and C was chests. Sister Barrow left me in B with instructions not to send for her unless I had to, and an assurance that there was nothing that need frighten me. I wasn't really frightened yet: I still had a certain confidence in my ability to cope with the ordinary events of the night, especially with a Sister behind me all the time.

I did not know then that there were no ordinary events in a head ward.

The hut looked reassuringly normal. There was a row of grey-blanketed beds stretching into the darkness on either side of a solid substantial kitchen table, and the lights, already shaded with red handkerchiefs, shone on the usual array of jugs and bowls and lotions. But the utter normality of the surroundings only intensified the horror of madness.

Fantasy should be clothed in fantastic garb, and should not stray among solid tables and rows of grey beds. Voices that speak of green teeth – millions of them – should speak in tones of awe or frenzied horror, not in the quiet matter-of-fact manner that is suitable for discussing the weather.

After I had seen the kitchen table transformed by the queer lucidity of delirium into an orchard, and the dressing pail become a policeman, I lost faith in my own power to keep things as I knew they really were and allowed my mind to go through facts as my body went through the ghostly visitants who thronged round the beds.

I became accustomed to shouts and alarms but never to a quiet and collected madness.

At the end of a week I had learned how to deal with many terrors and hallucinations, and I stood in the middle of the ward, with my back to the wall, and waited for a shout or a movement.

It came suddenly from a man beside me. He sat up in bed with a pointing finger and shrieked:

'They're at it again, Sister. Ow, fer God's sake do 'em in before they're on to me. Sister, 'ere they come; see all them rats.'

Instinctively I followed his pointing finger and saw, not rats, as I had almost expected, but the man in the opposite bed sliding his legs stealthily over the side of his bed, and I called to him as I ran:

'It's all right, old man, I'm coming.'

But he never looked at me, he just went on slipping his legs free of the bedclothes. I held his shoulders gently and told him in the correct soothing voice that it was all right – everything was all right. He looked straight through me – as if contemptuous of my fatuous remarks – I couldn't blame him, but I had to try to stop him from getting out of bed.

'It's all right, old man,' I reiterated wearily.

'It bloody well is,' he said, and fell back on his pillow.

'Ninety-nine, ninety-eight, ninety-nine, ninety-seven.' That interminable counting had gone on night after night. It disturbed no one. No one heard it except me and I didn't know if I heard it or not. I only knew that I was always conscious of numbers charging in ordered sequence through my brain.

'Ninety-six, ninety-seven, ninety-nine.'

Number Seven raised himself on his elbow and said in a quiet, prim voice:

'Sister, I must ask you to be so good as to address a few words to those boys who are troubling me.'

'Certainly, Mr Carson,' I answered. I knew these boys; they were a constant annoyance to us, they would try to steal the fruit from Number Seven's orchard. He had some special pears which had only borne fruit this year, and I was very firm with the boys. I walked straight up to the steriliser and, looking severely at it, said: 'Now boys, I've warned you once about stealing these pears and if I have to speak to you again about it I shall report the matter to the police, do you quite understand?' I wagged my finger at the steriliser.

'Ninety-nine, ninety-seven, ninety-eight, ninety-nine.'

'I shall undoubtedly report …'

'Mary, oh Mary, where are you?' It was Number twenty-four.

'Here I am,' I answered, 'just coming. I've put the kettle on for your tea. I knew you'd be in soon.'

Number Seven had a fixed belief that the ward was on fire and he sat up in bed and threw imaginary water over the flames. I helped him for a moment and then assured him that the fire had been quite put out, and he lay back at rest for a time.

'Ninety-seven, ninety-eight, ninety-nine.'

A slight sound disturbed me and I turned quickly. Bowers had got right out of bed and was squatting like an obscene China ornament underneath it. His head was a white rotating mass of bandages and one arm was missing. All the king's horses and all the king's men would never be able to put him together again, but he wouldn't die, if I could only keep him quiet and in bed. He would always be in an asylum, of course, but the whole world would be an asylum after the war – bound to be to take us all in. At the back of my mind I knew that it was midnight and that things would seem more reasonable in the daylight, but it was easier to relax the tension and allow my thoughts to chatter inconsequently than to hold on to reality.

'Ninety-seven, ninety-eight, ninety ninety, ninety-nine.'

I stopped aghast, conscious through all my being that the rhythm had changed. He had begun to hiccup, but I could not go to 'Ninety-nine' until I had got Bowers back to bed.

I tried to coax him in vain and at last sat on the floor beside him, and when the orderly officer came in I was playing imaginary cards with Bowers and listening anxiously to ninety-nine. The orderly officer was a new man with a chinless face like a rabbit. As I looked up from our cards, I realised that guest night had been too much for him, and he could not get down the ward to where I was sitting. I called to him that I would come in a moment, Sister wanted morphia ordered for numbers seven and eleven. He waved a feeble hand and said:

'S'all right, don' hurry, little girl.'

I coaxed Bowers back to bed with great difficulty and then joined my helpful medical officer.

He seized my hand and stroked it murmuring:

'Poo lil gal, poo lil gal, give them all four grams morphia and have a peashful night.'

It was quite natural in 'Heads', nothing could have seemed odd. I thanked him for his sympathy, led him firmly to the door, and hoped that he would fall down the steps. But I hadn't time to waste on guest-night casualties. 'Ninety-nine' might possibly have a flicker of consciousness before the end. I ran back to look at him, there had been nothing to be seen through the mass of bandages but two eye-holes and a gash for the mouth, but at last there was a change, a trickle of blood was dribbling slowly out of the gash and soaking the white bandage. Old ninety-nine would not count much further. The new rhythm was strangely disturbing:

'Ninety ninety ninety – hic – seven, ninety ninety-nine, hic, ninety hic, ninety hic.' He was obviously just going. Well, there wasn't anything to be done and it was no use disturbing Sister, she was having a heavy night in 'Chests'.

I walked to the middle of the ward and stood with my back to the wall again, peering in every direction. A noise at the far end, like the scratching of a rat, ceased as I looked round, then began again. I walked quietly down the ward, but half-way I was stopped by seeing that Bowers had begun sliding his legs over the edge of the bed again and was almost on the floor. I ran back and, while talking about cards and the game we had just had, managed to lift his legs into bed once more and tuck the clothes tightly round. Night Sister came in and I walked the length of the ward with her and agreed that it was quite a quiet night. At the end she said:

'A convoy is expected through. Have you many beds here, Nurse?'

'Six, Sister,' I answered.

'Well, let's hope they don't come till the morning. We need an occasional quiet night.'

I hadn't located the scraping noise in the corner, so I walked back after seeing Sister out and flashed my torch up and down between the beds. There was a little whimper from a young boy at the far end who had lost his leg and a bit of his skull. He usually lay blind and silent but now I saw that he was lying on his back, crying gently and waving the bloody stump of his leg in the air. He had carefully unrolled the bandages and thrown them under the bed, and every time he looked at the stump he whimpered again.

'Ninety-six, ninety ninety ninety, hic, ninety-nine.' The counting was stronger again; anyhow, it didn't matter; but Evans's leg did. I ran for the orderly and asked him to go and fetch Sister from 'Chests'. As I was getting the dressing tray ready I saw that the blood had oozed half over ninety-nine's bandage and again I told myself that it didn't matter. Bowers still eyed me suspiciously, but the clothes were tightly tucked in and it always took him five minutes to ease them loose enough to get his legs out. The others were tossing and muttering but safely in bed. I took the tray up to Evans's bed and the bucket for soiled dressings. In a minute Sister came breathlessly up the ward.

'Everything ready? Good. Having a hectic time in "Chests". Sorry I've had to leave you so much, but it's a quiet night here, isn't it?' She nodded towards Evans. 'Go and hold his hand and talk to him while I do his leg again. We'll have to move his bed up to the middle of the ward if he is going to be troublesome.'

I held Evans's hand firmly but gently in the manner one instinctively adopts as a reassurance. He looked at me wildly and cried like a little boy who has been scolded.

'Don't stare at him, Nurse,' said Sister impatiently. 'Talk! Tell him he is a good boy. Anything bright like that.' She had managed to renew the dressing by this time and was rolling the bandage on tightly.

I talked and talked – a murmur of banal conversation poured over his head, but Evans only whimpered again. He looked straight through me and was frightened at what he saw there and cried again.

'Ninety-nine, ninety-seven, ninety-nine, nine hic ninety hic.'

Sister looked up startled.

'It's changed, hasn't it?'

At that minute the orderly from A tore in.

'Please, Sister! Nurse says would you come at once, there's a haemorrhage.'

'Take this, Nurse.' She handed me the remains of Evans's leg and was gone.

'Mary, oh Mary, I want you.' The plaintive appeal in his voice was heartrending, even though I knew that it was quite unconscious and that I made a perfectly good Mary. But, before I could answer, the corporal opened the door of the hut and called:

'Four stretchers, Sister.'

The bearers tramped in, up the length of the ward, and then laid the stretchers on the floor and stood waiting, dumb with exhaustion and almost as indifferent as the patients. I stopped to fumble amongst the folds of brown blanket on a stretcher for the case sheet. It only said 'Gunshot wound of head', but a filthy bandage covered the whole side of the man's head and there seemed to be no response in his one unblinking eye.

I hurriedly rolled the clothes back from one of the centre beds which were kept for the most difficult patients, shouted to one of the orderlies to give an eye to Bowers who was trying to take advantage of the confusion to get under his bed again, and then signed to the bearers to bring the first man up. He lay unmoving and helpless, unable even to put an arm round my neck as I knelt on the bed and tried to lift him. Suddenly Matron slipped her arms in beside mine, said 'Now' in a quiet voice, and we drew the solid mass of filthy khaki on to the bed, folded the clothes over him and left him. The General [Matron] waited to help me till we had got our four stretchers in bed, then said abruptly:

'Can you manage, Nurse? Sister will be back soon.'

I was just going to say that I could manage when twenty-four gave a terrified shriek of 'Mary!' as if he had suddenly realised that he was deserted. I ran to hold on to him and old 'ninety-nine' gave a last triumphant shout of 'Ninety ninety hic nine' and was silent for the first time since he had come in three days ago. A breathless pause held us stationary for a moment, then Matron tramped out saying 'I'll send Sister.'

She had evidently just got out of bed and was in pyjamas and gumboots and an overcoat. I had forgotten that the night must be nearly over, but another pallid dawn had dimmed the lights and shone grey and cold through the windows. I sat down to write the requisition for a shroud before beginning to do anything for the new patients, and then Sister came back from the lower ward and we put the red screens round ninety-nine and began to lay him out.

I rolled him over gently towards me, and the unwieldy white roll of bandages that was his head suddenly fell on the pillow as if it had decided reluctantly to follow the body. There was a crash in the ward and I ran out from behind the screens. Number seventeen had found something to put the flames out with at last and had thrown a whole bottle of eusol on to the floor. I threw some imaginary water to add to the mess, and soon had him back again on to his pillows.

'Bring the dressing tray as you come back, Nurse,' Sister called from behind the screens.

'We'll have to do this head again. I'm sorry,' she added as I appeared with the tray, 'we can't let him go to the mortuary like this.' She cut through the stained bandage as she spoke, squeezed a handful of wet swabs, and said:

'Now, Nurse, lift his head a little.'

I put my hand at the back of his head and then dropped it and laughed and laughed. The funniest thing had happened. My hand had gone right through the bandages. There was no head there! And as I laughed Evans started crying again and his childish whimper cut across the noise I was making and I stopped. Sister ran and I followed. Evans had got his bandage off again and lay waving that awful bloody stump in the cold light of the early morning.

'We'd better finish old ninety-nine first, Nurse. Evans will be all right for a minute or two, and please don't be silly again, there isn't time.'

I murmured an obedient 'No, Sister,' and we went back behind the screens. I held what was left of that rolling head and then went to help to tie up Evans's leg once more. Sister looked at the light, which was filling the whole ward by this time, and said:

'Good Lord, we're late, of course. Go over and get a cup of tea before you begin on the new people, Nurse, and eat some bread and cheese with it, there's a long way to go yet.'

The night bunk was thick with the fumes of the oil stove and the smell of food and macintoshes. Everyone had eaten at some time or other and left dirty plates and crumbs, but only Gracie was finishing a cup of tea when I went in. There was still a little milk at the bottom of the tin. I snatched it hurriedly before Gracie could take it, scraped round for the last smear of butter and sat humped in a corner with my bread and cheese.

'Busy?' said Gracie at last. I nodded.

'"Heads" is pretty bad, isn't it?' Then suddenly she leant across and whispered: 'Look here, I've hidden a tin of milk on the top of the cupboard for emergencies. We could have some bread and milk if you can wait for a minute or two.'

I accepted gratefully and ten minutes later went back to B hut through the clear morning light. My mind had stopped chattering and I thought over what there was still to do and reviewed the happenings of the night. Even when fortified by bread and milk I felt sick when I thought how my hand had gone through the hole into ninety-nine's head. I had scrubbed and disinfected but I'd never feel clean again.

I stayed in 'Heads' for eight weeks, and at the end my only happiness was in remembering how few during that time had recovered enough to go home. It was not possible for me to attune myself to the existence of head wounds. Death has its own clean finality; but these men, whose admirable bodies lay inert and helpless at the mercy of a grotesque, obscenely rolling head, seemed a denial of everything beautiful and fair. And I was trapped in their horror. I saw and admitted the triumph of ugliness and evil, and knew that wherever I went afterwards, I would take my own Bedlam with me.

I came off night duty at the end of September and interposed a whole day and night of oblivion between the head ward and day duty. I spent the whole day in a luxury of relaxation that can only be experienced after months of tension and vigilance.

Matron had taken some trouble to arrange that Gratton should have her day off from theatre on the day that I came off night duty, and we could not afford to waste a moment of that golden opportunity.

We cleaned our shoes and powdered our noses and started out to walk to Hardelot for lunch.

Curiously enough Major Brewer suddenly appeared on the road in front of us walking slowly and obviously waiting for us. Theatre Sister had apparently told him that we were lunching at Hardelot and he wanted to come with us. It was a lovely day and we wandered quietly across country, enjoying the unlimited quality of the time ahead of us; the whole day was ours, and all the countryside was new to us and untouched by war. The rolling sand dunes crested by little dwarfed pine trees, the gentle cultivated fields and mud-coloured villages lay remote and innocent beneath a clear blue autumn sky.

We had a leisurely lunch in a real room with windows and a fireplace, and an unfortunate incident, that might have marred the day, luckily only added to our enjoyment.

Just as we had finished a mountainous omelette a feminine voice rang through the hall loudly demanding lunch.

'Good God! It's the Matron-in-Chief' [Miss Macarthy], said Gratton, looking round distractedly for somewhere to hide. But the Major's mind was evidently more alert than I had thought, or perhaps fear may have stimulated it, because in one movement he seized his plate, glass, knife and fork, and before the door could open he had jumped through the window into the garden and was sitting at a little iron-topped table with his back to us. The Matron-in-Chief came in and looked extremely suspicious when she saw us sitting there alone, but when Madame caught sight of the Major's innocent-looking head in the back garden, a faint gleam of amusement showed that she had a Gallic appreciation of the situation. We rose at once, of course, and stood to attention. Matron-in-Chief asked us a few questions about our movements and the unit to which we belonged, and we answered with painstaking conscientiousness. At length she departed – but only into the next room.

In a few minutes Madame returned with our coffee and with delighted gestures waved her hands at the rigid back of the poor Major. He daren't even come to the window for his coffee, but Madame had pity on him and, wrapping a large black shawl round her shoulders, she took his coffee out to him and a note scribbled on the back of the menu to say that we would start in exactly five minutes and would walk down the Boulogne road.

We met again successfully and congratulated the Major on his duplicity. It was all very amusing and childish, but the consequences of being found out would have been neither! Very probably Major Brewer would have been sent up the line and we should have found ourselves cleaning vegetables for sick Sisters at Abbeville or carrying trays to convalescent officers.

We celebrated our escape by drinking sirops in an estaminet, which only seemed romantic, rather than sordid, because it was so strange and dark, and then we went down to the shore and lay among the sand dunes watching the odd little birds that inhabit that coast.

At last it was time to start back to camp, and we reluctantly turned on to the road again and began to walk hard towards bed and supper. Just before we reached Camiers the lights of a car showed on a turn of the road ahead of us. Immediately we stopped dead and Major Brewer shot ahead and was walking 250 yards in front of us when the car swung past. It was the Matron-in-Chief again and, if she recognised us, she must have had an annoying ten minutes …

1916
Malta

Miss Vera Brittain

St George's Hospital, Malta

After her fiancé, Roland Leighton, was killed at Louvencourt in December 1915, Vera's friendship with two other young men gradually deepened through correspondence. Victor Richardson had been at Uppingham School with Roland and her brother Edward – and Geoffrey Thurlow was serving in the 10th Battalion Sherwood Foresters with Edward.

On 24 September 1916 Vera sailed for Malta with a contingent of VADs on board the hospital ship Britannic. *She was still grieving for Roland and wrote in her War Diary that leaving England was 'all part of the hard path which I have assigned to myself to tread'. At this time her brother Edward, who had been wounded on the first day of the Battle of the Somme, was training in England; Victor and Geoffrey were in France.*

On board the Britannic *the VADs were given a lecture by the sister in charge on the stringent rules they were to follow and the behaviour that was expected from them during the voyage. Many places were out of bounds and the girls were forbidden to fraternise outside their section of VADs.*

As these arrangements did not separate us from the medical officers as completely as the Sister had intended, she and the Matron of the *Britannic* nursing staff – a 60-year-old 'dug-out' with a red cape and a row of South African medals – ordered a rope to be stretched across the main deck to divide the VAD sheep from the RAMC goats; by this expedient they hoped automatically to terminate the age-long predilection of men and women for each other's society. After a few days, during which the more adventurous of both sexes had edged as near to the rope as they dared, and several others had regarded one another from a distance with eyes full of cupidity, the guardians of our virtue were astonished and pained beyond measure when one or two couples, being denied the opportunity of normal conversation on deck, were found in compromising positions beneath the gangways …

Tuesday 3 October
In the afternoon after sailing safely through three rows of mines we reached Lemnos, and anchored in Mudros harbour … We were told that on the Island are the graves of three Canadian Sisters, who died nursing in the camp hospital there. The place was

grim and sinister looking, yet there was a queer unaccountable fascination about it which would not allow me to take my eyes from it nearly all the afternoon …'

'The Sisters Buried at Lemnos'
('Fidelis ad Extremum')

O golden Isle set in the deep blue Ocean,
With purple shadows flitting o'er thy crest,
I kneel to thee in reverent devotion
Of some who on thy bosom lie at rest!

Seldom they enter into song or story;
Poets praise the soldier's might and deeds of War,
But few exalt the Sisters, and the glory
Of women dead beneath a distant star.

No armies threatened in that lonely station,
They fought not fire or steel or ruthless foe,
But heat and hunger, sickness and privation,
And Winter's deathly chill and blinding snow.

Till mortal frailty could endure no longer
Disease's ravages and climate's power,
In body weak, but spirit ever stronger,
Courageously they stayed to meet their hour.

No blazing tribute through the wide world flying,
No rich reward of sacrifice they craved,
The only meed of their victorious dying
Lives in the hearts of humble men they saved.

Who when in light the Final Dawn is breaking,
Still faithful, though the world's regard may cease,
Will honour, splendid in triumphant waking,
The souls of women, lonely here at peace.

O golden Isle with purple shadows falling
Across thy rocky shore and sapphire sea,
I shall not picture these without recalling
The Sisters sleeping on the heart of thee!

HMHS *Britannic*, Mudros
October 1916

Tuesday 24 October [St George's Hospital, Malta]
This is a most beautiful hospital, built on a peninsula of land running right out into the sea … The sea is right below the rocks but there is a delightful little bay which is quite safe and very shallow though full of large fish; here we have our bathing place, and it is so near that we can go down from our rooms with mackintoshes over our bathing dresses …

Wednesday 25 October
… There is no bathroom but just a hip-bath which everyone uses; there is no hot water of course laid on anywhere, but twice a week there is hot water in the boilers behind the dining-room (which is a large tent); you can then have a hot bath if you like to carry the water for it up to your room in cans. There is generally rather a rush for it. The meals here seem good, but will probably need a little supplementing with biscuits.

We all wear white shoes and stockings, low soft collars and Panama hats; no one seems very particular about uniform, unless you are unlucky enough to meet the Principal Matron. The difference between the stiffness and starchiness of the Nursing Profession in England and the freedom here is quite remarkable. No one minds whether you come into meals in your mess-dress or coat and skirt or indoor uniform and no one says anything if you are late. The Sisters treat you as friends and equals instead of incompetent but necessary evils whose presence they resent; in fact yesterday two Sisters helped me chase a locust out of my room with a mat and a tennis racquet.

You go on duty here on blocks instead of in wards; each block has an upper and lower floor with about 3 wards on each. Of course there are more orderlies than in England. At present the cases are chiefly dysentery, enteric and malaria, but they are going to be more surgical …

1916
Dardanelles, Persia, Romania, Russia and Mesopotamia

Sister Kathleen Mann

Hospital ship *Devanah* at Cape Helles, Dardanelles Peninsula and off the coast of Albania

The hospital ship Devanah *reached Mudros on 3 January and then arrived at Imbros two days later. A sports afternoon and then a concert were arranged over the next three days while all on board waited until they were needed at Cape Helles when the final contingent of men were evacuated. The ship left Imbros for Cape Helles on 8 January.*

8th

At 4.30pm a terrific bombardment took place near Gulf Ravine. The cannon fire was horrible, all big shells without a break. We could see the batteries firing until the smoke became too dense. Our monitors kept up a continual fire. It was horrible. Our ship vibrated with every shot. Stores have been leaving the shore all day, but huge quantities of stuff yet remain – ambulances, steam engines, gun-carriages, horses, mules and a lot of canvas. Down on the beach there are many things ready to be removed but quantities of stuff will be left behind. The railway in course of construction by the French still remains. No lights on shore last night. How they managed it is difficult to surmise. The only visible light was a signal on shore, for the use of the lighter. No lights on the ships removing stores, but we could hear the men shouting to one another, that was all, but many ships came up after dusk. The moon is a new one, so it is quite dark and the keen wind has gone down, leaving a quiet sea but it is still bitterly cold and almost impossible to keep warm. The *Salta* is still not full, her blue Peter is nearly at the top of the mast, the Red X lighter is loading at the pier. Then we shall start but we are to remain for the final finish up which is to be later tonight or tomorrow.

Had our first lot of patients at 11.30. I obtained two shell cases from the Captain of the lighter in return for a bottle of whisky.

Second lighter out at 2.30pm. Some bad cases but only about 150 on board.

Three head cases too ill to be removed on to beds so were left on the stretchers.

Four deaths soon after admission. Most of the wounded were from the battle we saw taking place yesterday.

Orders received this evening to leave as the *Asturias* would take our place. All very annoyed as we are not half full and there must be some reason. Colonel Warren Lowe packed up and is leaving us for the *Asturias* to see the finish up. We have varied accounts of the doings on the Peninsular. There are still 1,500 to be evacuated. Transports taking men on at 6pm. The final men will be off by 12.

Large quantities of stores, tents and ambulances are to be left behind but as far as possible destroyed. Our monitors will finish off a lot towards morning after the men have left.

On 2 Jan the Turks dropped a bomb with a message which said 'We are sorry the soldiers are leaving us', so they must have some idea as to what is happening.

Left about 7pm and steamed off so slowly but seemed hardly to move. At 9.30 we were still in sight of land and could see the flash lights at Cape Helles and the *Asturias* is visible. Our small boats had all been slung out in case they were needed for the transport.

12th

Reached Malta about 6am.

17th

We are to leave at dawn for Taranto Bay, southern Italy, and should there receive our orders which would be to take Serbian refugees or perhaps the Serbian Red X units, which we brought out from England.

18th

Reached Taranto at 12am. We were escorted in by a small Torpedo boat. An Italian Battery was practising firing at a target from her big guns. We took on water and received a visit from the Admiral and told to proceed to Avlona, Albania and there pick up refugees and wounded.

We wonder as to clothing for our refugees, as we have no extra stores. Took on no clothing at Malta. Shall be thankful to work again.

19th

Have sat on deck all morning in brilliant sunshine, how perfectly lovely it has been. We came within sight of glorious snow capped mountains about 10am and gradually crept up to them. Then an escort met us and we went round Avlona Pt quite near the rocks and saw the entrance to a cave and some lovely deep ravines in which trees were growing plentifully. Some parts of the mountains looked quite green. The sea was also a beautiful blue. As we rounded the Pt three different snow covered peaks came into view and perched on the top of the nearest was a small village and fort, the outline of which showed up against the sky.

There is a Red X Hospital on the beach, and we can see rows of khaki-clad people wending their way along very slowly. We think they must be refugees or soldiers, probably the latter, as transports are in, taking Serbian soldiers off to Corfu. There are two other hospital ships in, one a German prize of the Italians and the other a small Italian ship. It is a heavenly spot, so peaceful, with these lovely mountains all round and there are a few scattered houses dotted about. We have fixed on a very suitable title for us, namely 'Kitchener's Tourists' as that is what we feel like, just lounging in deck chairs on a very comfortable steamer slowly passing up the most beautiful coast line. But what we are in for we do not know. The scene will change and I feel will be a very pitiful one. This morning a plan was fixed on for housing numbers should we get them.

20th

In the afternoon all the Sisters landed which seems to have made rather a stir on shore. The Officials received them and showed them round. They returned with a black lamb and the Purser had a white one.

The Albanians seem to be a dirty neglected race and are I believe the oldest in Europe. They wear skins as coats and have dirty loose clothes under their sheep-skins. We heard that there was cholera about. The Serbian troops have retired rapidly over the mountains, instead of retreating slowly and holding the heights covering as much as 10 miles a day, it being too rapid for the Austrians to follow. It also wore out the boys so that on reaching the high snow covered mountains they went back and gave themselves up, and all now working on the land again.

About 18 miles over the mountains there are hundreds of starving men, there being no means of reaching them over the mountains. It seems very horrible when we have so much and to spare. Many more Serbs have arrived on the beaches and being taken off on transports. The other hospital ships have gone out so we shall soon have orders. We hear that we are to go up to Medua.

The Italians have claimed this Bay and mean we hear to hold it.

23rd

Last night the Captain had orders about 10pm to leave at once for Medua to take on refugees. We arrived at Medua about 8.30 and started to embark about 10am. It looked an absolutely uninhabited spot. Save for a few old buildings on the shore it is all mountains. We hear that the Austrians are 15 miles off and expected this evening. The only sign of life are a few straggling soldiers making their way along the beach. Church Parade is off for this morning. Orderlies gone to their wards. The sun is warm, but out of it bitterly cold. There are several sunken ships here. When the Austrians bombarded the place some little time back they were sunk.

5pm. About 1,000 on board. Rather over I fancy. The men are an appalling sight. Absolutely black with dirt and only skin and bone. Their clothes are just hanging in rags and SO dirty. As each boat came along side we could smell the men before they came on board. I would not have believed it possible that men could live under such conditions. All their clothing has been thrown overboard. It is more than alive. What a gruesome picture it is. Such a hopeless, helpless sad mass of people. I shall never forget it, the horror attached to it all. We have about 27 women and children on. Some are officer's wives with their families. A pitiable sight, some of the women clothed in mess garb and miserable little children. On the beach were some bodies of the men who had just dropped on the sand and could go no further. They remained there for the tide I suppose. But the worst side must have been the numbers of miserable men left for whom we had no more room, having then more than we had space for. They clamoured to come off, but our MO could allow no more. We are off with a not too comfortable mind. Our departure was accompanied by six shots from either a ship or shore. One passed directly over the stern of the ship. We did not discover the enemy ship but it has made us all feel a bit uneasy as they may be following us through the night. We started at 15 knots and our usual speed is from 13 to 14. We shall not slacken down until we leave enemy waters as we may have some followers.

Many of the men will die tonight.

Our Padre is a brick. He looked so business-like, clad in an overall. He bathed 50 patients and his description of the performance was quite funny. Armed with a scrubbing brush and large slab of soap all who came his way were scrubbed and making very little improvement on some, but on others good results. He is just splendid.

24th

I think we have kept near the Italian coast all night and after passing Brindisi came out into the Ionian Sea. It was very rough and to add to this we had to slow down and so rolled horribly.

The neglected condition of the men is terrible. Six died last night and the smell on the troop deck is enough to make anyone ill.

25th

Horrible discovery on going round. Found that two sets of the latrines were blocked. These people will throw down shirts and clothing and empty meat tins, blocking the whole thing and causing the latrines to overflow black into corridors and wards. One cannot stop them so have guards on.

These gaunt specimens of humanity seem to have lost all powers of thought and look so terrible. Their habits are so awful.

Messina Straights reached at 7am. A lovely bright morning. We went into Messina to take on water and remained all day. It is so pretty. Built on the side of low mountains which in some places are beautifully green. One street leading down to the harbour is wide and quite fine. The wrecked buildings remain in parts but some have been rebuilt. On a rock which is rather prominent is a pretty church.

Left Messina at 5.30pm and passed Stromboli about 8pm, quite near. We could see the outline against the sky.

Have had several more deaths, but on the whole the men are cleaner and we are more used to their horrible appearance.

26th

At 12.30 a message received that we were to go to Bizerta on the African coast and there leave these men. The French will have a camp for them.

Have supervised some more of the bathing which has been done by some Serbian Orderlies and the men are now arrayed in bright coloured pyjamas (very thin cotton ones) left over from the summer stock. Poor things they look cold but are certainly cleaner. Have cut up some flannel coats and shaped some children's frocks which the women are sewing. We cannot clothe this herd of people.

We had another gift from the Captain, of sweets for the Sisters. He is awfully kind. He gave me cigarettes for the men but they may not smoke below as we are so frightened of fire. I can only give out one at a time to the men on deck.

27th

Reached Bizerta, Tunis at 8am. The town reminds me of a French seaside place, with nice buildings and palms growing by the roadside. It looks fertile with plenty of green about. Most refreshing to see some green fields again.

More patients have died. As usual they do not seem to know what is to be done with us and our load. They have not expected us so must wait for further orders.

Most of the staff are off duty for the afternoon. They need to get away from the wards a bit.

Many patients on the decks but alas their only covering is a shirt and a blanket over their shoulders. They must be cold but we have no more clothing. All has been issued and they are quite keen to have some clean things. They are not quite so ravenous but some still hungry. All hollowed eyed. I wonder if they will ever make men again. There are some very old men amongst them.

28th

Returned to entrance of harbour to disembark the civilians and convalescents. Afterwards going up again to unload the rest. What a scene below stairs. The Sisters trying to grapple with the few cardigans, boots and socks they have. It seems almost like a market place. It poured with rain. Some of the men walked off, down the gangway in a cotton shirt, a pair of socks and blanket. Others had pyjamas, some could hardly drag along but still they managed. How terrible it looked seeing that unclothed lot go off as they did but we were helpless. Homeless beings with nothing left to them and not knowing if their own people were alive or dead …

Miss Sarah Macnaughtan

Red Cross Ambulance Unit, Erivan and Hamadan, Persia

As there was still no sign of the ambulances which had been trapped in the frozen river at Archangel in December, Sarah Macnaughtan decided to buy a car at Tiflis. After the car broke down she travelled with Mrs Wynne and Mr Bevan by train for the next part of the journey to Erivan. Her bad cough persisted.

20 January, Erivan

Today we have been busy seeing the Armenian refugees. There are 17,000 of them in this city of 30,000 inhabitants. We went from one place to another, and always one saw the same things and heard the same tales.

I am hearing of one million Armenians slaughtered in cold blood. The pitiful women in the shelters were saying, 'We are safe because we are old and ugly; all the young ones went to the harems.' Nearly all the men were massacred. The surplus children and unwanted women were put into houses and burned alive. Everywhere one heard, 'We were 4,000 in one village, and only 143 escaped.' 'There were 30 of us, and now only a few children remain.' 'All the men are killed.' These were things one saw for oneself, heard for oneself. There was nothing sensational in the way the women told their stories.

Russia does what she can in the way of 'relief'. She gives four and a half Rs per month to each person. This gives them bread, and there might be fires, for stoves are there, but no one seems to have the gumption to put them up. Here and there men and women are sleeping on valuable rugs, which look strange in the bare shelters. Most of the women knitted, and some wove on little 'fegir' looms. The dullness of their existence matches the tragedy of it. The food is so plain that it doesn't want cooking – being mostly bread and water.

The Armenians are hated. I wonder Christ doesn't do more for them considering they were the first nation in the world to embrace Christianity; but then, one wonders about so many things during this war. Oh, if we could stamp out the madness that seems to accompany religion, and just live sober, kind, sensible lives, how good it would be; but the Turks must burn women and children alive, because, poor souls, they think one thing and the Turks think another! And men and women are hating and killing each other because Christ, says one, had a nature both human and divine, and, says another, the two were merged in one. And a third says that Christ was equal to the Father, while a whole Church separated itself on the question of Sabellianism, or 'The Procession of the Son.'

Poor Christ, once crucified, and now dismembered by your own disciples, are you glad you came to earth, or do you still think God forsook you, and did you, too, die an unbeliever? The crucifixion will never be understood until men know that its worst agony consisted in the disbelief which first of all doubts God and then must, by all reason, doubt itself. The resurrection comes when we discover that we are God and He is us.

21 January

Today I drove out to Etchmiadzin with Mr Lazarienne, an Armenian, to see that curious little place. It is the ecclesiastical city of Armenia – its little Rome, where the Catholicus lives. He was ill, but a charming Bishop – Wardepett by name – with a flowing brown beard and long black silk hood, made us welcome and gave us lunch, and then showed us the hospital – which had no open windows, and smelt horrible – and the lovely little third-century 'temple'. Then he took us round the strange, quiet little place, with its peaceful park and its three old brown churches, which mark what must once have been a great city and the first seat of national Christianity. Now there are perhaps 300 inhabitants, but Mount Ararat dominates it, and Mount Ararat is not a hill. It is a great white jewel set up against a sheet of dazzling blue.

Hills and ships always seem to me to be alive, and I think they have a personality of their own. Ararat stands for the unassailable. It is grand and pure and lovely, and when the sun sets it is more than this, for then its top is one sheet of rose, and it melts into a mystic hill and one knows that whatever else may 'go to Heaven', Ararat goes there every night.

We visited the old Persian palace built on the river's cliff, and looked out over the gardens to hills beyond, and saw the mosque, with its blue roof against the blue sky, and its wonderful covering of old tiles, which drop like leaves and are left to crumble.

25 January, Tiflis
Last night I was invited to play bridge by one of the richest women in Russia. Her room was just a converted bedroom, with a dirty wall-paper. The packs of cards were such as one might see railway-men playing with in a lamp-room. Our stakes were a few kopeks, and the refreshments consisted of one tepid cup of tea, without either milk or lemon, and not a biscuit to eat. We all sat with shawls on, as our hostess said it wasn't worth while to light a fire so late at night. A nice little Princess Musaloff and Prince Napoleon Murat played with me. We were rich in titles, but our shoulders were cold …

On 8 February Sarah Macnaughtan was reunited with her car and two days later she left Tiflis for Baku and then continued, with her car, to Kasvin on a steamer. Here she met Captain Rhys Williams who was anxious to go to Hamadan in Persia and she offered to drive him there.

24 February, Hamadan.
I had always had an idea that Persia was in the tropics. Where I got this notion I can't say. As soon as we left sheltered Kasvin and got out on to the plains the cold was as sharp as anything I have known. Snow lay deep on every side, and the icy wind nearly cut one in two. We stopped at a little 'tschinaya' (tea-house), and ate some sandwiches which we carried with us. I also had a flask of Sandeman's port. I think a glass of this just prevented me from being frozen solid. We drove on to the top of the pass, and arrived there about three o'clock. We found some Russian officers having an excellent lunch, and we shared ours and had some of theirs. We saw a lot of game in the snow – great coveys of fat partridges, hares by the score, a jackal, two wolves, and many birds.

We passed a regiment of Cossacks, extended in a long line, and coming over the snow on their strong horses. We began to get near war once more, and to see transport and guns. General Baratoff wants us up here to remove wounded men when the advance begins towards Bagdad. The cold was really as bad as they make after the sun had sunk, and an icy mist enveloped the hills. We got within sight of the clay-built, flat Persian town of Hamadan about 10pm, but the car couldn't make any way on the awful roads, so I left Captain Williams at the barracks, and came on to the Red Cross hospital.

We are buried in snow, and every road is dug-out, with parapets of snow on either side. All journeys have to be made by road, and generally over mountain passes, where you may or may not get through the snow. One sees 'breakdowns' all along the routes, and everywhere we go we have to take food and blankets in case of a camp out.

Transport is the difficulty everywhere in these vast countries, with their persistent want of railways; so that the most necessary way of helping the wounded is to remove them as painlessly and expeditiously as possible, and this can only be done by motor cars. Only one of Mrs Wynne's ambulances has yet arrived, and in the end I came on here without her and Mr Bevan.

Yesterday I was in request to go up a pass and fetch two doctors, who had broken down in the snow.

I shall be working with the Russian hospital here till our next move. There are 25 beds and 120 patients. Of course we are only waiting to push on further.

26 February
I have begun to suffer from my chillsome time getting here, and also my mouth and chin are very bad; so I have had to lie doggo, and see an ancient Persian doctor, who prescribed and talked of the mission-field at the same time.

29 February
The last day of a long month. The snow falls without ceasing, blotting out everything that there may be to be seen. I think the snow was rather thicker than usual today. Mr Lightfoot [a member of the Consulate], and I went to Hamadan, plodding our way through little tramped down paths with snow three feet deep on either side. By way of being cheerful we went to see two tombs. One was an old, old place, where slept 'the first great physician' who ever lived.

The pass here is quite blocked and no one can come or go. My car has disappeared, with the chauffeur. The whole thing is a mystery, and is making me very anxious. There are no answers to any of my telegrams, and I am completely in the dark.

3 March
I think that to be on a frozen hill-top, with fever, some boils, three dogs, and a blizzard, is about as near wearing down one's spirits as anything I know.

I lie in bed all day here amongst these horrible snows. The engineer comes in sometimes and makes me a cup of Benger's Food. For the rest, I lean up on my elbow when I can, and cook some little thing – Bovril or hot milk – on my Etna stove. Then I am too tired to eat it, and the sickness begins all over again. Oh, if I could leave this place! If only someone would send back my car, which has been taken away, or if I could hear where Mrs Wynne and Mr Bevan are.

I have lost count of time. I just wait from day to day, hoping someone will come and take me away, though I am now getting so weak I don't suppose I can travel.

Of course, I ought to have turned back at Petrograd. But I thought all my work was before me, and in Russia one can't go about alone without knowing the way and the language of the people. Permits are difficult, nothing is possible unless one is attached to a body. And now I have reached the end – Persia! And there is no earthly use for us, and there are no roads …

Lady Kennard

Military Hospital, Bucarest, Romania

On 15 October 1915, the day after Bulgaria declared war on Serbia, Dorothy Kennard arrived in Bucarest following 'a wild wish' to get away from England. Although there was talk of Romania joining the war on the side of the Allies, to begin with Dorothy Kennard enjoyed the 'childishly simple' way of life in the city. Many Germans lived and were accepted in Bucarest but tensions grew and by November refugees from Serbia began to pour in. In the early months of 1916 rumours intensified that Romania would declare war on Germany and although there were preparations throughout the city, Dorothy Kennard wrote: 'hats still arrive from Paris ... and the clothes are wonderful, and even more wonderfully expensive'. In March a British Bureau was established to purchase large quantities of corn. This was impossible to transport back to England so it was planned to store the corn throughout Romania in granaries built for and sealed by the British Government. With the arrival of Spring in April the round of tennis parties, visits to the racecourse and parties started again in the city; but it was the women who were working in the fields in the countryside as the army had been mobilised and 'all the men are away digging trenches on the Austrian and Bulgarian frontiers.'

May 1916

There are three classes of hospitals in Bucarest: about a dozen permanent and well organised, attended by first-class surgeons. These have existed contemporaneously with the army and were instituted on French military lines, so as to be prepared for war, should war, by any chance, break out. In peacetime they serve as sanatoriums and civilian hospitals.

Then there are about ten auxiliary hospitals, which have sprung into being quite lately and which are in the process of organisation. They are awaiting stores and supplies from home, and will probably be in working order by the time that war comes to us, provided, of course, that their stock arrives satisfactorily. What they lack are efficient doctors and nurses. Of the former there are a few, mostly students, who have done superficial training in Germany or in France. There are no nurses at all. Even those who work in the established institutions are Roumanian amateurs now, because the women who originally ran them were Germans, who have lately been recalled to their own country. The Catholic nuns are really the most efficient amongst them, but they are limited in number and barely suffice for their own small charity concern, which has existed for years and which is financed by their Order in France.

The third class consists of all the supplementary adjuncts that are springing up daily all over the land, on private estates, in schools, and in private houses belonging to rich people in Bucarest. These are purely temporary concerns, and do not pretend to be anything else. In many cases only the covering sheds exist, so as to give them an excuse for a registration number. Beds and stores have, naturally, been ordered, but the people who are at the head of them are private individuals, and consequently ignorant of the first principles of medical requirements. Even the greatest optimists amongst us cannot count on them as anything but primitive dressing-stations for the future.

I think that everybody has at last realised the very urgent need for preparation and reorganisation which has held fire so long, but it is by no means easy to know where to begin. One cannot embark upon satisfactory activities when one is as lacking as we are in every form of material. Germany and Austria, who supply Roumania with all that she requires for industrial purposes, can obviously not be approached for these, her greater needs. And the Russian routes remain defiantly closed to all except the very irregular transmission of mails. A few small parcels arrive by letter post, but Roumania needs many shiploads of everything, from chloroform to aeroplanes, before she can even begin to consider their distribution.

Our days are spent in drawing up lists and posting them to England of things which we are likely to require. They are so vast that one becomes discouraged. Whether the things will ever reach us remains to be seen, but anything is better than inactivity, which is what we all suffer from nowadays.

July 1916

A month has passed and we are still here, still neutral, still on tenterhooks. There is no news from Russia, but troops are said to have crossed the Danube.

All the ladies have been requested to report themselves at the Headquarters of the Roumanian Red Cross. We Englishwomen can go and work where we like, and I have offered myself to one of the big military hospitals.

I was asked whether I had ever done any nursing, and was obliged to give a negative reply. But I was told that it 'did not matter', my hands would be useful. I work there feverishly every day trying to accumulate as much knowledge and nursing information as is possible. Nurses are even more completely non-existent than I had realised. There is not a woman in the place who knows the first principles of hospital training such as we have in England, and I feel just as competent as are any of the others to use lavish quantities of disinfectants and to do exactly as I am told. The doctor who is to be my immediate chief is a very clever man; he knows how to teach me my job, and now it is only a question of time.

August 1916

War is really coming. Our street today looks quite martial.

It is said that our first taste of warfare will be an aerial bombardment. I have ordered water to be kept in all the bathtubs from today forward, and am having a tap connection provided between the garden hose and the pantry. All the blankets are piled in the front hall. Perhaps in this manner we can ensure a slight protection against fire.

The prolonged waiting is hard. I have packed the silver away, also the china. I have tried to busy myself all day with absurd superfluities, and all the time I find myself listening.

Three German aeroplanes or one Zeppelin could play hell with this little town of trees and plaster. And Bulgaria is only one hour's flight away!

Later. Hurrah! The die is cast. All the telephone wires have been cut, the enemy envoys are to be packed off this evening, and mobilisation for active service begins at midnight. We have already been declared 'under martial law'. War will be declared in Vienna, a little bit late, by the Roumanian minister.

Later. Well! The passes are half taken, wounded are coming in, also prisoners. It is really war, and I am really in it!!!

Bucarest is quite calm. Orders have come round to extinguish all the lights in view of the Zeppelin raids which have actually begun. I had only one little green light burning in my house last night when the first one was signalled, and the police came and told me to put it out. I was so snubbed that I did not attempt a candle, and sat through the raid in the dark.

All the church bells rang wildly when the signal came through, and the guns were infernal. I counted twelve searchlights and tried to believe in the actuality of the happening, but honestly, if I had not hurt myself by bumping into a tin trunk in the dark, I should feel today as if I had dreamt the whole thing.

September 1916

I have fallen into regular hospital routine, and have been given charge of one of the pavilions into which our own institution is divided. Needless to say that I feel singularly incompetent, but am bound to acknowledge that it had become a matter of necessity to put some reliable person at the head of each. Most of the women who work there are young girls who have no notion of responsibility or method. They do not know enough to take the most ordinary of sanitary precautions.

I go at breakfast time every day till late at night, and only get home for lunch, and supper in the middle of the night.

Later. It has been a wild twenty-four hours! Today, at three o'clock on a sunny afternoon, I drove back to my hospital. In the open market-place, which is the halfway house, I noticed all the people looking up and gesticulating, and then for half an hour I was really in the war, for there were six Taubes overhead all dropping bombs.

As I neared the hospital, shrapnel began to fall. The bombs, of course, fell all round. I picked up one man wounded and unconscious and took him on with me in the car. A woman was killed at the gate of the hospital, and one man died on the doorstep. There are barracks just near by, and all the soldiers got out of hand and fired their rifles madly in all directions. Two men wounded by their own comrades were carried in to us afterwards. We settled down to work, and had three operations between four and seven. Just as we were preparing to go home, stretchers began to come in from different parts of the town where bombs had fallen. We worked on till 9.30, when all the operations were over. The wounded were all over the town, and all the other hospitals filled up too. The casualties were thirty dead and over a hundred wounded, for the streets were crowded when the Taubes came. The beasts flew round and round, thus hardly a quarter of the town escaped. All our airmen had gone to the front. The Taubes flew very very low, and I saw the pilot's face in one quite plainly as he turned.

I got home to find that five large pieces of shrapnel had fallen in the garden. Apparently the confusion in the town whilst the actual raid was going on was terrific.

The troops lost their heads and fired quite aimlessly, killing men and women before they could be stopped.

One couldn't be excited in the hospital, there was no time. If a doctor is cutting off things and calls out 'pansement' or 'acquaelacta' like a pistol-shot at you, you somehow find it even if you don't know what it is. One just works without the faintest understanding of what one is doing. After it was all over we collapsed, and sat in the model hospital kitchen with a petrol cooking-lamp for our only light (the electric light had been turned off at the main and we operated by candle illumination only), and drank hot tea and Zwicka and tried to recover. I don't feel that it is over yet; we shall have them back before the morning. They have only an hour to fly for more bombs. But twice in twenty-four hours is rather hard on one's nerves; I forgot to say that they came last night too, but I was too sleepy to get up and listen.

The bombs fell absolutely all round the hospital, but did not hit it, thank God! The populace is raging, and will probably lynch some German women who are still allowed to be at large. All the men are, of course, interned, in the hotels.

Later. They came again last night – six Taubes. That makes three visits in twenty-four hours. I was too worn out to move, though the whole house shook and the thuds sounded uncomfortably close. This morning I am told that they were all round us, and that the rest of the household spent the night in the cellar.

I was sent for very early by my doctor chief and we worked feverishly, the surgeons only half dressed in their uniform, myself in ordinary clothes, as there was no time to get into overalls. Twenty women and children are laid out in the mortuary. I have ceased to be affected by corpses, but I hate amputations.

It had ceased to be surprising this afternoon when those devils flew back to us again just after we had got to the hospital after lunch and were well started on an operation. But this time we nearly had a panic with the wounded. I stayed on in the ward with the helpless cases, for they said: 'If you will stay with us, we are not afraid.' The lightly wounded were sent to the cellar.

As I write it is about 6.30, and, according to the time the Taubes take to reload, they should be back by seven. Something from outside should be done to help us, for this has become a bombarded town and is defenceless. Our own aeroplanes are needed at the front, but some French aviators are expected today, which will make us feel a little safer. The hospital, standing as it does in the centre of a military quarter, is an objective for the raids, and I must honestly confess that I don't like going back there a bit. But we now have a dozen really serious cases which require hard nursing, and one knows that if one did not go perhaps no one else would.

The peasant soldiers who are brought back wounded from the front are paralysed with terror born of ignorance of the operating-table. It is all so wonderful to me! To see the big muscles cut away and through, to see a horrible wound grow daily less painful instead of a life lost through gangrene. A man pumping blood three days ago from a main artery is today eating heartily and getting well. Contrary to all existing regulations, I have procured permission to give hot tea and a cigarette after the operations when the men ask for it themselves and no active injury can result. It saves their morale and quietens their nerves. They have the wonderful recuperative power of undeveloped nervous systems, and many can stand almost anything without anaesthetics.

Curious! A month ago I felt faint when I saw blood or smelt a nasty smell.

Later. One bomb fell over our garden wall and smashed all the kitchen windows.

People have been hurt quite near our house; a bomb fell in the street killing three and wounding two who passed there.

I went round to the hospital to find that a patient had been killed in his bed in pavilion number three. The men there are clamouring to be moved, and if this sort of thing goes on the whole place will have to be evacuated, though there is no alternative site where greater safety can be provided. But a panic would be fatal. It would spread to the town and bring about a rush for the trains.

The streets did not offer a pretty sight. Several dead horses lay about, and a horse bleeds prolifically.

It's an odd life; one has to think how many are standing it hourly in the trenches. No one can realise a real air bombardment until they have been in it any more than I did before I saw it. I am frankly frightened and had no appetite for lunch.

Later. We have had two days peace and feel much better, but my nerve has decidedly gone. One does not realise the horrors properly until a raid is well over. Three of the poor legless fellows who were brought into the hospital died.

The Red Cross flags have been removed from all the hospitals, and the men are slowly regaining their nerve. The doctor and I carry harmless doses of bromide and dole it out to people who look as if they need it.

All the wounded in my pavilion call me 'Little Mother' now, and I have grown to love each individual man.

October 1916

The Germans were just – waiting. Waiting their own time, and that time came. We hardly know ourselves what has happened or how far and fast our army has retreated, but we know that things are very serious from the complete absence of reliable news.

The passes are obviously falling with incredible rapidity, and the wounded are coming in in hundreds.

We now have thirty-five cases in each of our wards, planned to hold fifteen. They are packed like herrings, poor wretches, and lying two in a bed. We keep one room for gangrene cases; but what is one room? And there is no real operating-hall. Still, one does the best one can. And the doctor is a hero.

Almost all the recent arrivals in the hospital have been operation cases. We are treating three trepanned heads, and all are going to live and think again. Sometimes I can hardly credit the fact that this woman, indifferent to blood and white bones and gangrene horrors, is myself. I had been inside one hospital in my life, and that when I was the person who was ill. One of the men in pavilion four has lost his knee-bone, but there is a possibility, apparently, of screwing one on. And another has a beautiful new jaw of gutta-percha. Once we saw him smile, and the whole room rocked with the laughter of the others. But the doctor and I are very proud of him.

The town is beginning to panic, and I don't blame it. I was told today that we shall probably have to pack up and leave in forty-eight hours' time, to spend the winter in – well, we don't know where, but in the snow anyway!! And this not because the

Bulgars have crossed the frontier, but because the Germans really have rushed the passes and are marching rapidly towards us.

We all had champagne tonight for dinner. Stocks are low, but if the Germans are really invading us – well, we certainly don't intend to leave anything worth having.

Every time I go to the hospital nowadays the soldiers smile with pleasure and say: 'So you have not yet run away?' They will be left behind, I suppose, poor wretches; and one can do nothing. Still, in a way they will be better off than we are. For really the prospect does not smile. All supplies of necessaries in the town are fast giving out. A great many of the shops are shut, and people rush about the streets looking distracted. Apparently we are going to lack soap, food and fuel, so we shall be dirty, hungry and cold.

We are now living in a house that is completely stripped of all but the barest necessities. Every time anybody wants anything, it has to be unpacked from the place, usually unfindable, where it was stowed away. It is now a week since we were told that we were leaving in forty-eight hours, and we are still here.

The French General Staff is expected hourly, as are the Russian troops. On the whole, the population has recovered remarkably well from the recent panic.

The hospital still claims most of my time, but most of the original patients are convalescent, and few have come in just lately.

I have never spent an odder day. We packed jam and sugar and all available soap into every spare corner. We all frankly forgot our lunch until past two and then found nothing in the house, so went without. We were told that we had twelve hours to finish up in and that the boxes would be called for at midnight. Of all the many terrible packings that I have done on Eastern caravan journeys, this has been infinitely the worst.

I know that I will wish that I had sent none of the things which now seem indispensable and that I will need all which I left behind. I have racked my brains to think of a place for three precious bottles of champagne, and have decided to stow them in a hold-all with the family eiderdowns. The lined trunk is stuffed with jam – jam that came from England, and possibly the last that I shall ever eat. I get occasional attacks of maudlin sentiment over small possessions which I am obliged to leave; on the other hand, I am abandoning articles of considerable value without a qualm.

We have just heard that there are 30,000 people waiting at the station. There is only one station. If this is true, we have decided that they can take our luggage, that the Germans can arrive in their thousands, but we will not move into a crowd like that unless we are pushed there – and pushed hard.

The cook has appeared quite ready to start with six dead chickens hanging on a string from her arm. She says that they will be useful. We are going to dine off cheese and go to bed to wait for tomorrow.

Later. We woke to find the luggage gone. My bed was funny: a little travelling cushion and myself upon it, covered with a dust-sheet and a fur coat. Everybody looks tired. And now we have been told that we are not going today and that it may not be necessary for us to go at all. I have told the cook to prepare two of her chickens.

The luggage returned to us at eleven with the message that all heavy baggage leaves tomorrow. And now we don't know whether this means 'no luggage van with us' or a 'trunk van on our train'. It is an important point. Should one keep necessary things back for the train and there turn out to be no van - O dear! I am tired. And the unpleasant fact remains that all our linen, clothes, blankets depart into vague and unknown space at five o'clock tomorrow, and that we get left with nothing except the clothes we stand up in, four dead chickens, and a pot of jam which I unpacked and opened this morning when the trunks came home.

I went back to work after lunch, and found that a wounded Austrian prisoner had just been brought in. I asked him how they felt about the war in his country, and he answered in German: 'Oh, it is sometimes a good war and often a bad one. I want to sleep.' That is the way we all feel. The Queen is evacuating her hospital, and now perhaps they will have a try to do the same with ours.

A few English refugees turned up at our house today.

The streets are empty – not a cab is in sight. All the shutters are drawn in the shops, and the only sign of life is to be found about the hospitals. The weather is wonderful. Brilliant sunshine gives glow to the autumn tints, and the whole world is clean – smelling of recent rain and wind. When I think of the cold and the snow and the unknown miseries that are before us all, of the disease which is bound to come, of this happy little town as I knew it first, barely a year ago, I want, like the Austrian soldier, to 'go to sleep.'

November 1916

We are still sitting quite solidly in Bucarest. Luckily, however, our luggage never left us, for the panic quietened with incredible rapidity and we were told that all danger was over. The Germans were repulsed at the frontier during the days that we got no news and have not advanced since. The French General Staff has arrived and installed itself in a manner which gives us confidence most disproportionate to the small amount which reason tells us that it is humanly capable of accomplishing. A British aviator flew over in his aeroplane from Salonika, and this gives us the cheerful feeling that we are in touch with our own army. This despite the fact that a conquered Serbia lies between.

Our hospital is full up again with new arrivals, and I work there daily. The men are dears, and I have discovered that a few parcels of cheap sweets distributed make up for long hours of almost unbearable suffering. The few amongst them who can read invariably choose the Bible or prayer-books from the literature at their disposal. Unfortunately I don't know enough of the language to ask them consecutive questions about their experiences, but I doubt whether they would be capable of coherent answering. All look dazed and worried when fighting is mentioned.

We have been entirely without news again for a week, and somehow we envisage from this disturbing happenings in the near future.

We have been strongly advised to keep all belongings packed in case of a sudden emergency, because the next time the Germans advance in force they will be so near that we shall have but a few hours' notice, and it will not be a false alarm.

Later. We are now completely stranded in an almost deserted town, for our belongings have actually left us. Indelibly branded upon my mind is a moonlit picture of a Government servant perched high on a mountain of trunks piled in inextricable confusion at dead of night into the motor lorry that finally arrived, at half an hour's notice, to take them away.

Bucarest has become a veritable Tower of Babel. The streets are full of foreign uniforms all rushing in different directions and looking very busy. We are told that further quantities of French and British officers are due, also detachments of motor ambulances and Red Cross units. But the difficulties in the way of their actual movements are stupendous. A British Red Cross hospital, complete with twenty-eight doctors and nurses, has indeed been heard of somewhere on its way out from home, but they are all stuck somewhere on the road and quite untraceable.

I am told on all sides that the chloroform will shortly give out, even though it is most sparingly used. As for the ordinary hospital requisites, they are simply non-existent.

Later. The news is bad again, and the advancing Germans are reported to be in the plains and well over the Austrian frontier.

Later. The order has come to start, and to start as soon as possible, for Jassy.

I went to the hospital for the last time, though the men did not realise it a bit. They have not been told that the Germans are within marching distance of the town. I hated leaving the men who were making good recoveries; one has learnt to take such a personal interest in the hard cases and to know all their little idiosyncrasies so well that one has grown fond of them as individuals. They seem so forlorn somehow, and stranded.

News has just come of a steady German advance and that the need for haste is very urgent …

Miss Yvonne Fitzroy

Scottish Women's Hospital, Medjidia, Romania

In February 1916 Dr Elsie Inglis and her Scottish Women's Hospital Units were repatriated from Serbia. In May she received a request from the Serbian Prime Minister to take a SWH unit to Russia to be with two Serbian Divisions. These had been recruited in the south of Russia from Austrian Slavs who were unable to return to Serbia and had deserted to the Allies.

Dr Inglis's Unit of seventy-five women included Mrs Haverfield's transport column, Ellie Rendel, a medical student [qv], Margaret Fawcett, a nursing orderly [qv] and Yvonne Fitzroy, another nursing orderly. They left Liverpool on 29 August 1916. The hospital staff were known as the 'Greys' to distinguish them from the Transport column who wore khaki and were called the 'Buffs'.

The news that greeted them when they arrived at Archangel on 10 September was grim. The joint Serbian and Russian army fighting on the front in Romania had lost 1,000 men. Dr Inglis telegraphed the committee for extra medicines and the unit continued to Odessa and two weeks later left for Medjidia, the Russian headquarters in the Dobrudja district of Romania.

They went via Reni on a journey which normally took between five and six hours but the train moved slowly and halted for long stretches of time and they eventually arrived at Reni after travelling for four days and three nights. From Reni they went by steam-launch down the Danube to Czernavoda and then by train to Medjidia. Yvonne Fitzroy was a nursing orderly in 'A' Hospital.

30 September. In the train
We woke to sunrise, tea and biscuits, and arrived at Tchernavoda [Czernavoda] about 2, and beheld the great bridge over the Danube which carries the railway line from Constanzia on to Bucharest.

We began to unload at once, and to our astonishment found an Irishman [an officer called Bryson] serving in the Russian Army in charge. There are two Russian Infantry Divisions here and one Cavalry. This section of the Front is under the supreme command of a Russian General. The Russians and Serbians have borne the brunt of the fighting, and have done very well.

About 6pm forty Russian soldiers turned up, and the equipment was all got off by 9. I was checking in the hold most of the time. We were bustled into a train, and left about 10, reaching Medjidia just before 11. We dozed upright in the train for the rest of the night.

1 October. Medjidia
Both Units are to stay here for the moment, but later Hospital B is to move to another point 12 miles away. We are 10 miles from the firing-line, and we could hear the guns most of the morning. In the afternoon we went up to our Hospital, or what is to be our Hospital, and scrubbed until a party of gorgeous-looking brigands arrived who proved to be white-washers. They have given us part of the barracks, a very good building on a hill right above the town. Next door there is a Russian Red Cross Hospital, and behind more barracks full of soldiers, dogs, puppies, pigs, cattle, and other oddments.

We all slept in the train. I found a spare bit of floor space where anyway I could stretch. Half dead.

4–9 October. Medjidia
Men came in on Wednesday. We were at it without a break from 7.30 that morning until 1.30 on Thursday morning, then on again from 7.30 until 8.30 that night. At the end of it a mail saved our lives.

Between filth and wounds the men's condition is indescribable. They are coming back in thousands; our Transport have been working absolutely heroically; and bringing the wounded in is no joke, especially at night in a strange country and over these roads.

It has been the biggest rush of wounded they have yet had. By shoving the mattresses close to each other, and putting others in every available corner, we made room for every man we could, and still the cry of the Authorities was for more – more – more. In the Russian Red Cross Hospital next door two and three men were shoved on a single mattress just as they came in, the dead and the living sometimes lying side by side for hours. Even in our own wards, where British prejudice dies hard, and where every patient was in the end undressed and washed, the crawling uniforms, the dirt, the smell, the groaning men, or those still more terrible, lying in an inert silence, and last but not least the heat and the flies, made of the world a sufficiently ghastly chaos.

Thank Heaven we are beginning to see daylight at last; in the wards there is something approaching order, and the men who are well enough look happy and friendly. There are not any trains available so we cannot evacuate our men for a day or two. All except the desperately wounded are sent on at once when possible. The nursing conditions are something of a revelation, but what we haven't got we invent, and what we can't invent we do without.

We got a mail on the 5th. It was our last night in the top wards before we moved into tents, and was too blessed. And camp next night was wonderful. The tents are pitched on the open ground about 200 yards away from the Hospital, two in each, and single ones for the Officers. Below the Mess Tent and Kitchen Tent and two Bath Tents. The nights are chilly, but very fine and clear; you are away from the sights and sounds and smells of Hospital, and there never was such a moon or such stars in all the world before. Sometimes shadowy troops singing shadowy songs move up to the Front all night; sometimes they come and camp quite close, pitching tiny canvas tents and lighting fires; always there is a flaming sunrise, and in the early morning the steppe looks soft and big and the town below is hidden in blue mist from the marshes.

10 October. Medjidia

Hospital B and all the Transport but two moved on. There were streams of reinforcements and stuff going past us up to the Front all day, and an enemy aeroplane attacked the station. This was our first air-raid, and we were too busy even to look, though I did bolt out for a second when I was supposed to be occupying myself with something quite different. We all jumped when the first bomb went off, and then tried to look as if we hadn't!

11 October. Medjidia

We hear there is to be a big battle in five days. Wards very hot, and the flies awful.

13 October. Medjidia

Feeling rotten, off duty at 6. We've all had this sort of collapse, and put it down to the dust and the flies. It is impossible to keep either off the food.

14 October. Medjidia

I was sent to bed. A piping hot day, and we were bombarded by aeroplanes. Altogether there came twelve machines, and at times the bombardment was heavy. Two soldiers were killed in the courtyard of the Hospital, but there is said to be no serious material damage. One of our own Orderlies was wounded, and several civilians were brought in.

The Russians tried anti-aircraft guns, heavy guns, and machine-guns; it was all very noisy, but the aeroplanes sailed away unhurt.

16 October. Medjidia

Back on duty. The Transport have brought about thirty strange tin beds from Constanza. We erected these for the 'worst cases', and they make a great difference – to our backs at least. They must also add to the entertainment of the 'worst cases', for they have a nice little habit of collapsing at odd moments. Also they are covered with garlands of flowers and pictures of lovely ladies.

We evacuated a good number of patients, so the wards were much lighter.

17 October. Medjidia

Collapse of the Staff. Only one Sister on duty on my ward.

My birthday. We had a wonderful mail, and I received a present of chocolates when I woke up, and a further present of cigarettes and cakes was sent over from Hospital B. Mrs M. [Mary Milne] made me a wonderful scone, and three of us picnicked happily on Trajan's Wall, watched the aeroplanes, and tried to ignore the unavoidable proximity of a decomposing horse. It was a very nice birthday indeed.

18 October. Medjidia

We had an awful night, as the wind arose, and twice B and I had to sally forth in our pyjamas to hammer in tent pegs and rescue the kitchen stove. The three Bath Tents were blown flat, and most of the Mess and Kitchen Tents blown away.

19 October. Medjidia

A bad aeroplane raid at Hospital B, and they were bringing in wounded civilians to us all day. Ghastly. The flash of the guns at night is very clear now, and the sound continuous. Our 1st Serbian division has done splendidly, but has been so cut up it has been withdrawn, and for the winter we shall be nursing Russians.

Some of the Cossacks of the Imperial Guard camped here for the day, and the troops streamed up to the Line without a pause.

We have erected a 'Sick' Tent for the Staff. Hospital B and the Transport sent over their invalids.

20 October. Medjidia

An aeroplane bombarded us in the morning, and the guns are very clear.

As I went on duty after tea there came a message from the Serbian Headquarters ordering us to evacuate all our men at once and to follow ourselves in twenty-four hours.

The news came as rather a shock, and we got the men off sadly enough. Later we were visited by the Russian Commander-in-Chief, who told us it was true the Army had fallen back, but that we and the Russian Red Cross Hospital were all he had to depend on and the wounded pouring in. So of course Dr I. [Dr Inglis] said we'd stay only too thankfully. Our superfluous equipment is to be sent to Constanza by train, and we are to work as a Field Dressing Station and evacuate (if it becomes necessary) with the Army. There is a rumour that the line to Tchernavoda is cut. The bridge has been hit by a bomb, but not irreparably damaged.

A tiny mail wandered in in the evening.

21 October. Medjidia
The Russian Hospital left. We spent a long day packing and getting the stores off. They are to go to Galatz, as Constanza is not now considered sufficiently safe.

We struck camp, and all the men were evacuated, though a good many new cases passed through to be dressed on their way back from the Front. These were mostly walking cases, as the more serious are now sent further back. But it was interesting work dressing these weary men who had toiled in on their own for the most part.

I went twice down to the station with the baggage in the evening, a perilous journey in rickety carts, through pitch darkness over roads crammed with troops and refugees, which were lit up periodically by the most amazing green lightning I have ever seen, and the roar and flash of the guns was incessant. At the station no lights were allowed because of enemy aircraft, but the place was illuminated here and there by the camp fires of a new Siberian Division which had just arrived. Picked troops, these, and magnificent men.

We wrestled with the baggage until 2am, and went back to the Hospital in one of our own cars.

I dropped on to a mattress in the ward just as I was, as we may have to leave ourselves at 5. Six of the Unit are to accompany the equipment to Galatz, but mercifully I am not one of them.

22 October. Medjidia – Saragea
We were woken at 4.30 and breakfasted on a small bit of bread and butter and Tchi. There were no orders from Headquarters and the guns were incessant and sounded nearer. We spent a lazy morning, and about luncheon time got orders to evacuate at once. The majority are to go to Galatz by train with Dr C. [Dr Lilian Chesney], the rest (self included) are to go by road with Dr I. and work with the Army as a clearing station.

The train party got off as quick as possible, and about 4 a big lorry came for our equipment. We loaded it, seven of us mounted on the top, and the rest went in two of our own cars. The scene was really intensely comic. Seven Scottish women balanced precariously on the pile of luggage, a Serbian Doctor, with whom Dr I. is to travel, standing alongside in an hysterical condition, imploring us to hurry, telling us the Bulgarians were as good as in the town already. Dr I. quite unmoved demanding the whereabouts of the Ludgate Boiler, somebody arriving at the last minute with a huge open barrel of treacle, which, of course, could not possibly be left to a German – oh dear, how we laughed!

At last we started with orders to make for Carlo Murat. In the town our driver took us out of our way to pick up an Officer, and in so doing we missed the others, who thought we were on ahead. The road to Carlo Murat proved to be only mud and quite impossible for a heavy lorry after the rain, so we had to give up the idea of getting there and decided to push on to the Military Headquarters at Saragea.

We heard later that Medjidia fell the afternoon after we left.

The whole country is in retreat, and we had an extraordinarily interesting drive. Behind we could see the shells exploding, and the sky was alight with the glow of burning villages. On our right a bigger glow showed the fate of Constanza, which fell today. The road was indescribably dilapidated, and crammed with refugees, troops, and transports. The retreating troops seem mostly Roumanian; I gather the Russians are protecting our rear.

The peasants are a picturesque lot, not of course purely Roumanian, as the Dobrudja was so lately a Turkish province. Ponies and oxen are harnessed into their little springless carts, all their household goods are packed inside, and they are followed by terrified flocks of sheep, pigs, and cattle. The peasants trudge along, going – one wonders where?

It was showery at first, but turned to a beautiful night though very dark. Our progress was slow, as the lamp refused to burn, but we cheered the way with frugal rations of biscuits, jam, and cheese. Though lost we have at least had the intelligence to get lost with the food!

We reached Saragea about 10.30 almost too tired to speak, our lorry deposited us in the mud by the roadside, bade us a tender farewell and – left. But the General of Division was very kind, invited us into Headquarters and refreshed us with black bread and Tchi.

We ate amidst a chaos of maps, Generals, messengers, and field telephones. The men looked anxious to breaking-point, but their kindness to seven lone females is unforgettable. Our kit they stuck under a form of shelter in charge of a sentry, and we groped our way through deep, deep mud to a house where we were given two rooms. Mud floors, hard but clean.

23 October

We scraped the surface dirt off our hands in filthy water, and then set out in search of news and breakfast. The endless procession of troops and refugees never ceased to tramp past all night, and there was no news of the Unit. Meanwhile the General had sent to Hirsovar, on the Danube (I think a distance of about 60 kilometres), for two lorries to fetch us and our stuff. A very nice Russian boy gave us boiling water and half a loaf in exchange for treacle and cigarettes; P., I rather fear, looted four eggs, which we hard boiled, and so breakfasted handsomely. The rest of the morning we spent dealing out treacle. The soldiers very soon discovered it, and fell out as they marched past, bringing everything, down to their water-bottles, in which to carry it away.

About eleven o'clock Dr I. and three of our Transport cars drove up. Having invented every awful fate for us, her relief was immense when she found us sitting by the roadside drinking Bovril. Orders to evacuate at once came to the village, and the Staff moved off.

It was a pretty heart-breaking sight to watch the people stripping their little houses and packing what they could into some tiny cart. The women sobbing, and the men dogged and inert. Here and there on the road, of course, there were moments of panic in which they lost all self-control …

The unit continued to retreat over the following twelve days until they reached Ismaila. They were then divided into three sections. Yvonne Fitzroy and her group were sent to Braila which was 'one vast dumping ground for the wounded' who poured in every day. There were only seven trained doctors in the town. 'There were still men lying about in empty houses with their uniforms on and the horrible smell of sepsis from their wounds', Dr Inglis wrote. As there were no adequate hospitals, public buildings were taken over. An operating theatre and wards were opened and the unit worked under intense pressure for several weeks. Towards the end of November the Germans crossed the Danube and Bucharest fell on 6 December. Dr Inglis was told that French sisters were to take over the hospital at Braila and her unit was to move on 'to form a large dressing-station near the front'. Yvonne Fitzroy continued to write her diary.

6 December. In the train
Packed. We are only to take bed-bundles with us, which is rather a relief, as I gather we are bound to retreat before very long. We got into our train about 7pm. It consists of one coach and one truck for the equipment, so five of us arranged to sleep with and on the latter. It was a quaint scene when we had all settled down, but we made ourselves quite comfortable on the bales and we wrapped everything we possessed round and round us.

There were no windows, so for the sake of light the door had to be open by day and it froze hard just after we started. Wednesday night we slept in the train. It was somewhat disturbed and chilly, and we did not leave Braila until 8 on Thursday morning. About 10 we made ourselves an excellent breakfast of Tchi, bread, sardines and chocolate. The weather was very cold, and we kept going most of the time across a desolate flat landscape. All day we improvised excellent meals (a distracting amount of chocolate was produced), and we danced breakdowns at intervals to keep warm. Reached Ciulnitza about 5. It is nothing but a large station full of wandering rumours to the effect that Bucharest has fallen, and that our being allowed to stay is uncertain.

Dr I. had us all out to sleep in a sort of waiting room place. It was quite the funniest night I have ever spent. Half the soldiers in the place had apparently been accustomed to live there, and so would burst in at odd moments to fetch their belongings. B. was next to the door, and it was her business to prevent them – if she could – so, whenever I opened an eye, there she was capering about the room in her pyjamas, pursuing some bewildered foreigner, and shouting: 'Ide – ide – (Go, go) – oh, you fool, why don't you go, Ide, ide,' while the Unit howled with mirth and Dr I. vainly tried to assert a sense of outraged propriety.

8 December. In the train
Breakfasted at 8, after which Dr I. went off to search for the authorities. We walked up to the Aerodrome, and found five small French machines and three big English just arrived. They all had orders to evacuate at once. Bucharest has fallen, all communications are therefore cut, and the Army is falling back and will take up this position tomorrow.

Back to the station for luncheon. Food is running very low. Dr I. announced that our orders were to leave. What wounded they are able to move are being taken farther back.

The Russian Red Cross people at Braila can have known very little of the situation up here. We are to go back to Ciura. So we packed ourselves once more into our truck, and watched the aeroplanes depart. They looped the loop over our train, and waved farewell. We had orders not to leave our carriages, and news came through that everyone was to be out of the place before 5, as the station would then be destroyed. So we spent the afternoon watching train after train, each with its crowd of refugees and soldiers, creep away. At 5 to 5 it was almost dark, we were still lying in the station, and eight trucks of explosives had just been hooked on. A young and quite presentable Roumanian Officer had been helping us to open our methylated barrel for cooking purposes, when huge flames were seen leaping up alongside our engine. He dashed forward to see what was happening, and instantly the place became a seething mass of jumping, screaming humanity. The Officer came running back, shouting to us to shut the truck doors. We hauled him in, and slid the door to. It must have been touch and go to take our train with its load of 'obus' within a few inches of what proved to be a blazing oil-tank. As soon as our carriage was past, we got the door open again. The horizon was in a blaze, oil-tanks, granaries, strawstacks, everything burnable was set alight. It was very terrible and very beautiful. Peasants, men, women and children were running alongside the train in a panic, trying to clamber into the already overcrowded trucks; others had given up the struggle, and collapsed by the side of the line, or had settled down into that familiar dogged tramp with the blazing sky behind them.

The Officer came as far as Slovosia with us. By rights, it is an hour's journey, but we took three. Our guest was really interesting and quite tolerant and intelligent. The great hope of the Roumanian Army was, he said, General Avarescu, who gave up the command in the Dobrudja before the fall of Constanza, in order to take the supreme command in the Carpathians.

We gave our guest supper. Soup, bread and cheese, bread and sugar, bread and sardines, chocolate and cigarettes, the last of our private supplies, but all, we felt, in a good cause.

9 December. In the train

We waited most of the morning for the train to go on, and by 3.30 were approaching Tanderei (the junction where the line to Braila branches off from the main line to Tchernavoda), and feeling very bored and cold when I saw an aeroplane planing down towards us. She was hovering quite low, and apparently just over our engine, when we heard a loud explosion, and realised she must be German. The whole place became alive with soldiers. The enemy followed up with a smart machine-gun fire; the French Officer, who was travelling with Dr I., leapt out of his carriage, shouting: 'Tirez, tirez, donc!' and two more loud explosions followed. We made one dash for the bales to try and find bandages and dressings, the Russian Army remembered their rifles, and the aeroplane was driven off. In the station we found that the material damage was small, and the casualties only one horse killed and two men wounded. The aeroplane returned, and dropped two more bombs, but was driven off easily.

Our engine-driver felt so shattered that he actually hastened our departure, and we went much comforted by a drink of hot soup provided by some Russian Sisters.

We did not reach Ciura until 10.30pm and then only to discover it had been evacuated at midday, and that we were to go on and try our luck at Faurei.

10 December. In the train

Woke up after rather a miserable night. The world was very cold and rather hungry. At some wayside station Dr I. found a goose, a duck, a hen, and half a pig. Our Russki's cooked them for us, the pork not half bad, and we got a liberal supply of bread and sugar. The water is pea-green, but the Russian Red Cross people again came to the rescue with soup. We move infinitesimal distances at long intervals, and are told we are just about to get into the congestion! Saw a long column of artillery retreating across the plain. All tucked up by 8pm.

11 December. In the train

A very cold night, but the truck woke in excellent spirits, and we had good Tchi for breakfast. After that we got into the saltmarsh district, and could get nothing but salt water, which was misery. Reached Faurei soon after 1, and found nothing there but mud, trains, and orders to go on to Braila. All the trucks from the north come in covered in snow.

Arrived late at Braila.

12 December. Braila

We woke in a siding to brilliant sunshine. The water supply is off, so there are no baths to be had – rather a blow, as I have not moved out of my clothes from my fur coat downwards for five days.

At the Russian Headquarters Dr I. was told that we should probably proceed to Traian, some 25 kilometres in the direction of Faurei, there to work as a dressing-station.

Met Colonel Griffiths, the Head of the British Oil Destroying Mission, and he lent us his room at the Français for the afternoon. It was rather fun, as the Officers of his Staff were running in and out all the time, and were very interesting. It seems that everything now depends upon holding the railway junction at Buzei, east of Ploesti, where the lines from Braila and Moldavia meet. The Germans are making a big offensive movement there, and it is just a chance whether or no the Russians will arrive in time to hold it. The loss of the line will probably mean the evacuation of Braila and Galatz.

Many tons of grain have fallen to the Germans, but, thanks to the British Mission, no oil.

At tea we heard that owing to the serious news from the Front our departure was to be delayed, and meanwhile the Russian authorities had provided us with two empty rooms in which to sleep. They are in a house perched on the cliff above the Danube, with a heavenly view. We got our camp beds and bundles, and passed a decidedly chilly night.

13 December. Braila

Grey and wet. The streets inches deep in liquid mud. After tea Dr I. announced that the Buzei line was not to be held, and in consequence we are to start work at Galatz and leave tomorrow. Glad at least to have something settled.

I got some hot water out of the other inhabitants of our villa, and we went to bed very clean and happy.

14 December. Braila
Heard definitely after tea that the congestion on the line was too great to allow of our going today, then hardly had we got back to the house and erected the beds than an order came that we were to go at once. Packed in a fearful hurry, and went down to the Station. There we sat in a waiting-room full of Officers from 5pm to 5am. Quite the most appalling night I have ever spent. At last the train turned up from the Port, and I tumbled into the truck.

15 December. In the train
We woke soon after 9 to find ourselves just outside Braila, and spent the whole day in the train crawling along at intervals. At about 7.30pm we arrived at Barbosi, and the Commandant of the station gave us an excellent meal of potatoes cooked in oil. A Roumanian officer, on his way to the Front with stores, contributed some tinned meat. He and a friend paid their respects to Dr I., and then visited us in the truck and stayed until 11. They made lovely Turkish coffee, and told us the story of their lives, which was – dramatic! We all parted sworn friends.

16 December. Galatz
Reached Galatz about 5am; 15 miles in 36 hours! A tiny mail awaited us, but it was good to get. Spent the rest of the day getting clean. I am billeted in a dear little house with five of the others. Sambo, our terrier, is here. He was with the Transport for a time, then returned to Galatz with a Hospital B Orderly. He is the most perfect gentleman I have ever met.

19 December. Galatz
Hospital B is to evacuate to Odessa tonight with the British Red Cross Unit. We are to stay here. The Russians say they will not take the responsibility of getting us away, but nevertheless would like us to stay. Am glad.

20 December. Galatz
A Russian success is reported between Faurei and Braila and four guns taken. This evening huge guns passed us on their way up from the quay to the town defences, some parts drawn by teams of not less than twelve oxen.

23 December. Galatz
We visited our new Hospital. It is in a dark and dismal slum between the port and the station. We slithered through much mud and found a fair-sized house that was once a Greek School and rejoices in the name of Pappadopol! Until we can find rooms we are to be quartered on the first floor. There are no drains, and we were decidedly peevish after viewing the new premises. The rest of the Unit and most of all the Sanitary Inspector even more so. Our belongings were brought down in ox-wagons. Twelve in our room – Orderlies I mean, not ox-wagons.

24 December. Galatz
Having developed a violent toothache I slept badly, and am as cross as the tongs. We

begin work in Hospital tomorrow. Sister C. is suspected of diphtheria.

I orderlied for Dr I., and asked to stay on for another six months.

The guns in the Dobrudja direction very clear all day. No one seems to know for certain whether or not Tultcha has fallen, but rumour has it that our Transport are back at Reni. Tultcha is important in that it commands one of the branches of the Danube delta, and, in consequence, an access to the Black Sea.

25 December (Christmas Day). Galatz

No work to be done except for the Sanitars [Russian Orderlies], who were kept busy stuffing mattresses. Everyone was rather too obviously cheerful, and I spent the afternoon with the Dentist and made my toothache far worse.

They have flung a pontoon bridge across the Danube here, and the Dobrudja guns sound nearer.

A mail came in, but there was not one letter for any of us – all for Hospital B and the Transport! It was bitter.

A most wonderful spread awaited us at tea, and we played games and chanted carols far into the night. I'm sure the Russkis think we worship strange gods indeed!

To bed on 30 grains of Aspirin and two Somnytics, I should imagine a record.

26 December. Galatz

We were woken at 2am by a terrific explosion, followed by two less violent. It proved to be a Zeppelin – our first night raid – and the bombs were very near.

The Dentist later, but he did no good.

News is bad and plans uncertain. Tultcha fell last Thursday or Friday, and our Transport are believed to be at Ismaila.

27 December. Galatz

Everyone busy getting the mattresses made and stuffed. I had a large tooth removed and am thankful.

Iliatchenko, the chief of the Russian Red Cross in these parts, visited the Hospital. He said that in four or five days they will know whether or not it is possible to hold the line from a point between Issacea and Macin in the Dobrudja, up to Buzei, where a battle is now raging. If Macin falls Galatz must follow in three or four days' time, in which case we are to move north to Folteste, which lies at the head of a pontoon bridge on the Pruth, and set to work there. The Transport have done very good work in the Dobrudja.

Commander Locker Lampson's Armoured cars have all turned up here. They say Galatz will be bombarded from two sides, and blown to little, little bits. Today the guns were incessant.

We moved into our billets in a wee cottage 50 yards from the Hospital.

28 December. Galatz

I am to have a ward to myself, and am absolutely thrilled. The second upstairs ward is nearly finished, but mercifully there are no wounded yet, and we ought to be quite ready by tomorrow. There is a rumour of a Russian victory …

Miss Frances Eleanor Rendel

Scottish Women's Hospital Unit, Medjidia, Romania

Scottish Women's Hospital Unit, Field Hospital, Bulbulmick, Romania

Scottish Women's Hospital Unit, Ismaila, Russia

Ellie Rendel was in her final year as a medical student when she wrote to her mother on 23 August 1916:

> *You will probably think me quite mad when I tell you that I have decided to go to Russia for six months with the Scottish Women's Hospitals people. We went to see the war pictures at the Scala on Monday night and as a result of that I felt it to be my duty to offer my services to Dr Inglis [qv]. I never thought they would be accepted. As a matter of fact she, or rather her deputy, Dr Chesney, jumped at the offer, as it appears that they are very short handed and find it exceedingly difficult to get people. The Russian government have asked for four units from this country. The British Red Cross and St. John's Ambulance are providing two and the SWH the other two.*

During her months with the unit Ellie Rendel was entrusted with much of the responsibility of a fully qualified doctor.

The unit of seventy-five women, which included two orderlies, Miss Margaret Fawcett [qv], and Yvonne Fitzroy [qv], left Liverpool on 29 August 1916 and arrived at Archangel on 10 September. The women continued their journey to Odessa nine days later. When they arrived they were told that the Serb division had been in action with the Russians and the Romanians (who had recently joined the war), and casualties were heavy. Dr Inglis was asked to take her unit to the front. The Serb headquarters was at Bulbulmick, a village behind the front line, and it was decided to open a hospital in barracks at Medjidia, the Russian headquarters in the Dobrudja district of Romania, some ten miles away. 'It was no good in the world talking about regular Field Hospitals to the authorities until they had tried our mettle. The ordinary male disbelief in our capacity cannot be argued away; it can only be worked away', Dr Inglis wrote later.

After caring for a continuous flow of wounded at Medjidia – more than half Russian soldiers – Dr Inglis so impressed the Russian medical department and Serb headquarters that she was asked to open a field hospital at Bulbulmick. Here a constant stream of wounded were nursed until the Austrian army advanced even further and the field hospital was evacuated. As conditions became worse the unit was sent to various other locations.

Ellie Rendel was a prolific letter writer to her mother, father, sister, and various friends, and wrote her first two letters during the voyage on board HMS Huntspill.

7.9.16 [to her mother]
The Unit is under the command of Dr Elsie Inglis. It is divided into two sections.
1. The Motor Transport Section under Mrs Haverfield. This consists of:
A First class drivers
B Second class drivers
C Cooks
D Secretary
E Interpreter

Uniform – Khaki
They almost all have short hair. They are popularly called 'The Buffs'. They are very smart and very conceited. Mrs Haverfield is a great stickler for discipline, obedience, etc., etc.

The Hospital Section under Dr Inglis
Uniform: grey

It consists of:
Doctors
Administrator
Matron and Assistant Matron
Sisters
Orderlies
Sanitary Inspector
Secretary
X-Ray assistant (myself)
Cooks
Laundresses
Interpreter

The doctors names are:
Inglis – Surgeon
Chesney – Surgeon
Potter – With the Motor Transport Section
Corbett [Dr Catherine Corbett, an Australian] – Medical

We have come a tremendous round in order to escape from torpedoes and mines. At first we skirted along the coast of Ireland and then we made for Iceland. We do a zig-zag course the whole time.

7.9.16
Dear Betty [her sister],
This is a wild adventure I am on. It reminds me in some ways of our camp life at Studland. So many of the women here have belonged to semi military organisations such as the Women's Reserve Corps etc in which they do a lot of saluting, that the

military spirit has crept in – much to the annoyance of the Sisters who have already begun to rebel.

Dr Inglis likes a great deal of deference paid to her as head of the unit, and she goes in for roll calls, cabin inspection, etc., and at roll call she has given the order that we are to say 'Here Ma'am'.

Some of the Unit are already rather upset by this and there are one or two grumbles. The officers, i.e. the doctors, Matron and administrator are accused of being too much on their dignity, etc. You can imagine the kind of thing. The Secretary, Sanitary Inspector and myself feel secretly that our claims to authority have been a little overlooked. Otherwise we loyally and wisely uphold the higher command. Anyway we have deck cabins to ourselves which is something.

The Sisters – as in military hospitals all the nurses are Sisters here – are the oddest collection of old dug-outs. Most of them apparently were private nurses and haven't been near a hospital for years. They look anything but smart. There is actually one old and toothless harridan who rouges shamelessly. The Assistant Matron who is rather a bright spot told me that they had found it very difficult to get nurses. All the best ones have been snapped up long ago. These creatures will never have much authority over the orderlies. The orderlies are active intelligent educated specimens. The Sisters are essentially uneducated. Some of them go in for flirting openly with the ship's officers.

20.9.16

Here we are still in this dirty old train. We can't possibly get to Odessa now before Friday 22 September. We have had to stop at every station all the way from Archangel and we have had to wait for every train on the line. It is only a single line and there are quantities of Red Cross trains and goods trains so our progress has been slow. The last few days it has been getting warmer and we have been able to sit on the trucks which hold our motor cars. But it is still cold at night. I haven't undressed since we left the boat and washing is very scanty.

At every station that we stop at Dr Inglis jumps out and waves a letter given to her by some official at Archangel. She talks in English and very bad French and stamps her foot and shakes her fist. All the railway officials come and shake their heads and our interpreters are kept hard at work. The result is that they promise that the train shall go on in 15 minutes and it invariably stays for two or three times as long. This morning we were kept for 5 hours in a station. We couldn't go for a walk or do anything interesting because we were told all the time that we were going off in ten minutes.

It is a very odd life and we are all getting a little tired of it. It's not so bad in the daytime. We make our own breakfast which consists of a slice of bread – generally black – and butter and a cup of very primitive tea made in a saucepan and with no milk. Lunch we have at a railway station at any time between 12–3. The food provided is generally very good – cabbage soup, meat, mostly veal and vegetables and coffee or tea.

Tea we make for ourselves, and it is the fashion to have tea parties. Biscuits, rolls, apples, chocolate are bought at exorbitant prices at stations. Supper is handed round by the orderlies. It consists of rolls and butter, baby chickens (cold) and cheese sometimes.

The Sanatorium
Odessa
24.9.16
We arrived at Odessa on Thursday evening 21 September. We were met by 40 carriages lent by residents and driven at a gallop by most wonderful horses to our present place. It is a large open air nursing home for nerve cases. It is very comfortable with a large garden and an open air dining-room.

Since we have been here we have been very well treated. We have been fed in the most luxurious way. The English residents have had us to tea etc and tonight we went to a gala performance at the opera where we were given boxes and received by a grand-duchess.

Everyone here says we shall perish with cold so the authorities have agreed to give us leather coats.

We are off tomorrow 25 September at 6pm. No one knows how long we shall be in the train.

The train
28.9.16.
Here we are in the train again, and no one knows when we shall be able to leave it.

We are now going south and going to rather an exciting spot I believe. We are having lovely weather, and the country is hilly and wild. During the day we sit on the trucks and walk about the countryside while the train is held up. It is really quite a pleasant existence. Our uniforms are already in rags. Dr Inglis refused to have new ones made in Odessa because she thought there wouldn't be time!

The authorities promised to buy us fur coats but I am glad I didn't trust them and bought one for myself. All they have done is to buy skins which are to be sewn together when there is time and sewn into our greatcoats. As our greatcoats are already on the small side this is not a very practical scheme. Besides there will never be time to do this. If I ever do get a chance I shall make mine into a sleeping bag as the blankets provided are made of paper and we have no beds and the nights already are very cold.

The Barracks
Town in Roumania [Medjidia]
5.10.16
We came here from the boat by train on Saturday evening 30 September. The town from which we came [Reni] was quite deserted. Everyone had fled and the shops were boarded up. Aeroplanes visit it daily and drop bombs in order to destroy a bridge in the neighbourhood.

The day after we arrived here i.e. Sunday, the order was given for women and children to leave the town and all day long waggons full of luggage and refugees went northwards. We were told that a big battle was going on about 15 miles away. We had our first taste of camp life that day. We had to sleep four in an ordinary railway carriage not meant for night journeys for 3 nights and there wasn't a drop of water to be had for washing.

We got our meals in a miserable little canteen for soldiers in the town. Breakfast consisted of bread, no butter, and some very weak Russian tea with no milk or lemon. The bread was black and heavy.

This is a vast barracks perched on a hill and a very good mark for shells. It was filthy dirty and had to be cleaned and whitewashed by us and Turkish prisoners. It consists of two vast long rooms one on top of the other and a few odd store rooms. The first floor room we made into a ward. The beds are made of sacks put in rows along the floor. The beds almost touch and there are 100. The upper room is our bedroom and dining-room. It contains 75 camp beds in 4 long rows. There is a semi partition down the room. There is no other furniture in the room except an upright deck chair between each bed. The walls are whitewashed. There are no carpets or rugs. There are no mattresses or pillows provided. We each have three army blankets and a rug and they have now brought us each a sheep-skin. The room is warmed by day by two stoves but it is very cold by night. There is no water supply. All the water has to be brought in from a pump. In some marvellous way an operating theatre has been made, a dispensary, a kitchen and a place for washing in. We have all worked like niggers unpacking the stores and arranging things.

Yesterday at two o'clock before anything was ready patients began to be brought in. They came in batches up to 3am. By that time we had 100 patients. They were in a very filthy condition but they had had first aid dressings very well done by Russians. It was rather a nightmare because we had nothing really ready. As soon as possible we are going into tents which will be cold but more comfortable. Here we have to eat sitting on our beds and it is all rather messy.

Dr Chesney is doing her best to get her part of the show moved on and made into a real field hospital. It would be much more interesting. There are too many doctors here for my taste.

We have just been inspected by a Russian general who has given medals and crosses to all the patients. All the men who are going to die get crosses. Most of our patients are Russians so far. Tomorrow we are going to open another ward in an outside building.

13.10.16
Camp B [Bulbulmick]
Roumania
Dearest Mother,
To my great joy Dr Chesney was sent here on the 7 October to start and run a field-hospital. It is a good deal nearer to the firing line than the other place which is being run as a clearing hospital.

In this camp we are only 12 people all told i.e. Dr Chesney, Miss Henderson, the administrator, Dr Chesney's assistant = me, four Sisters, four orderlies and a cook. It is great fun here for me. I have a tent to myself and Dr C introduces me to all the officers who come as 'Meine Colleague Dr Rendel'. I have also had my salary raised to £100 which is extremely generous of the SWH.

The whole camp here is under canvas. We have 7 tents for sleeping in. A mess tent. A tent for doing dressings in and a large hospital tent. We have to be ready to move backwards or forwards at 2 hours notice. The only drawback to all this is that so far we have no patients. The guns go on spasmodically but it is believed that our people and the enemy are bringing up men and ammunition for a big affair. However there is still a good deal to be done arranging the camp, etc. We all go about in breeches – skirts are put on for tea if officers are expected.

Dr Chesney is a great character. She is extremely kind to people she likes and very rude to people she dislikes. Luckily for me she is very friendly to me.

We are having lovely weather. It is like a hot English August in the day and very cold at night. The country all round is flat and rather wild, with little deserted villages with all the shops boarded up. The only excitement we have is a daily visit from an aeroplane.

19 October
Enemy guns became louder. At 10.30am aeroplanes again bombed us. One of the Sisters was hit on the arm by a piece of bomb but she escaped with a bruise and a hole in her coat. Guns were much louder. 4.30 news came that things were better, but we were to sleep in our clothes and all our personal luggage was packed. 11pm wounded men were brought to us. Between 11pm and 5.30am, 200–300 wounded came in.

20 October
7.30 am. All the wounded were sent off to Medjidia. 8 am we were ordered to evacuate. We left Bulbulmick at twelve o'clock and were taken by our motors to a little village about 8 miles to the rear. There we put up three tents. We slept in our clothes on the ground.

21 October
We sent off all unnecessary luggage including beds, pillows, stores and all our tents except four. We kept the mess tent, two small tents and a hospital tent. A box of emergency rations, a few cases of provisions and a small quantity of hospital stores. At 2pm an orderly galloped up with bad news and at 4pm we were ordered to retreat. We started at 5pm. We, i.e. Dr C., three sisters, four orderlies, our cook and myself. We were under the orders of Dr Stanovitch the head of the first Serbian Lazarette. He had 120 men under his command and about 40 wagons. We each climbed on a wagon – already piled high with equipment and started off – destination unknown. It was then almost dark and there were no lights. The guns were going hard the whole time. We went in the direction of Constanza. At 11pm there was a violent thunder storm and rain. At 1am we stopped and pitched our mess tent. We all slept in this after eating a meal of bread and marmalade.

22 October
Got up at 6.30am and watched processions of Serbian and Roumanian cavalry and artillery. We were in the middle of a huge camp of Russian and Serbian soldiers. We left at 12 midday. This time two in a wagon. After we always sat in the same wagons. We halted for an hour in the afternoon and then drove on. It was a lovely evening and we watched Constanza burning. All round the horizon we could see burning villages.

The guns were very loud. We drove on until 12.30 mid-night in the direction of a place called Karamagat. Our object was to cross the Danube and get into Russia. But except for Czernavoda there are no bridges in the Dobrudja and we had to depend on the chance of getting steamers or of crossing by a hypothetical pontoon bridge.

23 October
Left at 9.30am and got into a stream of refugees. The roads were blocked with peasants fleeing with all their worldly goods including cattle, ponies, geese, hens, etc. and with soldiers retreating. All kinds of rumours were flying about. During that day we heard that Constanza had fallen. As the day went on the crowds of refugees became more and more disorganised. Roumanian troops dashed down the road in complete confusion. They flogged their horses and shouted and behaved disgustingly. Our Serbian doctor told us that no one knew where head quarters staff was and that he had had no orders or communications from them for two days. In the evening we lost our way and wasted about three hours going bang in the wrong direction. We camped at 12.30 midnight.

24 October
Left at 10am and got to Hirsova, a town on the Danube, at 5.30pm. We heard there that Medjidia and Czernovoda had fallen, that the disorganisation was complete and that no defence could be made. The Roumanians had started to run away at once and had been running hard ever since. The Serbians fought most wonderfully and have been, owing to those miserable Roumanians, almost destroyed. Four thousand or so are all that are left of the first division. There were no wounded for us to attend to because they had to be left behind for the Bulgars and the Bulgars are not taking prisoners. Dr Stanovitch came to see Dr C. that evening. He told her that he had been ordered to consult with her if he was in a tight place. He said he was in a very tight place. That the position was very serious. It was impossible to communicate with the staff as no one knew where they were. It was impossible to cross the river at Hirsova as the barges were all too crowded already. He didn't know the country or the roads and his only plan was to follow the crowd and hope to find a pontoon bridge at a place called Iskaktcha. As far as he knew there was no reason why the Bulgars shouldn't swoop down on us at any moment, as there were no troops between us and them.

25 October
Left Hirshova at 10am and drove until 2am without a halt. Our food was rather sketchy that day. We lived on ship's biscuits and bully beef.

26 October
Started at 9.30am and halted at 6pm on a plain overlooking some hills near Machin. The Bulgars were the other side of the hills and there was no one between them and us. We rested there for three hours and went on from 9pm to 11.30am next morning without stopping. Luckily the night was fine though cold. We were able to go a little faster here because we had by this time got clear of the refugees. But we never managed more than 3 miles an hour. Roumanians running hard passed us all night.

27 October
About 10am we came to Iskaktcha and found a pontoon bridge which we crossed and got safely into Russia. We camped at 8pm at a place called Karagatch. It was a beastly night, cold and windy and very wet. The rain dripped through the mess tent and we had to hammer in the tent pegs at intervals during the night.

28 October
Spent the morning washing some of our very dirty clothes. For nine nights we had not undressed and our washing had been almost nil. In the afternoon we moved into a little house in the village. It was clean and dry although cold as there was no fire and we had to cook over a camp fire in the garden. We stayed here for three nights, put up the hospital tent and had two or three patients.

31 October
We trekked again to a small village about 12 kilometres away. Spent the night in a delightful little cottage in which there was a fire.

1 November
Trekked again from 10am till midnight with a halt of an hour. It was very cold and a beastly day, and the roads were very bad. We got in too late to cook anything and there was no water to be had anyway.

2 November
Moved on from Bolgrad to a small village 12 miles away.

3 November
Arrived at Ismaila at 3pm and were given our present quarters. We have been here ever since but we may move again shortly.

I wish we were going back to the front but it's not very likely that we shall do so just yet as the poor Serbs need a rest badly. Everyone says that they fought magnificently. The Roumanians made no attempt to stand up to the Bulgars, and the wretched Serbs were left to do the best they could. The news is now much better. The Russians have sent a large army to the Dobrudja and Czernavoda has been retaken.

I gave an anaesthetic the other day entirely on my own, and to my great joy the man was not sick afterwards.

[Letter of 4 November from Ismaila]
We are settled here possibly for three days – possibly 3 months. Four rooms have been commandeered for us in a house.

The four orderlies sleep in one large room. Dr C. and I share a room, the three Sisters have the third and we eat in a fourth. We have no beds, or mattresses or pillows, but I am getting quite hardened to sleeping on the floor.

We get rations of meat, butter and bread. The bread portion is sometimes rather meagre as it is difficult to get.

The Unit is now split into 3 lots – some are at Galatz – others at Braila – and we are here. Until today we didn't know where anyone else was and communication was impossible.

We are opening a hospital here tomorrow. The Serb doctors are to be in charge of the medical cases and Dr C. in charge of the surgical.

We have no clothes or possessions here as all our kitbags were sent off in a hurry to Galatz. Most of us had a change of clothes with us but we have had to do a good deal of lending and borrowing.

21.11.16
Ismaila
We are getting quite a number of patients in our hospital now. I have five under my care!

We are learning Russian industriously from one of the Russian doctors attached to our Lazarette.

In return we teach him English.

At present we are living very well because the chief cook of the Unit is staying with us for a week. She really belongs to Dr Inglis's Unit but she has been lent to us while our two very amateur kitchen orderlies are having a holiday in Galatz.

Mrs Milne, the head cook, is a perfect marvel. She makes the most delicious dishes out of nothing. Food here is very scarce and dear and we are supposed to live on our rations which consist of meat, bread, milk where there is any and eggs when they can be bought. We are allowed to add to this occasionally, i.e. we get apples and quinces from the market and we still have jam and marmalade and sugar.

21.11.16
Ismaila
Dearest Louise,
We live a happy party of nine in four rooms and we haven't yet quarrelled. We are as civilised as we can be but even doing our best we can't help being rather piggy. Washing is a difficulty. Dr C. has a rubber bath and she and I have one every other night. The hot water comes from a kettle and the supply is apt to be inadequate. Our lamps are apt to go out for lack of petroleum and there is not a candle for sale in the town. Our kitchen orderlies who cook for us are the merest amateurs and not very clever ones either. They do their best but their only idea in life is to make a stew.

The two nursing orderlies we have with us are not bad, in fact they are very capable etc. etc. but they are very Scotch and one of them sits next to me at meals. The three Sisters are the most hopeless people you can imagine. Dr C. is the one bright star in this company. She is very clever and amusing and kind but she has the devil of a temper and can be quite ruthless on occasions.

4.12.16
Ismaila
Dr Inglis is starting a hospital for Russians at Isakcha, a little Roumanian village on the other side of the Danube and about 2 hours journey by steamer from here. Dr

Chesney is going there tomorrow to consult with her about our future and I am to be left in charge here! Luckily there isn't very much to take charge of.

It is getting very cold here now but there is no snow. This miserable house is like the Arctic regions. There is no wood to be had and no means of warming it.

In the afternoons Dr C. and I go for a walk from 2–4 to keep warm, and we have now explored all the country round about. My Russian is getting on very slowly.

Our only amusement is having tea in the café. But one can't depend on that. Last Sunday we went there and there wasn't a thing to eat in the shop. We had to be content with black coffee. There was no milk or sugar.

11.12.16

We have just heard that Bucharest fell 3 or 4 days ago and that 5 of our Unit have been taken prisoners. But we don't know their names.

Dr C. is going with one of our party to Odessa in two days time to try and make arrangements there for a base hospital until the Serbs go into action again, when we go with them. The rest of us are to follow with the Serbians next Sunday 17 December. It will be a loathesome journey. We shall have to drive to Belgrade and it will take us two days. From there we go in a military train to Odessa. It will be very boring. We now have nothing to read and have exhausted all topics of conversation. Two of the Sisters are not on speaking terms with each other – otherwise we have no quarrels. It must be rather awkward for the Sisters because they share a room and sit next each other at meals.

18.12.16

Belgrade

We left Ismaila at 8am on Sunday 17th. It was dark and very cold and disgustingly muddy. We each sat on an ammunition cart beside the driver and we drove along about 2 miles an hour. The news is very bad and I should think it is quite a question who gets to Benderi first, ourselves or the Germans. Braila has fallen and Galataz is evacuated.

When we arrived here we found to our great joy some English Naval volunteers with armoured cars and an ambulance. They had just escaped from the Bulgars and got here about the same time that we did after fleeing more or less all night hotly pursued by Bulgarian cavalry. They told us that aeroplanes visited Ismaila yesterday – the day on which we left.

19.12.16

We arrived at the station, which is 7 miles away from the town, at 10am, and were then told that our train would not leave until 10pm at the earliest. All we could do was to put our rugs etc in the waiting room and fill up the time by eating and drinking and talking to Russian officers. One of the officers gave us an account of a terrible scene in the Duma which ended in the fall of the Russian premier. This man heard it from a friend of his who was a member of the Duma and had been present. He was very mysterious about telling us and insisted on walking up and down out of doors so that he could be sure no one was listening. If what he says is true, and I think it is, the situation is very serious.

24.12.16
Odessa
Found to our great joy that Dr Chesney had managed to get a hospital here.

The news is bad and everyone seems to think that Odessa may have to be evacuated shortly.

For the moment we are just starting a hospital for 100 beds here. It is an ideal place as it has just been fitted up by the Russians for a hospital and everything is new and clean. They had no medical staff ready to work it and we have come along in the nick of time.

Our outfit was not designed for city life and after camping and trekking and living in hovels for 3 months we feel most terribly shabby and ragged …

Miss Florence Farmborough

1st Letuchka (Flying Column)

10th Field Surgical Otryad of the Zemstvo of all the Russias

Throughout 1915 the Germans continued to advance and the Russian army was forced to retreat. The flying columns set up their dressing-stations wherever possible – and then dismantled them and followed the retreating army as the situation deteriorated.

In October 1915 Florence Farmborough had a month's leave in Moscow and then returned to her unit at Chertoviche.

In May 1916 the Russians began an offensive against the enemy army, successfully pushing them back westwards. The flying column once again found suitable places for hospitals and dressing-stations in strategic towns and villages and continued to nurse the endless stream of appalling casualties. At the end of May, Florence Farmborough's field hospital was at Buchach on the Eastern Front.

28 May. Buchach
We arrived in Buchach at 6pm. We passed many Austrian trenches, interspersed with the trenches hastily dug by the pursuing Russians; they, needless to say, were recognisable by their general untidiness and slight depth. A great battle must have raged here, for the earth looked blackened and bruised and the trees too bore the marks of devastation.

Trinity Sunday, 29 May
Unexpected instructions were sent to us. We were to open and equip a new lazaret for wounded in another district of Buchach. We left after dinner and drove to the appointed premises, where all the rooms were in a terrible state of disorder. It took us some time to get everything straight and clean. At last all was ready; and not a

minute too soon, for ambulance-vans were making their way up the street; about thirty wounded men were deposited in and around our station. We unpacked all the necessary equipment and prepared ourselves for some hard work.

Monday, 30 May
The Red Cross Otryads, stationed in Buchach, are leaving and our Unit will be the only one left in town. We already have requests from the 41st and 47th Divisions to accept and attend to their wounds. Firing is continuing intermittently, but there is no further news from our Front.

I went into the garden for half an hour this morning. It was a brief respite, but in those thirty minutes I had seen something which steadied my nerves and refreshed my mind. It was the flowering beauty of the Austrian countryside. How strange that men should want to kill each other in springtime! How monstrous that war can exist when all the world is in blossom!

Tuesday, 31 May
During the afternoon the news was flashed round the Unit that, on our Southern Front, a great victory had been won. Whole regiments of Austrian soldiers had given themselves up and the town of Chernovits, in the Austrian province of Bukovina, was about to surrender to General Lechitski, the Commander-in-Chief of Russia's 9th Army. The good news was, naturally, very heartening; we went about our work in high spirits.

Later in the evening a message was received that about 100 wounded were on their way to us. They arrived around 11.30pm. We bandaged them, fed them and sent them off in our motor vehicles. Some of them were so exhausted that they fell asleep while we were still cleaning their wounds.

Sunday, 12 June. Buchach
During the last week work has been strenuous at times. We have had several deaths, but many of the men were fatally wounded and only came to us to die. I was on duty all day yesterday. Two of our operated patients died; both operations – one head, the other stomach – were exceedingly difficult, but there was just a slender chance. Once again, the valour of the men of the 102nd Vyatski Regiment has come to our notice; the Regiment has sustained dreadful injuries and nearly a whole rota [company] has been wiped out. The enemy had broken in on both flanks and our men, practically surrounded, were fighting the Austrians face to face; many of the wounds we dressed were inflicted by bayonets and the butts of rifles.

When the operations were over, the patients would be set apart in a room, tent, or barn, with a Sister and orderly in attendance. One of our ambulance-drivers was brought to us yesterday evening with a very badly wounded leg. When I saw him I sensed that there would be trouble, for he was a Tatar and I knew that Tatars had many strong convictions and strange prejudices.

Among our transport-drivers were several Tatars, sturdy, reliable men, who kept themselves somewhat apart from their Russian comrades. Being Moslems, they were scrupulous in observing their holy days and their diet. There were so many of them in our Letuchka that at times special food would be prepared, and one of the large 'drums-on-wheels', our mobile kitchens, allotted to these soldiers, who would go hungry rather than eat the food forbidden by their religion.

Kulja, our driver, was a quiet middle-aged man, a very devout Moslem. When he came to himself, our head doctor told him quietly that his leg would have to come off. He shook his head: 'No!' emphatically, 'No!' He would never allow his leg to be amputated. The doctor told him that he would wait until the next morning and hoped that by then he would have changed his mind; otherwise his life would be in jeopardy. Had he been a Russian, the situation would have been easier, but with a Moslem it was a different matter; they had rules which might prevent the amputation of a limb against the owner's will. The morning came and the doctors told Kulja in plain words that, unless his leg were taken off, he would certainly die, for gangrene had set in. Again he steadfastly refused an amputation. 'Good,' he said, 'I will die willingly, if Allah so wishes. The will of Allah be done.' He died in the evening, exactly 24 hours after he had been brought to us. I was with him at the end. He was quite happy: his simple faith never wavered for a moment. We hear that one of our Base hospitals is to be transferred to Buchach; we are glad, because our wounded men will be spared a long journey. A new prekaz [order] has been issued to the effect that all Austrians in the districts near the Russian Front Lines are to leave their homes and go eastwards to Trebunovski. All must go – old and young. I watched a sad procession of them pass through Buchlach; their carts were overladen; they carried what they could, driving their cows before them. I had often seen such endless streams of broken-hearted homeless people during 1915; nevertheless, I once again felt compassion for these helpless multitudes, driven from their native villages and forced willy-nilly into strange surroundings under a strange, hostile Government.

Thursday, 23 June

Many wounded arrived – both Russian and Austrian.

A doctor and a Sister have already gone to our new punkt [post] near the Fighting Line. They may send for a few more of our Letuchka tomorrow. I am living in hopes that I shall be included.

Friday, 24 June. Barish

The much wished-for summons came; I was called to join our team at the new first aid post.

After dinner we started off in our motor to Barish, an hour from Buchach. Arriving at 4.30pm we found the forerunners of our Letuchka installed in a partly demolished house near some devastated Austrian trenches. We distributed among them their belongings which we had brought with us, replenished the drums of sterilised material and filled the ample cupboards with lint-rolls, bandages, surgical instruments, first aid packets and general equipment. The Austrian trenches, as ever remarkably well-constructed, were smashed and shattered; wire entanglements tangled and trampled; strips of uniform-cloth were still caught up in the barbs. Craters pitted the ground on all sides; shells were piled here and there in heaps; a motor plough stood derelict in a nearby field. There were patches of dark-stained earth where men's blood had drenched the soil; bits of torn paper, oddments of cloth, battered mess-tins, a crushed furashka [peak-cap] littered the ground. And there was one corner, canopied by the broken branches of decapitated trees, where stood many groups of wooden crosses. No names were inscribed – there had been no time.

Saturday, 25 June
News reached us early this morning that our 37th Division had twice broken through the enemy lines only to be beaten back each time. Intermittently, news filtered through from the various Fronts. A great victory was reported near Balanovich, with many Germans taken prisoner.

Friday, 1 July
We hear that the British Army has smashed through the German First Line in the Somme territory, advanced many miles and taken over 14,000 prisoners.

Important instructions have just reached our Unit: two Sisters, two Brothers, two surgeons and a dozen hospital orderlies are to be sent to the Front tomorrow. To my indescribable joy, I am to be one of the two Sisters.

Saturday, 9 July
We returned to Barish this morning and a relay team of workers has taken our place. It will be difficult to give a coherent account of the happenings of the past week. We were in the thick of it and there was no time to think, much less to write. We turned day into night, night into day; and only a level head like the one on Alexander Mikhaylovich's broad shoulders could tell which day of the week it was – and he had to consult his pocket-calendar more than once!

The past, gloomy year of 1915, with its hopeless defeats, culminating in the great Spring and Summer Retreat of the Russian Armies, was stamped with unspeakable tragedy, suffering and frustration. It was warfare at its cruellest and worst.

Now the tables have been reversed. Instead of retreat, it is ADVANCE! We traversed the Austrian countryside – still showing signs of springtime's generous flowering – and we revelled in the knowledge that our Russian armies, and those of our brave Allies on the far-Western Front, were gaining success after success. But as we followed in the rear of our advancing troops, the trail of devastation left by war was painfully visible: we passed through deserted villages and hamlets, many of them riddled by shells and blackened by fire; an isolated chimney or half-demolished wall stood mutely forlorn on a devastated landscape. Dead, or dying, horses were lying by the wayside. Broken gun-carriages, or other vehicles, blocked parts of the roads. Trampled wire-entanglements and shell craters studded the ground on every side. Often the trees themselves would indicate the proximity of a recent battlefield; blasted, bent and broken, with their branches drooping in untimely decay, their trunks seared and jagged – dumb victims of man's inhumanity to man … and to Nature.

And the battlefield! – I saw the battlefield in all its grim reality, for we were following closely in the footsteps of our advancing troops and ever ready to tend the wounded and dying left behind in their wake. We did not enquire as to the nationality of the helpless man, nor did we seek to distinguish the colour of his uniform; we saw

– and I thank God for it – we saw only a suffering human being, who needed our help; and we gave it of our best, without discrimination.

I cannot pretend to describe all that I experienced at the small Red Cross station alongside the vanguard of our troops, for it was there that I became acquainted with a new aspect of warfare which, although savouring of victory, was no less savage and terrifying than the dark days of disastrous defeat. On the battlefields, all natural features had been blasted into nothingness and there remained only scattered vestiges of the hideous scars inflicted by lethal weapons and the spoors of wild, flying feet and staggering, stumbling bodies.

Twice had our men rushed headlong into the attack; twice had they been beaten back; yet a third attempt had left them free to occupy the deserted trenches of the enemy. But the loss of life had been appalling. Some had received no outward visible wound; their hurt had been inflicted on mind and spirit; and those we were powerless to aid.

The badly-wounded received an injection without delay and were carried to the 'sorting-house', where operations were immediately performed – stomach and head operations being in the majority. As the fighting became more intense, the wounded lay massed outside our temporary dressing-station, waiting for attention – countless stretcher cases among them. A few would crawl inside, beseeching the care they so urgently needed.

We were working day and night, snatching a brief hour here and there for sleep. In the evening the dead would be collected and placed side by side in the pit-like graves dug for them on the battlefield. German, Austrian, Russian, they lay there, at peace, in a 'brothers' grave'. Swarms of flies added to the horror of the battlefields and covered the dead brothers, waiting in their open ditches for burial, as with a thick, black pall. I remember the feeling of horror when I first saw that black pall of flies *moving*.

Wednesday, 20 July
We have all been working round the clock. Yesterday, we started at 5am, and went on steadily until five o'clock this morning. We have been told that over 1,130 wounded have passed through our Unit in the last two days.

Thursday, 21 July
Yesterday, too, we worked all day with only a few minutes' respite to drink tea or swallow a few mouthfuls of food. I am very tired and my feet and legs are aching so much that I am wondering just how long they will be able to support me.

The patience, the sustained endurance of the heavily-wounded is heart-rending. They may be in the same position for hours, seldom asking for anything, unless it be 'Water! Water!' If anyone should ask me what I consider the outstanding qualities of the Russian soldier, I would have no hesitation in replying: patience and endurance.

In one nearby yard, some 800 men are awaiting transport; it is, we know, dangerous to keep them so close to the Front Lines, but there is no alternative. They, poor souls, seem content enough; they think that, because they are in the hands of Red Cross Sisters and doctors, their safety is assured.

Saturday, 23 July

We have begun to notice the rapid development of both gangrene and tetanus resulting from flesh-wounds. It has been confirmed that enemy shrapnel are often filled not only with bullets, but with particles of rusty metal, nails, even fragments of shrapnel picked up on the battlefield. These, covered with any filthy substance, become more than ordinarily lethal. Even a small flesh-wound, little more than a scratch or graze, can prove fatal; and once the jaw is firmly locked and the spasms become more frequent, there is little medical skill can do, except to keep the doomed man under morphia sedation. We have had several bad cases in recent weeks of lockjaw; one of them had laughed at his slightly-gashed left arm – already showing signs of inflammation – and said that he was lucky that his arm had caught the splinter and not his heart! He said that he had had dozens of similar scratches at home and had taken no notice of them, but he had come to us, because his Sergeant-Major had sent him; and, he joked: 'You know what sergeant-majors are!' But after three days he had ceased to laugh and his frightened eyes were dumbly asking what had happened to him. It had been such a small scratch. We placed a wedge between his upper and lower teeth, so that his tongue could be moistened at times with a tiny swab. He died silently.

So, from now on, every soldier with a flesh wound will receive an injection of serum anti-tetanicum. Should they rebel, we shall warn them of the grim alternative! We hear that this new treatment will save thousands of lives and we thank God that such a remedy has been found in *time*.

Cholera and typhoid have taken toll of many, both military and civilian; even a smallpox scare flared up for a few days.

We are saddened at the thought that there has been no advance and that the valiant efforts of our men have met with no results – only casualties, casualties, hundreds and hundreds of them.

Lady Muriel Paget

Russian Red Cross Field Hospital, Eastern Front, Russia

By the outbreak of the First World War, Lady Muriel Paget, daughter of the 12th Earl of Winchilsea, and wife of the baronet scientist and inventor, Richard Paget, had spent nine years running soup kitchens for desperately poor mothers, children and the elderly in deprived areas of London. She was delicate and suffered from recurring ill-health, but in the spring of 1915 she was deeply influenced by a family friend, Sir Bernard Pares, who had been with a Red Cross unit attached to the Russian 3rd Army and witnessed the appalling suffering of the peasant-soldiers as they retreated before the Germans during the winter of 1914. He told her of the huge number of casualties and the great need for field hospitals and medical equipment. Muriel Paget was 'determined that she should do something about it' and became honorary organising secretary of a committee set up to recruit the staff and gather equipment for what was to become the Anglo-Russian Base Hospital in Petrograd. This was housed in the Dmitri Palace under the auspices of the Russian Red Cross. Illness kept her in England when the unit left in November 1915 and prevented her from becoming the director of the hospital when it opened at the beginning of 1916.

She eventually arrived in Petrograd in April 1916 and immediately started to organise a field hospital to operate behind the Russian front lines. Eventually the field hospital was comprised of two units both housed in tents – a mobile field hospital or lazaret, with up to 120 beds, and a casualty clearing station which was supported by ambulance carts. On 10 June the field hospital, administered and supplied by the Russian Red Cross, left Petrograd in a special train of 37 coaches which contained over 100 horses, 125 sanitars [Russian orderlies], 44 transport carts and ambulances, 2 mobile kitchens, and English doctors and nurses from the Anglo-Russian Base Hospital. There was little need for the field hospital when it arrived at Voropayevo but later at Lutsk Muriel Paget had her first taste of the real horror of war:

> *the casualties lay in their hundreds, in the public squares or the gardens, not bandaged or drugged but still in the first agony of their fresh wounds. There was the raw and featureless mass of flesh that had once been a face … the bleeding stump projecting from tattered, blood-soaked coat or trousers. The dying lay beside the dead, their faces black with flies; waiting, hour after hour, till the nurse or the surgeon could come to them. The day was hot and the stench almost unendurable …*

Two days later Muriel Paget returned to Petrograd, leaving Dr Andrew Fleming, the commandant of the Anglo-Russian Base Hospital at Petrograd, operating at Lutsk. She wrote that 'the day I left he asked for a trephine to operate upon a man's head, and was given a chisel instead. I am sending cables from Petrograd begging for more motor ambulances. We really want a hundred, to work in connection with our dressing-stations …'

The field hospital was transferred to the Galician border as part of the 8th Army and in July Muriel Paget spent a month with the hospitals at the Eastern Front during the second phase of General Brusilov's offensive. On 28 July Russian troops took the east Galician border town of Brody and 40,000 Austrian soldiers were captured. Russian casualties were heavy. Both Muriel Paget's and Florence Farmborough's [qv] field hospitals received hundreds of wounded men.

On August 12 Muriel Paget sent an impulsive and hastily written letter from Petrograd to her husband.

I am just back … still rather dazed after a very strenuous month at the front but am well and a few undisturbed nights will be all to the good – lately I have either been travelling at night or wakened by air raids at early hours of the morning – It is good to realise that you are all peacefully at home and that there is another existence besides the hell on earth. There was a continuous stream of mangled human beings on stretchers passing through our two hospitals during the guards advance – When I wrote last we were just going to Rosiche from Lutsk to join the field hospital with the guard – and the second morning I got there we were woken up at 4.30am by a bomb – whiz bang – that fell in our compound and killed two of the patients in the next hospital – 4 tents were peppered with shrapnel. That day we had two officers and several men brought to us, some of whom had air bomb wounds – at 4.30 we had the big air raid – I saw the five brutes on the sky line looking like gnats, as they came nearer they circled over the town and in line formation came over our camp – I was near a farm building and about 30 soldiers and I got inside and then the bomb fairly buzzed down and we expected to be scattered but luckily escaped – A man in a tent in the military camp was killed – one of our sanitars had his head blown off and two more men in the Rodzianca hospital were so badly wounded they died – We were extraordinarily lucky that none of our patients were hit – but as you can imagine they were very much unnerved after being wounded in the morning by bombs and then to be in a raid in the evening – 80 people were killed in the town and large numbers wounded – We saw one house in a blaze and found after it had been set on fire by incendive bomb and there had been an explosion of munitions that had been unfortunately stored in it – Several people were burnt and others who went to save them were killed and injured.

Our motors were near our camp and three bombs were dropped either side of them, the two chauffeurs were v. funny about it and said they lay on their faces and their legs flew up in the air behind as result of shock.

I went down to see the Red X and military people and found old whiskers (Gen. Willemenof) standing outside his house in which all the windows had been broken – I told him it was a shame to leave hospitals so near the station and the staff – We were one of three hospitals together under canvas – and asked if some of the patients suffering from shock could be removed and he said no – Col. Roddsianka whose wifes [sic] hospital was next to ours said he would ensist [sic] on its being removed to a place a few versts away and I said we would do the same if he did – I then had a council of war with our Drs and Ignatieff [Boris Ignatiev, the Russian Red Cross Administrator of the Field Hospital] and said we ought to move if possible because of the patients who could not be put in safety during raids – the staff could get into dug outs.

In spite of Williemenofs calous [sic] refusal of permission I started off at 11.30am, on advice of Drs, with three officers and 3 men and Hans (our mechanic who had been previously wounded) and took them in motor ambulances to Lutsk – The officers were all pretty bad and refused to have operations at Rosiche – one they thought would haemerrage [sic] on the way so fervently praying that it would not be necessary to use it I armed myself with a tournequet and for two and a half hours was wedged in between the stretchers in an ambulance trying to calm a boy who could luckily talk French and who was terrified that he would never be brave again – his friend was on the other side of me and they had both been lying asleep together near their battery when a bomb was dropped and wounded them both. An ambulance is v. uncomfortable conveyance when one is well and I pity the wounded who are jolted along in it – just when we were leaving Rosiche a sentinel stopped us and I thought was turning us back but it turned out he was only ordering us to put out our lights as a Zeppelin was expected so we had to bump along a road v. much broken up by passing of heavy artillery and bomb holes, in the night! When we got to Lutsk about 2am I went and woke Dr Jefferson [the neurosurgeon at the Anglo-Russian Hospital in Petrograd] up in his tent and we took the patients to a hospital in the town to get permission to take them on to ours [the second Field Hospital], which was granted and beds were made up for them.

You never saw such a heartrending sight as the outside of the hospital that night – as far as you could see wounded men were lying in rows and heaps in the courtyard and along the roads, half naked many of them and it was quite a cold night – Quite by chance a chauffeur and 4 of our Sisters arrived just after we did, from Petrograd en route for the Field. They slept in the motors and I was put in the Night Sisters' bed about 4am and slept till I was woke about 9.30 by an aeroplane raid but no harm was done.

We went back to Rosiche that afternoon and found the hospital had not been moved and that as the old whiskers had hinted that the English were frightened there was no question of moving but I sent a polite message to say that English and Russian Red X methods of working were different – that our staff were there to do whatever work was required but that I thought more consideration might have been given to the wounded – I knew that none of you would think we were cowards and that you and the children would hate such a thing being said as much as I did – As a matter of fact we had good dug outs made so that our only anxiety which was a v. real one was for the patients. We splattered our tents with mud and covered them with branches to conceal them as much as possible from view.

I arrived back to find our tents were full of patients – Harmer [Mr W. Douglas Harmer, Senior Surgeon at the Anglo-Russian Hospital, Petrograd], and Fleming hard at work which they continued for 4 nights and days with very little cessation – and there was great strain on the nurses and we were much understaffed as 2 nurses and a R [Russian] Dr were at our forward dressing-station in the line of fire.

You can imagine the scarcity of nurses when I tell you I was given charge of the officers' ward for two days with two sanitars to help – and had one v. anxious case of amputation of an arm – gas gangrene – and the poisoning was spreading – he is living still although Harmer said he could not live more than two days – I found the officers v. exigeante [sic] and fussy, poor dears, but I didn't mind. What worried me was the difficulty in getting food the first two days. Ignatieff had gone to dressing-station and left chaos re catering and I had to go to the kitchens and take all my patients' meals – I had a spirit lamp in the tent to heat milk etc. and gave them eggs beaten in milk and my gas gangrene man had half a bottle of brandy the first day.

A woman with an abdominal wound from a bomb was brought in and we had to put her in the mess tent, a darling little girl of 3 called Ola was sitting quite unperturbed on her mother's stretcher and I had her in my tent as well as a R sister to sleep for two nights and did not get much rest, especially as we were disturbed by air raids at 6am – and had to bundle Ola down to dug out – she didn't seem the least surprised and was much more annoyed when I gave her a bath – v. necessary and the hair combing was not too pleasant – A little brother had been wounded in the head by the same bomb as the mother and we thought he had been killed and did not dare to tell the mother, and then we found him in another hospital – such a joy – he is about four and is now walking about in white hospital suit – we hope he and mother may live.

I don't turn a hair at all the horrors seen in the operating and dressing rooms, but when children are brought in wounded I can't bear it.

It is 2am now and I have scribbled this for a nurse to take home in hopes it will get through all right, but a more coherent letter will follow Monday – I went to the dressing-station a few versts from the Stochardt (don't know how it is spelt in English) river and came in for a night attack by Germans, though I was quite safe in dug out and only heard tremendous cannonading – A spy let off a rocket in our village to show exactly where the divisional staff was.

I sent the two nurses down to help at F.H. and stayed in case any wounded came through in the night with R Dr, but they didn't and the whole of that night there was a retreat of troops – changing position – I ran like a rabbit when shrapnel came in my direction but it is nothing to the air bombs – When our transport went to the dressing-station a German aeroplane followed it and shot at it with maxim gun.

When rush of work was over I came back here [Anglo-Russian Hospital, Petrograd] and will tell of my journey next time – there are many difficulties and complications re Drs and I just long to come home and see you all but may face things better tomorrow – meanwhile all my love … am almost asleep.

Our hospitals were really wanted at front, all serious cases from neighbouring hospitals brought to us for operations, great compliment …

Miss Dorothy Seymour

Anglo-Russian Hospital, Petrograd, Russia

Dorothy Seymour was the daughter of General Lord William Frederick Ernest Seymour, a granddaughter of an Admiral of the Fleet, and a Woman of the Bedchamber to HRH Princess Christian. Although socially she moved in illustrious circles when serving abroad as a Red Cross VAD, she also experienced the hardship and discomfort of hospitals near the front line. Between November 1914 and June 1916 she served in hospitals in Wimereux and Versailles.

On 9 September 1916 she left Newcastle in the troopship Jupiter *bound for Bergen in Norway, en route to Russia. She was sent to the Anglo-Russian Hospital in Petrograd, which was housed on the first floor of the Grand Duke Dmitri Pavlovich's baroque palace. The ground floor was occupied by the Grand Duke, who was a favourite nephew of the Tsar. Family retainers and friends lived on the top floor. During her time here Dorothy Seymour was often entertained by Russian aristocrats and prominent members of the British diplomatic community.*

6 September (Russian date)

The hospital is beautiful in many ways, but a lot of people hate it and a lot like it. Lady M [Lady Muriel Paget, the first Administrator, qv] and the Matron are both away at the field station at this moment and everyone likes both of them. Personally I am in luck as I'm in what they call the bandaging room so have always plenty to do, but some of the other VADs have a deadly time. The nurses seem a very nice lot and we are awfully well treated by them. Everything is beautifully done here, our rooms like little cabins all in one huge vast saloon and I've got next to a window so am in luck. Everything very clean and a home sister who takes endless trouble to make one comfortable, our hot water bottles filled at night and hot water in the mornings, the food excellent and plenty of it. In fact I don't see why they all grumble, but they do, mostly I think because they imagined that they were going out to tea every day and the Russians have other things to do.

Petrograd is very smelly, very large and very unwarlike, much more so than London. Also the ordinary Russian seems to take very little interest in the war.

The Russian Soldier 'officers' we met travelling etc are awfully interesting and so extraordinarily pleasant. Four of them gave up their carriage from Tornea to all of us and travelled in the passage as if it was the most ordinary thing to do.

21 September (8th)
The men in hospital are so comic. All like children of six, very few able to read or write, but all able to sing in parts which they do every day. They are taking a huge interest in teaching me Russian but every man pronounces every word differently so I'm in a nice jumble.

The hospital is in a most beautiful palace. It is really lovely but all the tapestry covered up with wood. Wonderful fireplaces and ceilings and doors.

We have been very busy so have only had about an hour off each day so I haven't seen much but the view from the window is lovely. One of the small rivers or canals from the Neva goes just past and the Dow Emp Palace all pink just opposite and alongside a lovely green carved wooden palace.

10 September
I had a half day yesterday and went all along the Neva. Perfectly lovely, a huge wide stretch of water and palaces the whole way.

I saw Maud Hoare yesterday and him. Their accounts of the difficulties of food etc out here are very funny. Luckily being Red Cross we are very well fed.

Politics are thrilling out here but it's difficult to get a grasp of them at all, it's such a glorious muddle.

22 Sept. (4 October)
I see more of the Russians than English people. Lady G.B. [Lady Georgina Buchanan, the British Ambassador's wife] is very sniffy about who she invites and has a deadly household, so nobody takes much notice of her.

It's so odd there being no trace of the war here, heaps of men about, dinners and plays going on, the only thing no man changes for dinner which is supposed to be because of the war, but it's the only sign except the prices of everything which are ruinous.

The canals are all filled up with barges bringing wood to burn as there is no coal here. Even the railway engines burn wood.

14 Oct.
Admiral Phillimore has been here again and took me and the Lindleys to the Ballet, quite lovely. I've dined out every night this week. It's lucky the work is so light. Tonight I am having dinner with the English Naval Attache, Captain Grenfell.

It's been beastly weather the last ten days, rain and trying to snow, but it's lovely again now and a hard frost. The Neva rose yesterday because the wind was in the south and it rained and all the canals overflowed and swam into the streets.

The great amusement here is to take the cripples out for drives. An expensive amusement but some have been in the same ward 9 months as no one takes these men out or gives them teas and they love it. The isvoscheeks are only made to hold two at a pinch, but that's dull for them to go out one at a time so I take them out two sitting bodkin with crutches and stiff legs sticking out in all directions.

I do wish you could see them all singing and dancing in the evenings. The orderly is the shape of a very prize pig but dances the most marvellous steps and hops and jumps.

4 Nov.
Still heaps of people doing nothing and we are badly wanted in Odessa but organisation is so bad that we can't get there. I went to a gorgeous ballet last night. The night before I dined with the Hoares. Very amusing party, Roumanian Minister, French Ambassador, Russian Admiral and a very elegant and totally brainless English attache.

Yesterday we had a wonderful day. Went to Tsarkoe Selo [The Village of the Tsar] and had a special ticket to see it. A wonderful palace and a new church the Tsar has just built that made one feel like being in the Arabian Nights. It's the most wonderful place I've ever seen, positively made one gasp with the beauty of it as one got in and such luck to see it as very few are allowed in. The whole thing is looked after by the Tsar's special regiment of huge Cossacks and they were hanging about guarding every stone and outside each blade of grass that the Tsar might ever walk over, and one enormous, very old man with a long white beard, a brilliant red Cossack coat and an enormous top heavy fur cap, all white astrachan, on his head, walking round to see to everything.

I feel so ashamed of jaunting so much but it seems different out here somehow and unless one did one would never hear a word of war news, as nothing gets into the papers and it's only what one can glean from meeting people that one can go by. No Russian ever mentions the war, it is so odd, but of course everyone else talks of nothing else and the men in hospital always talk of the war and what they think of it. Anyhow one is being useful out here by giving them the one bit of kindness they ever get in their lives. I took one boy out for a drive the other day. He is a cripple for life and has been in the same ward ever since he was carried in last March. So with enormous excitement he was carted downstairs and into an isvoscheek and we drove about Petrograd and he'd lived all his life in the middle of Siberia and never seen a large town and was so overpowered by all he saw that his eyes nearly walked out of his head and he pinched my arm black and blue.

12 Nov.
I am so far having luck with Sisters. I was with an awfully nice woman till she went on nights and then two days with a most objectionable lady and every prospect of remaining with her when two men got desperately ill, both of whom had been in the ward where I had been and they were moved into a small room together, with a very nice nurse in charge and luckily she wanted help and I was sent to her as I knew the

men already, so I'm having a most peaceful time with her as she's a real nice woman, not the least like a nurse and both men take up all our time looking after them. One, alas, I don't think there's a chance for, the other is mending.

Lady Sybil Grey [who took over as Administrator from Lady Muriel Paget] and I had luncheon with Captain Grenfell the other day. She is a nice person.

I'm dining with Maud Hoare this evening. I had a comic dinner-party at the parson's the other day. I wasn't looking forward to it at all and went feeling virtuous, to find a house crammed with Russian treasures, furniture, prints, ikons, drawings, carpets and silks, a real gorgeous medley, so unparson-like.

15 Nov.

I went to a lovely Russian opera the other day, *Igor*, and to dine with the Lindleys last night. We've just sent off a party to Archangel to help them. Isn't it appalling? I do wish I'd been one of them.

21 Nov.

There's plenty of news but none writeable, but we are fairly living here, no day without some excitement, sometimes sheer rumour, sometimes only too true.

It's really got cold at last, the Neva and canals beginning to freeze over and everything so pretty.

Tonight, alas, the French Ambassador asked me to dinner, but I can't get off duty till after 8 so had to refuse. Instead I'm having dinner with Admiral Phillimore who is here for one day.

1 Dec.

The Empress has just sent word that she wants me to go down and see her one day soon. It will be very interesting as she is busy making history that will count large in the future and I want to see for myself what she is like. It will be too annoying if they start a revolution before I have time to get down to see her.

The old Empress's lady in waiting sent and asked me to tea with her the other day. Such a nice woman, Countess Olga Heyden. She first called on me in pomp with a royal carriage, and the royal footman, clothed in scarlet dressing gown and gold lace and a cocked hat paraded the hospital looking for me, which has upset the whole company, most of the nurses thinking it was Admiral Phillimore in his best uniform.

17 Dec.

The interview I told you was likely is now not the least likely to happen as she is not seeing anyone just now, an amazing fairy tale the reason like the middle ages.

I saw Lord Hindlip the other day. He's out here for a week at the Hoares and has been King's Messengering everywhere lately so we really heard the news at last.

Last night Lady Sybil took me to the Barraclicka concert, awfully fascinating and quite wonderful.

26 Dec.

Dined with Mrs Lombard and met Dmitri Pavlovitch [The Grand Duke] – beautiful to behold, vastly conceited, but superb in glorious youth and dash. Talked of many intrigues. Gather something big is afoot.

28 Dec.
We have Xmassed and are still doing so. We had an awful Xmas dinner that took hours, the whole staff dining together, which as we saw each other all day and every day was most funereal as no one could think of anything to say to each other. Tonight there are mawkish theatricals for the benefit of the people who have been nice to us and asked us out etc.

Last night a little Russian Admiral sent me tickets for *Shaliapin*, such luck as it's perfectly impossible to get them anyhow else as they are all booked months ahead and he was singing in *Boris Goudonoff*. It was too heavenly. I didn't know anyone could sing like that and he is so magnificent as well to look at.

There's real snow now to stay and sleighs and everything looking lovely.

The hospital has filled up with some bad cases, three blind, that are all very miserable. They are so bad, poor things.

30 Dec.
Rasputin was killed by Dmitri Pavlovitch and Prince Usonpoff [Prince Felks Yusupov, a relation by marriage of the Tsar] at six this morning after a night of very noisy revelry in this Palace. No facts known – great mystery – Prince Usonpoff takes all blame – also had it put into evening papers: 'This morning after high revelry left life Gregory Rasputin'. That is all. Dmitri and Usonpoff came into the hospital to have a wound in Usonpoff's neck dressed. In mad spirits …

Miss Marjery Swynnerton

No. 3 British General Hospital, Basra, Mesopotamia

Marjerie Swynnerton lived in India and when the war started she trained as a nurse in a nursing home in Mussorie. She served in various military hospitals in India from April 1916, until at the age of twenty-two, she was sent to No. 3 British General Hospital in Basra, as a temporary army nurse.

Alas for my excitement, the Home Sister knew nothing about my arrival. I was an enigma. I explained about missing the convoy. She was not interested, what was a temporary nurse?

The huts were long prefabricated ones chopped up into sections to form rooms for the Sisters. They were designed for the heat, as there was a gap of six inches or so between walls and floor, to allow for wind.

At that moment the wind was frightful, cutting cold and sandy, freezing my feet. I just leant against the wall as the room was empty and still did not feel depressed. This was really 'Active Service'.

At last an Indian servant brought my kit: my trunk, my hold-all and somewhere along the route I had signed for, and been given, my camp kit. This was a large green canvas bag containing my bed, a chair, a canvas bath and basin and a small round canvas bucket.

The Indian who put up the bed had the end of his turban hanging down, an insolent gesture in India, and also answering back when I spoke to him sharply about some small thing.

So off I went to the Home Sister and reported him. 'Oh', she said in English to the man, 'Ali, you mustn't be rude to the Sisters, and if they are rude to you you must come and tell me.'

This was the first puzzling chink, to me, of the cracking of the British Raj. Speaking in English was bad enough, but telling Ali to come and tell her if the Sisters were rude!

Then the bugle went for the midday meal. I was directed to the dining hall and told to sit anywhere. So I did – then told I must not sit there as it was the Senior's table – then at the next, reserved for someone else. Finally I found a nice, humble place where no one spoke to me.

In fact no one spoke to me, except for some orders, for two weeks. The food was nearly always bully beef, rice and dates, the bully beef sometimes cold and sometimes dressed up as rissoles or hash. We had rice instead of potatoes. The dates were in great lumps and had to be prised apart, and many were the stories that were told of Arabs trampling down the dates with their bare unwashed feet! The Red Cross provided comforts which included bottles of claret which were shared out at the meal. All water was suspect, heavily chlorinated and tasted vile and smelled worse.

There were only a few 'Temporary' nurses from India and we were bitterly resented by the QA's at first. They looked upon us as 'young chits' who received the same pay as they did; that was the bitter pill, after all their years of training and experience.

To mark some difference for all to see, the first step was to order us to tie our caps back. This made a sort of butterfly at the back of our heads and made us look very attractive which had not been the idea! We were also to be called the 'Voluntary Aid Detachment', or VAD's, in future.

I was told to report to the Sister in charge of three huts. Each hut had about 32 or 36 beds. After a time we became friends but for about two weeks no one spoke to me in those wards except the patients – except to order me about. My first orders were to go from bed to bed, one hut after the other, to tidy beds and get the sheets the right width at the turnover. The right width was the width of the bed-board exactly. It was winter and I do not think I have ever suffered so much from the cold as I did getting those beds and sheets straight. That awful wind, the 'Shamal' was at its height; it cut right through one and the sand in the rough red army blankets and mostly unbleached sheets cut my fingers and nails to pieces. My chilblains were frightful. The wind is said to blow for 40 days and 40 nights.

I shall never forget my gratitude to a walking patient who rather adopted me. He would bring me a basin of hot water to soak my frozen hands. That treatment was not the best for chilblains but it did thaw out my hands. Sometimes he would sneak me a hot mug of cocoa from where the sisters and MO's were having their elevenses and laughing and having a great time. The man's name was McNamara. I hope he is in heaven if no longer here.

Another job I was detailed for, because no one else liked to do it, was to be on duty in the large tent where the walking patients had their midday meal. In that cold they were only too pleased to wear their thick hospital blue but a red tie goes with that costume and I had to stand at the entrance and not let anyone in without a tie properly tied!

I was very nervous at first; it was not very pleasant to send someone back for his tie when he had only one arm or leg, or looked like death. However, they soon realised that it was I who would get into hot water, if they had no tie, and I had no trouble on that score.

But there was great trouble of another kind. The British Tommies did not want to sit with the 'blacks' and the blacks did not want to sit with each other.

The blacks were not Indians; we never saw them. They were negroes. Some, from the West Indies, were cultured, educated men, more fastidious than many a British soldier with their array of toilet articles on their lockers – tooth brushes, sponges, talcum powder, etc.

Some were just wild savages from the Gold Coast or Nigeria, brought to work on the Inland Waterways. Cups and saucers, cutlery, etc., were something they had never seen at that time, and their table manners were simply non-existent.

So the two lots of negroes, who looked exactly alike, had to be found separate tables. The poor West Africans died of pneumonia like flies in that cold. Some were in the medical huts where I tidied the beds.

One called Accra did not die. We called him Accra as none of us had any knowledge of the Gold Coast. In his delirium he had climbed up the high central pole in the hut, thinking it was a coconut palm, and had to stay there as pulling him down might have been too rough on his heart. He came down eventually and recovered.

The Sister gave him a bag of Red Cross comforts to take away. These included a gaudy pair of pink striped pyjamas. He was delighted, and put them on over his drab khaki. All the West Africans, in spite of some very dirty habits, were great favourites as they were always ready to smile and were grateful for everything done for them.

Kut, under General Townsend, had fallen in April 1916, and we still had some who had been through that hell, and had been sent down as totally unfit. However ill they were, they were the lucky ones, as of the 13,000 odd made to walk into captivity 70 per cent had died or were to die. With no medical attention, hardly any food or water, they had to struggle through burning hot deserts, terrible mud when it rained, flies, sand, mosquitoes, with dysentery, malaria and sunstroke. But what was feared most was the deadly enmity of the marauding Arabs.

It was their Moslem duty to kill 'infidels' and any poor, sick soldier who fell away from the main body of captives would be tortured, killed and sometimes mutilated. They even crept silently into the camps and stole the boots off the exhausted men and any other kit they could find. The apathy and indifference of the Turks to the terrible misery of their captives roused many of their German allies to protest at their treatment at some places en route.

The siege of Kut, which had lasted 5 and a half months, was still being talked about. 'The most heroic muddle in our history'. And although everything had improved so much in Mesopotamia, we still did not have enough blankets for the patients in that cold wind. We had some Valour stoves at intervals down the wards but they were inadequate owing to the draught from the gaps under the walls of the huts built for hot weather only.

One day my eldest brother, Dick, turned up at my ward. I did not even know he was there in Mespot. He had been very ill with malaria and lying on the deck on some boat. He said that conditions had been frightful. Men had died on each side of him and there had been no one to take them away or to attend to the living. He was in an Indian Regiment. He was on his way on leave to India. He presented me with a very pretty Persian rug which I used on top of my bed to keep out the cold.

Perhaps it was my brother's visit which now tipped the scales in my favour. Anyway, from then on I was treated normally and even allowed to have my elevenses with everyone else. We VAD's were now called 'Very Adorable Darlings' and were becoming rather spoilt.

In our off-duty time, we would hire a bellam – a kind of canoe – and go shopping. Basra is full of creeks – No. 3 BGH was on Ashar Creek. Flies are one of the plagues of Mespot. It was horrible to see hundreds of flies clustering unnoticed round the eyes, noses and mouths of young Arab children. They are sticky flies and very difficult to discourage, but the Arabs did not seem to mind them.

Another plague is mud. When it rains it pours, and the rain does not sink into the earth, instead all the sand and mud comes up to mix with the water so that the land becomes like runny, sticky porridge. One day I had gone out with a very tiny sister (we had to go out in twos). Somehow, she tripped and fell into this frightful brown mess. It was quite a job to pull her out and, luckily for her, we were not far from the Sisters' Club where we were able to clean her up.

Christmas was now upon us and we gave a Fancy Dress Dance at the Quarters. I went as 'Eve of the Tatler' and scored quite a success. A gunboat, I think the *Moth* was in harbour, and the officers came to our dance and then invited us back on board.

Just about this time, a terrible tragedy occurred. A boat full of real VADs and their Matron had just arrived. They had been at Salonika and had had a very horrible time after the Dardanelles fiasco.

The ones I saw were jolly, pretty girls and everyone was out to invite them to parties and to make a great fuss of them and they had invitations en bloc to all sorts of things.

They were all invited to a big dinner party down the river at a place called Mohommerah and a motor launch was sent to fetch them. They never arrived. Their launch was cut in two by another boat in the dark and most of them were drowned. It was my unfortunate task to sit with the half-demented Matron who had been rescued, as the sodden piles of clothing were brought in for identification.

Just as I was going to the burial service for those whose bodies had been recovered, an officer from the 7th Hussars whom I had known at Meerut turned up and wanted me to go out with him. He was extremely annoyed when I could not go …

Miss Ida Jefferson

Desert Hospital, inland from Basra, Mesopotamia

Ida Jefferson trained as a nurse and joined the Queen Alexandra's Imperial Military Nursing Service at the outbreak of the war. After serving in a hospital – a day's journey from Bombay – in the hills near Nasik, India, her unit was sent to Mesopotamia. They were taken on bullock carts from Basra to the desert hospital.

Soon after our arrival we experienced our first sandstorm, and it was very unpleasant. It was unbearably hot and many of our number were very soon patients themselves. One had to walk up and down hastily to create a breeze to enable one to breathe more freely. It was almost suffocating. A very dry heat. We settled in as comfortably as possible, but, at first, the heat, lack of water and fresh foods, affected us all.

There was an intense number of drawbacks to our comfort, but we all agreed that the worst was the terrible heat. The patients, many of whom were heatstroke and sunstroke cases, suffered terribly. The sanitary arrangements were the best under the circumstances but very far from what we had been used to in India. We were now on active service undoubtedly. Many of the staff were down with malarial and sandfly fevers, and as we had 3,000 beds in tents – the shortage of staff – badly off as we were at the best of times – made matters rather worse, but we all did our best and tried to be cheery and bright and make the best of things. Later on, we had more water supply and a few fresh food stuffs, but chiefly our food was tinned. Even the butter and the milk! Butter was very difficult to keep cool. It was, in fact, impossible. As things eventually improved, however, ice was manufactured for the 'Heat' cases, for treatment, and iced water for spraying the tents and floors. Even the tents would catch fire from the intense heat of the sun. We had so many tent wards.

Considering all the inconveniences, everything was most marvellously arranged. We were nearly always full up with cases, from Kutby Hospital Train in the desert. The orderlies and doctors were splendid. Doctors worked in shorts and carried sunshades between the wards and had to wear red spine pads just the same as all the staff. They too wore goggles and none of us dare go out without a toupee, not even for a second.

We had a temporary wooden Mess, and one night one of the curtains caught fire. There was no glass in the windows and soon the hut was ablaze. It was noticed by one of the Night Sisters and the 'Fire Brigade' all turned out. This consisted of most of the staff. Luckily it was at a time when we had more water. I was fast asleep and almost the only one to miss the fire and very amazed to find no Mess next morning.

The jackals often kept us awake at night, especially so at first, with their howls, but we soon got used to them. The Arabs had to be watched carefully and guards were around for our safety, but I remember an instance of one of the guards being knifed by one. The English were not popular up there. There were Armenians and Turkish prisoners very near, in barbed wire defences.

Some greenery of a sort was fastened to the outside of the tents containing the worse cases of illness, and this was sprayed continuously by natives, to keep them cool. I have known the temperature 125 degrees in the shade, when we were on duty.

In the hot weather the heatstroke cases were pitiable, and we all had to work with scanty clothing and change frequently owing to intense perspiration.

I was a patient myself at times, with malarial and sandfly fevers, of which illnesses one has to have a secondary attack, all very unpleasant indeed. For the Night Sisters, mud huts were put up, and very nice and cool they were for day sleeping. The only inconvenience was the sandy floor through which came the sand rats to disturb one's rest. These I kept down, when on night duty, by feeding well, as I found, that by leaving food on the floor, the rats would eat and be content to run away again. I once did waken to find that I had been lying on a few baby ones. There was a hole in my camp mattress where the mother rat had snugly made her nest.

After being in the desert hospital nearly a year, I was invited to go out to a native town, Kuwait, further inland, with another sister, and two officers, who were going out on 'inspection' duty.

We all started early in the morning to make the day as long as possible, and because the journey was a tedious one and our conveyance a Ford car. We had a driver who knew the way, otherwise we should never have found tracks in the desert. It all appeared as one vast space to me and I really am amazed that anyone can find a way through. Ford cars are very suitable for driving through sand and the thick mud of native towns and villages.

We passed carcasses of camels as we travelled further inland. The route was very uninteresting, so we were glad to arrive near the gates of the native town of our destination. Passing through the gates, our friends asked the way to the residence of the Englishman who was living there.

He was dressed as a native, telling us that he found he was more popular when he did so, and he made us very welcome indeed, as he saw very few visitors. He told us that he rarely saw an Englishman and never an Englishwoman. After showing us round the native town and the bazaar, followed by dozens of curious natives, he took us up to visit the Sheik, a very friendly old man, who could speak no English, so our kind friend acted as interpreter. The Englishman was teaching English to a grandson of the Sheik and this boy was very pleased to talk with us and air his English. We were invited to sweetmeats and tea or coffee, all of which were very sickly, in a room full of sweet scented plants and flowers, and precious carpets, and we made every effort to take of everything, in order not to offend the Sheik. We were told that he was very much in favour of the English and their ways, though so far he had made no change in his life there. After tea he invited the other lady and myself to visit his harem. We were taken along by the small grandson, and being the first Englishwomen to enter, were naturally hailed with much chatter and noise by the wives and their women relatives, of which there appeared to be a considerable number.

I believe there were about sixteen wives, some of them quite young and some very lovely indeed. The latest and youngest one was very lavishly adorned with anklets and bangles, and her robes seemed very gay. Their quarters were quite spacious and off a very large courtyard, and seemed very wonderful and full of precious embroideries and carpets.

We visitors could not speak Arabic, so we did not understand what was being said, but the grandson translated and he told us that one of them was very curious to know why we were travelling in a car alone with gentlemen who were not our husbands. It was very strange to them. News evidently travels fast in a harem. They asked us to take off our hats and stroked our hair and faces. It was all very embarrassing and rather amusing.

With great difficulty we made our way out of the harem and back to our friends who were quite concerned about us, wondering if we had been added to the number of wives, as we had been away a considerable time. On leaving, the Sheik made us all gifts.

Our journey back was uneventful, except for the jackals, who got in front of our car lights, and at times blocked the way. It had been a wonderful and unforgettable experience and one I should not have like to have missed, as it does not often happen that an Englishwoman sees the inside of an Arabian harem.

In the hospital our food consisted chiefly of boiled rice and bully beef done up in various ways, and tinned vegetables, butter and milk – no fresh foods. I have never been able to enjoy tea made with tinned milk, so tea was always an abomination to me. We could buy tinned chocolates, biscuits and 'Macconicie' vegetables from the stores if we cared to do so. There was little variety. Lime juice made from fresh limes is quite refreshing and we had fruit from India occasionally, but no potatoes.

At Christmas time we decorated the wards with dyed newspapers and wool, made into snowballs. The newspapers were dyed with coloured inks and then cut into streamers and they looked very nice indeed. Many of the patients were quite ingenious at decorations. We sent to India for any cakes, jellies and such things we might need, to come up by boat. We had no green stuffs such as holly or evergreen, but there were plenty of cigarettes and tobacco and we had whist drives and gave prizes and also had sand bran tubs.

The good fellowship everywhere was amazing and all worked to the utmost for the common good. All persevering and making the best of things. One hardly ever heard a grouse about personal discomforts, but just accepted it all, waiting for better things.

There were lots of compensations. We had lovely evening river picnics up the River Shat-el-Arab and up the Tigris and Euphrates, and also drives in the cool of the evening by the river banks. There were glorious sunsets and one could lie on the sands for hours watching the magnificent change of tints in the sky. Everyone had a share of these things as there were cars for the use of the hospital staff and we took our outings in turn.

As we sailed up river in the evenings we met lots of native craft, and it was interesting to watch them. There was good shooting of wild birds too, on the shores; we would often land and have our picnic on shore under some shady date palms, to the various records of a gramophone. After the work in the intense heat of the day it was a very welcome change indeed.

At one time a patient came down the line with smallpox, into my ward. We had to be isolated at once, as soon as it was discovered. Later, a smallpox hospital was opened across the river, in Persia, to accommodate other cases as they occurred.

We visited the wives of the Englishmen who were working for the Persian Oil Company. They had nice cool stone-built houses on the river banks, but must have been very lonely, especially before we arrived, as they were practically the only Englishwomen, except, of course, Miss Gertrude Bell, secretary to Sir Percy Cox up at Baghdad, or Lady Cox. They had electric launches to visit one another by river. Some of them managed to build sort of tennis courts and others got up games, dances or parties.

A Sheik's palace was turned into a convalescent home for sick staff. It was situated in a beautiful shady part of the Shat-el-Arab river, below Basra. The early morning until noon, and after tea in the evenings were full of hard work, except when we had our off duty. In the afternoons we rested as far as possible, but I am afraid that the orderlies had to be on duty where they were needed. Many of the staff from time to time were ill, myself included. After being ill for some time and then convalescent at the Riverside Hospital, I was again transferred to India, this time for health reasons …

1917
France and Belgium

Miss Dorothy Higgins

Anglo-Belgian Hospital, Rouen, France

The early weeks of 1917 continued with bitterly cold weather, which affected the garden and made life in the hospital very uncomfortable and difficult.

17 January 1917. Bonsecours
We have snow and frost and rain and sleet by turns and damp fogs squeezed in between. We have got our stove (paraffin) now: we call it 'Stuffy' as it stinks somewhat. However it warms our little dog-kennel nicely. I don't suffer from the cold except for chilblains, but these are very tiresome: my left foot is absolutely blobby with the beastly things and as you know I never have chilblains at home. However electrical treatment is excellent for them and so I am now giving myself a dose of electricity every day.

We are forcing bulbs with fair success in the sechoir. The sechoir be it known is a big hut full of stoves and drying linen. In it under the windows I have a shelf which the hospital carpenter put up for me. It is about a yard wide and 3 or 4 yards long. So it is almost like a greenhouse and we find it awfully useful.

24 January 1917. Bonsecours
All we can think or talk about is the cold. We have 8 degrees of frost in our barracks and everything is frozen as hard as a board. Even the flowers in our vases freeze solid. Little currents of ice-cold air pour through the cracks in the boards and the only really hot place is bed! We are on strict ration of coal too as it is almost impossible to get hold of in France. The frost and cold have increased steadily during the last ten days and we have all sorts of frozen water taps and things. All the rheostats for the electrical treatment are liquid and we spent ages this morning thawing them before we could start work, and the damp towels too were just like blocks of wood.

7 March 1917
I have been arranging our new tool-house and potting shed and looking over our seed-boxes and stores of sand and leaf-mould ready for our consignment of seeds.

Monday afternoon I was just tidying up in the electricity room and glanced out of the window and saw columns of smoke pouring up. I went outside to see it and flew back telling Tim and Nick that there was a fire close to our hut. So we all tore over and found the sechoir and the magasin with the Swede's quarters (medical gymnasts and masseuses) blazing. We had orders to clear our hut completely and the doctors and soldiers set to work to help us. In about 10 or 15 minutes all our clothes, books, china, camp beds, packing cases, tables, chairs, everything was thrown out of the windows and carried to a clear space farther into the hospital. We never expected to see half our things again. Then the roof of the garden house (thatched) caught fire just about 10 feet from our huts and we thought that all was up. They were certain our hut would burn next. Suddenly up came the British Army fire brigade (a ripping motor fire engine belonging to the base) and it got here before the village fire brigade or the Rouen fire brigade!!! They certainly saved us and thanks to them our hut was saved, though it was jolly well scorched at the far end. Two of my patients worked like angels for me. The job was afterwards to go round and pick out one's things from the strips of ground where everything had been placed higgledy piggledy. I got these two boys to collect all our things and put them in the electricity room. It was a long way, but I could lock them up and there was no danger of anyone stealing anything. I think it is due to that that we have recovered all our things, at least not all, but a great many. Of course we were told to make claims to the Belgian Government for our losses.

What no amount of restitution can set right is the loss of our garden. I say loss for it is nearly dead. There must have been a hundred people trampling on the four beds. Another one between our hut and the Mess was full of daffys just beginning to peep and it has been literally ploughed up.

I suppose we shall get it right in time, but following on the record frosts and bitter cold, which have already frozen and killed many of our treasures; it is a bitter blow and has grieved Tim and me more than anything. The sight of it is simply heart-breaking.

29 April 1917

We are awfully busy in the garden just now. We did not plant any yew trees by the summer-house. They are too expensive and we shall just have to risk people annoying us by staring in!

The weather is delightful. Tim and I have been slaving with the last of our seeds. Will you please get me some giant sunflower seeds – 1 pkt and some more (2 or 3 pkts) mignonette to plant for succession. Our Darwin tulips and narcissi in round beds look awfully healthy and it is wonderful to see the results we have in our packing case frames. Our chief trouble is cats and dogs. There is a perfect plague of them. They take a shortcut across our garden to the Mess kitchen to scavenge and frequently inter some succulent morsel in our flower beds. We are going to have rabbit wire put up but things move slowly in a military establishment.

20 May 1917

The garden is beginning to look lovely. I have a round bed of pink Darwin tulips underplanted with forget-me-nots which are a sight. I have had another very pretty bed with yellow jonquils and forget-me-nots: the jonquils are over now.

My sweet peas are tall and healthy: we have four double rows in various stages of growth. The annuals are doing pretty well too. The camassias are beginning to come out and look delightful.

5 June 1917
We have been busy in the garden since Tim came back from leave. We have four flourishing rows of sweet peas in various stages of progress but I have never known the annual seeds germinate so badly. Nothing has done its best and many have not come up at all. The camassias are just over. They were very fine. Our two formal beds in front of Matron's door were a sight. One had narcissi and forget-me-nots in it and the other had Darwin tulips and forget-me-nots. The bulbs had been presented by a late member of the staff. The Darwins were as fine and tall as one would see anywhere and the forget-me-nots did well too. They really were a sight, set in a small strip of carefully mown and rolled turf which we call a lawn by courtesy. My roses are very *malheureuses.*

The ramblers are fairly all right but some of the dwarfs have only just broken! Some of them were so trodden on after the fire that I had to cut them down level with the ground and others were all but frozen to death …

Sister K.E. Luard

No. 32 Casualty Clearing Station, Warlincourt, France

Sister Luard continued to work on the ambulance train through the bitterly cold winter of 1915, collecting the wounded – many suffering from frostbite – from La Bassée and then from Neuve Chapelle. On 25 March she wrote:

> *There was a day or two after Neuve Chapelle when the number of wounded overflowed the possibilities of 'collection'; the stretcher-bearers were all hit and the stretchers were all used, and there were not enough medical officers to cope with the numbers (extra ones were hurried up from the Base Hospitals very quickly), and if you wanted to live you had to walk or crawl, or stay behind and die …*

She remained on the train through the Second Battle of Ypres in April and the Battle of Festubert in May, vividly recording these days and nights. In June she was sent to a base hospital near Béthune and after four months went up the line to take charge of a casualty clearing station at Lillers. Seven months later she was in a hospital at Barlin, just behind the front line at Lens, where she remained until October 1916. During the following months Sister Luard was in charge of a casualty clearing station behind a quiet sector of the line.

In March 1917 Sister Luard's Unit was transferred to the 3rd Army, south of Arras, in readiness for General Allenby's Spring offensive. The new casualty clearing station of tents and huts was still under construction when the unit arrived. It was on the top of a ridge, about six miles from the line, behind Gommecourt some 500 yards from the railway halt on the line connecting

Arras and Doullens. There were already two casualty clearing stations close by. The weather conditions were appalling – hard frosts, blizzards, snow and torrential rain.

Saturday, 10 March. The frost has broken and left us in a quagmire, but the icy blast has gone. The roads are bad enough, but our camp is unspeakable. The original field sticks to your feet and gradually works towards your knees, and if your shoes are not anchored on by puttie straps you leave them behind. Tomorrow I shall tackle it in my ammunition boots.

Sunday, 11 March. The DMS [Director of Medical Services] rang up the Colonel last night to say that we should have to be ready to take in patients in three days, so things have had to get a hustle on today. The Engineers have sent 60 men to finish the wards and get on with the theatre, the kitchen and the road for evacuation. Neither the water supply nor the lighting are done, so both will have to be improvised at first. It takes a lot of labour to bring up water by man-handling and to store it in tanks.

There is to be a new Surgical Specialist, who coped with the Somme last summer, so we ought to do well. We've had a busy day equipping one of the Acute Surgical Huts and putting finishing touches to the Mess arrangements.

Monday, 12 March. It poured cats and dogs all night and you can't imagine the state of the camp. No one could who hasn't wallowed in it.

It is one person's job to run a Mess at the Back of Beyond, and I have this Hospital (700 beds) to run for night and day, with the peculiar difficulties of a new-born unfinished camp, and emergency work. For the Mess you settle for a rice pudding, but there is no rice, and the cows have anthrax, so there's no fresh milk, and the canteen has run out of Ideal milk. Well, have a jam tart; lots of jam in the British Army, but no flour, no suet, no tinned fruits, no eggs, no beans or dried peas, not one potato each. But there is bacon, ration bread and tinned butter (when you can get it), jam, marmalade sometimes, cheese, stew, Army biscuits, tea, some sugar, and sometimes mustard, and sometimes oatmeal and cornflour.

Also we have only 1 and a half *lbs* of coal per head per day, so when that is used up you have to go and look for wood to cook your dinner and boil your water. Everybody is ravenous in this high air and outdoor life, and so as long as there's enough of it, you can eat anything. None of them I hope will grumble if we can work up the true Active Service spirit, but it is an anxiety.

We have got to build and run our own Hospital laundry with 7 Permanent Base men as laundresses – when the water is laid on. So far we have only 70 beds and mattresses – all the rest will have to be on stretchers. I've bagged some lovely crates that the pneumatic-wheel stretchers came in, as linen cupboards. The CO and the Sergeant-Major go and steal planks from the road when I want boards for ward-tables, and I have stolen the trestles myself. The days aren't nearly long enough for all the scrounging that has to be done and prevented.

Saturday, 17 March. No sign of any buds out anywhere in these parts. I've got a plate of moss with a celandine plant in the middle, and a few sprouting twigs of honeysuckle that you generally find in January, and also a bluebell bulb in a jam tin.

We have got some flour today and a cauliflower, also some more coal.

The Hospital is developing daily in every direction. Now the mud is drying up and the roads beginning to be under control again.

Tuesday, 20 March. The gale last night was terrific – our compound was a wreck this morning. In spite of the wind deliberately picking up wooden posts and heavy canvas tenting (which yesterday were the walls of the compound) and bashing them savagely and regularly against the part of the hut next to the head of my bed; it didn't succeed in keeping me awake.

Sheets of rain all day and more mud.

Orders came this morning to be ready to take in large numbers of wounded at short notice, and guns are busy again. All departments immediately got a hustle on and this evening the CO wired that we were ready. The kitchen is not going – some water laid on – wards equipped and theatre improvised in one of the Dressing Huts, as the real new one isn't quite finished; 1000s of *lbs* of dressings are stocked, but they soon run out. Lotions, dressings and clothing will all run out, I believe, because things take so long coming up and have so much red tape to get through first. Our official strength is 7 Sisters – far too few for any battle, but this will become obvious.

Wednesday, 21 March. It is still snowing and yesterday was the first day of Spring. It is *unspeakably* vile – biting wind – driving snow and deep slush. We can still hear the guns but nothing like so close as before. I believe this group of CCSs clear the wounded now from the Arras area. The RE are still building the theatre and laundry etc., and until they clear out altogether we are only to take any overflow from the other two CCSs, which has not yet occurred, so we go on improving the detail of the Hospital all day – and expecting to be – but not being – called up all night.

Friday, 23 March. There is a crater at every crossroad, and every main road is exploded every 300 yards. The wells are poisoned, the apple trees cut down and the houses wrecked and burnt; bridges and railways destroyed.

We have been living on bully and beans for three days – it is rather good; bacon, jam, margarine and milk are all tinned, but we have very good meals out of them.

Monday night, 26 March. The QM paddled me round all his soak-pits, incinerators, thresh disinfectors, ablution huts, bath huts, laundry, etc., etc., this morning. They are primitive but clever.

Tuesday, 27 March. At last we've taken in our first convoy, no hitch so far. The two new Sisters arrived in the nick of time, and the posting of Sisters and Orderlies seems to be working out all right. We have a particularly nice set of Medical Officers. The CO and I and the Sergeant-Major meet and compare notes in our endless rounds and severally help each other out of holes. Sometimes I want a fatigue party from the Sergeant-Major or he wants one from my men, or the CO claims both lots or the QM wants them for unloading lorries, but we all get it done in the end.

It has been the usual poisonous weather again, biting N.E. wind, driving storms and deep slush. We take in from 6am today to 6am tomorrow – in rotation with the other two in this group. Our bombardment is still going on, and they also are shelling hard round the Arras pivot, into us in their old trenches.

Wednesday, 28 March. We are bombarding them harder than ever; it is a continual din. We took in another Convoy in the night and had a busy morning, but a train came before tea, so our first venture is admitted, operated on, treated and evacuated within 36 hours; all but the worst Surgicals and the Medicals unfit to travel, and a handful of walking-cases, soon fit for duty. One of last night's is dying of shock, in spite of strenuous efforts to pull him back. I've already had to begin writing Break-the-News Letters to the wives and mothers.

The Hospital is to be kept as empty as possible for the Strafe.

Friday, 30 March, 10pm. It stopped raining in the afternoon and changed back to the beautiful icy wind we get so much of.

The CO and QM are making preparations for possible thousands: so am I.

I managed to get a sack of potatoes for 17 francs today for our Mess; great rejoicings; tinned milk is still very scarce, and cows' milk does not exist.

The RC Padre has come but not the C of E yet. One of my best Orderlies is a Lay Brother of the Society of the Divine Compassion. He is helping me fix up the mortuary and the church tent.

Tuesday, 3 April. We're in the middle of terrific work. All the casualties from the attack on Hainy and Croisilles came to us; we hadn't nearly enough Sisters to go round and it never stopped all day and all night and all today till 5pm.

So many die that I shan't possibly be able to write to their mothers, and some have no trace of next of kin.

I had to run a ward equipped for 14 officers and had to get 28 in, on stretchers on every inch of floor, some badly wounded; they were all angels of patience and uncomplainingness.

Wednesday, 4 April, 10.30pm. Reinforcements are coming in – two more Sisters today, that is 13 altogether, and there are now 13 MOs and 2 Padres, and 40 men coming tomorrow. 12 Nursing Orderlies came the other day. There is still a 'team' to come, consisting of four people, one surgeon, one anaesthetist, one Theatre Sister and one Theatre Orderly; a brainy scheme – one team to each CCS.

We've had a very full day getting ready for tomorrow's take-in, opening new lines of tents and getting stock up, and patching up the too-bad-to-travel, of whom there are many.

We are running a Preparation-for-Operation Ward tomorrow, to which all operation cases are to go from the Dressing Hut, and from there to the theatre and then to the wards.

The increased Mess makes extra work and catering is appallingly difficult. We all eat whatever comes, whether cold or hot, raw or cooked, nice or nasty, and do very well on it. The kitchen range is made of petrol tins, cement, and draughts. Thank Heaven, it has stopped snowing and blowing, though it still rains a bit.

Thursday, 5 April, midnight. Just got to bed after my last round. Had a very big take-in, but not so many bad ones.

The Preparation-for-Theatre Ward has been working very well. It is to this ward that every stretcher-case is sent from the Dressing Hut, except those who are so slightly wounded that they can be sent to one of the Evacuation Wards to be dealt with at a Base Hospital. Here the number of battered men, generally from 50 to 60, never seems to grow less, as although they are carried when ready to the operating teams in the theatre, their places are continually filled by others.

All the layers of sodden or caked stiff clothing are cut off, pyjamas or long flannel pinafore gowns put on, taken from a blanket and screen enclosure kept heated by a Perfection Lamp. Hot blankets, hot water bottles, hot drinks, subcutaneous salines and hypodermics are given here, as also in the Resuscitation Ward to which all the apparently hopeless cases are taken. When the stretcher-bearers come from the operating teams for their next case, you have to be careful to send the most urgent before the ones who may have been waiting longer.

It often happens that no MO can be spared for this tent, so a great deal of responsibility is thrown on to us, and only the Sisters with nerve, experience and sound judgement are any good here.

Once when I was cutting off a split boot of a man wounded in the head, chest, and the other thigh, half his foot came off in it – a detail overlooked in the Dressing Hut and the Field Ambulance with all his other injuries.

It has been sunny and windless today, a blessed change, and bright moon tonight. It is all a ghastly business, but they take it without a word and it is grand to see the apparently dying men come to life again. And it is bringing out the best of everybody, from the CO to the man who does the lamps.

Good Friday, and pouring cats and dogs. Had a train today, but the whole of one Acute Ward are too bad to go.

A boy with his face nearly in half, who couldn't talk, and whom I was feeding, was trying to explain that he was lying on something hard in his trouser pocket. It was a live Mills bomb! I extracted it with some care, as the pins catch easily.

(Battle of Arras. Easter Monday, April 9th 1917)
Easter Tuesday, 10 April. The 3rd Army went over the top yesterday and a wire came through by midday that we'd taken Vimy and 34,000 prisoners and, Sir Anthony Bowlby [Senior Consultant with the rank of Surgeon-General] says this morning, 30 guns. The Cavalry are after them, and the Tanks leading the Infantry, and all is splendid, but here are horrors all day and all night. The three CCSs filled up in turn and then each filled up again, without any break in the Convoys: we take in and evacuate at the same time. The theatre, Dressing Hut, Preparation Hut and wards and tents are all humming – the kitchen goes on cooking with a Day Staff and a Night Staff, and the stretcher-bearers go on stretcher-bearing, and the Mortuary Corporal goes on

sewing up corpses in canvas. The Colonel carries the lame walking-cases on his broad back, and I look after the moribunds in every spare second from the Preparation Hut, which is (during take-in) the stiffest corner of all, and Sisters, MOs, NCOs, Orderlies, Convalescent Men and Permanent Base Men, all peg into it. We meet for snatching meals and five-minute snacks of rest and begin again. All are doing 16 hours on and 8 off and some of us 8 on and 6 off.

Evacuation has been held up today for some hours and the place is clogged. The wards are like battlefields, with battered wrecks in every bed and on stretchers between the beds and down the middles.

The Padre [the Reverend Eustace Hill] is wonderful; he fills hot bottles with his one arm and gives drinks and holds basins for them to be sick, and especially looks after those poor ghastly moribunds. The theatre team have done 70 operations in the 24 hours.

The transport of wounded is extraordinarily well worked out over all these miles. The walking-cases come in lorries and buses and the lying-cases in beautifully electric-lighted motor ambulances, which look like the lights on the embankment as far as you can see down the road, and the stream to the three Hospitals never ceases.

Of course we've had snowstorms and icy gales all the time.

Friday, 13 April. The DMS came today and said the Push was held up by this extraordinarily inopportune burst of bad weather. It blew and raged madly all Wednesday night, and there was deep snow in the morning. Last night and today we have been getting the poor boys in who have been lying out in it for two days, and many of them have died since of the exposure and gas gangrene.

The DMS said that Sir Anthony Bowlby (who has been here every day lately) has reported very well of this Unit – that the arrangements were excellent, and things going well, and that the report had gone in to HQ.

The Strafe is over for the moment, and we are full of the leavings, the most tragic part, though dozens who have been evacuated will die, too.

We have some Germans in; several have died.

Saturday night, 14 April. A grey, stiff, frozen man who was wounded on Monday, was brought in today; he had been kept alive by drinks in a trench and found and brought in last night. We got a pulse into him after some hours, and warmed him till he thawed and felt too hot, but one leg was hopelessly smashed and of course had gas gangrene and he died this evening.

On the other side of the picture there are many glorious 'resurrections', smoking cigarettes and eating chicken and reading magazines. They have lots of champagne and eggs and oranges and jelly, and everything to make them buck up. It has been a fine sunny day at last, but windy.

Sunday, 15 April. Early Service in the Church Tent at 7am. The Padre has made it very nice with a red and white reredos and our own altar-cloth. It has a Communion rail made of trees, and there is a duckboard with stretcher pillows to kneel on.

We've had a very busy day, some of it very disheartening. The theatre people have the longest hours, and for the Surgeons the greatest strain of work, but for the Sisters it is much less harassing and wearing than the work in the wards, cutting off the caked khaki and the clammy socks and heavy boots, with the incessant cries of 'Give me a drink' or 'Sister, I do feel bad', and the everlasting saline infusion and men being sick or delirious or groaning or haemorrhaging.

Tuesday, 17 April. We have had a lull the last two days, and everybody has been off duty long enough to go for a walk in relays and pick Lent lilies, cowslips, and anemones. Operations and funerals still continue, but the wards are not so full. I believe another stunt is expected tomorrow.

Today we have had no bread, but only 'dog biscuits'. At breakfast, with no porridge, and at tea they are rather a blight, as they are so hard they take hours to eat, but we manage to consume enough to support life!

I got about 60 behind in writing Break-the-News Letters the first few days of last week, and have never caught them up, but manage now to work them off as they occur, every 24 hours.

It poured and galed all last night and most of today with the usual alternations of heavy rain, snow and sleet, with a driving bitter wind. What the men in the trenches, and the wounded, are like you can imagine. I have never seen anything like the state they are in, mud caked on their teeth and under their eyelids.

Sunday, 22 April. This continued bombardment is shaking the earth tonight; it is on the same scale as on the day before Easter Monday. The Hospital is almost empty, ready.

I took some Lent lilies to the cemetery this evening; it is rapidly spreading over a high open field; there must be nearly 2,000 graves there now, since it began last June. There was a sunset and a young new moon showing.

No one knows when we shall fill up again but it can't be far off, with this din.

(2nd phase of the Battle of Arras. 23 April 1917)
Monday, 23 April, 10pm. We have filled up twice, and they are hard at it again over the road; we come next.

Tuesday morning. Some of the men say they were picked up and looked after by Germans, so we are being extra kind to the Germans this time.

There is in Hospitals an understood arrangement that all Germans (except when their lives depend on immediate attention) should wait till the last British has been attended to, for dressings, operations, food, blankets, etc. It is only kept up in a very half-hearted way and is generally broken by the MOs who are most emphatic about it in theory!

Tuesday 10.30pm. It has been a pretty sad day, 12 funerals.

They are not taking-in so fast tonight over the road and we hope to work it through the night with a single theatre team. They are very tired.

We had butter for tea today.

A German Sergeant-Major died in my Moribunds Tent today. Two given-up boys whom no effort of yesterday or last night would revive in the Moribund Tent, seemed to me not hopeless this morning, and after more resuscitation they are now both comfortably bedded in one of the Acute Surgicals, each with a leg off and a fair chance of recovery. The others, with torn kidneys and spleens and brains, are no good. The people who have been coming in all day are the left-outs in German dug-outs, since Monday, starved, cold, and by some miracle still alive, but not much more. This last 300 has taken 16 hours to come in, so the lull is beginning and probably the CCS over the road will be taking-in all tonight and the other all tomorrow, instead of all of us filling up every three hours or so. It is piercingly cold again and looks like rain.

Thursday, 26 April, 10.30pm. No take-in and no evac. today: just slogging along with the remains. My two resuscitated boys in the Moribund Ward are all right and we've got two more today who were pulseless, now operated on and bedded; one, a gas gangrene, is having the new Flavine treatment and stays with me, but he's going to do all right.

Icy cold wind all day. We shall be due to take-in tomorrow morning, the first that come back from Over the Top.

Friday, 27 April, 4pm. The attack came off all right, but 'he' (as the enemy is frequently called in these parts and in the communiques) didn't wait for it! He has gone back another 5 miles, so all those hundreds of our casualties are saved and there's nothing doing. Isn't it splendid?

My dear little resuscitated Suffolk boy got GG above the amputation and died this afternoon, and the other boy has had to have the other leg off now. The gas gangrene boy left is going wrong today, but the moribund head cases are smoking pipes and eating eggs and bread and butter!

In one ward there's hardly a man with two legs.

Monday, 30 April. We have had a whole week without snow or rain – lots of sun and blue sky. I went for a ramble after tea yesterday to a darling narrow wood with a stream at the bottom between two hills, a quarter of an hour's walk from here. Two sets of shy, polite boys thrust their bunches of cowslips and daffodils into my hand. Also banks of small blue periwinkles like ours, and flowering palm. Absolutely no leaves yet anywhere and it's May Day tomorrow.

Wednesday, 2 May, and another dazzling day. Hospital almost empty tonight after evacuation, ready for a Strafe.

Thursday, 3 May, 11.30pm. They went over the top this morning and have been pouring in all day. We are now taking in for the third time today. The fine weather makes a huge difference to the conditions of the whole thing. Their accounts vary as to success or failure.

Tuesday, 8 May. We have had a comparatively slack time the last two days, very little doing. Lots of noise but few casualties.

We have begun taking marquees down with a view to moving …

Miss Vera Brittain

24th General Hospital, Étaples, France

During the early spring months of 1917 at St George's Hospital, Malta, Vera Brittain enjoyed the leisurely life of tennis parties, dances and long walks, which came with lighter duties, as most patients were convalescents. In April her world was shattered once again when she received a telegram from her brother, Edward. Victor Richardson had been seriously wounded on 9 April at Vimy Ridge. Four days later she heard that Victor's left eye had been removed. On 1 May Vera had two cables. The first said that Victor had lost the sight in his right eye – the second, an hour later, told her that Geoffrey Thurlow had been killed in action on 23 April at Monchy-le-Preux. She and Geoffrey had become very friendly through the letters they wrote to each other once a week and for a little while she had wondered 'what it would all lead to'. She sat on the rocks in front of the night quarters to think through the sad situation and decided to return to England. She left Malta on 22 May 1917 and arrived home five days later. She spent the next ten days at Victor Richardson's bedside at the 2nd London General Hospital, Chelsea. He was blind and struggling to learn braille but the prospects of recovering from his wounds seemed good. However, on the morning of 8 June he told his nurse that he had experienced a small explosion in his head during the night. He deteriorated rapidly and died the following day.

A few weeks later, on 4 August 1917, Vera Brittain and a small group of VADs arrived at the 24th General Hospital, Étaples, to boost the staff coping with ever-increasing numbers of casualties, including German prisoners. A British Expeditionary Force base camp was situated a mile from Étaples, a small fishing port fifteen miles south of Boulogne. Eight hospitals, consisting of wooden huts, tents and marquees, stood at the northern end of the camp. The nurses lived in bell tents and canvas or wood huts. These were separated from the main part of the hospital by a main road along which a continuous flow of troops and vehicles passed on the way to the front line. The military cemetery, a short distance away, was 'a forest of wooden crosses stretching right down to the sea, and each long mound a mass of gay-coloured flowers – nasturtiums, marigolds and iceland poppies …'

At the end of the hospital complex German prisoners were nursed in separate marquees. Vera was assigned to Ward 29 – the German acute surgical ward – where most of the patients were dying.

9 August 1917. There is a theatre attached to the ward where we have anything up to 18 or 20 operations a day … The operations are mostly amputations, chests, abdominals and heads. Any bad operation case goes immediately into our ward … The hospital is frightfully busy all through … Malta changed my ideas about the amount an individual can be capable of and responsible for, but this changes them still more. Even in the 1st London after the Somme push I have never seen such bad wounds as these Germans have … It is hardly possible to feel any antipathy towards one's patients in practice however much one may in theory; they are far too ill and utterly

dependent on one for that … Our own men are very good to them; they come in to see them and give them cigarettes and fetch them drinks …'

The German Ward
(Inter Arma Caritas)

When the years of strife are over and my recollection fades
Of the wards wherein I worked the weeks away,
I shall still see, as a vision rising 'mid the War-time shades,
The ward in France where German wounded lay.

I shall see the pallid faces and the half-suspicious eyes,
I shall hear the bitter groans and laboured breath,
And recall the loud complaining and the weary tedious cries,
And sights and smells of blood and wounds and death.

I shall see the convoy cases, blanket-covered on the floor,
And watch the heavy stretcher-work begin,
And the gleam of knives and bottles through the open theatre door,
And the operation patients carried in.

I shall see the Sister standing, with her form of youthful grace,
And the humour and the wisdom of her smile,
And the tale of three years' warfare on her thin expressive face –
The weariness of many a toil-filled while.

I shall think of how I worked for her with nerve and heart and mind,
And marvelled at her courage and her skill,
And how the dying enemy her tenderness would find
Beneath her scornful energy of will.

And I learnt that human mercy turns alike to friend or foe
When the darkest hour of all is creeping nigh,
And those who slew our dearest, when their lamps were burning low,
Found help and pity ere they came to die.

So, though much will be forgotten when the sound of War's alarms
And the days of death and strife have passed away,
I shall always see the vision of Love working amidst arms
In the ward wherein the wounded prisoners lay.

5 December [after being transferred to an Acute Medical Ward]. Never in my life have I been so absolutely filthy as I get on duty here …

Sister A has six wards and there is no VAD in the next-door one, only an orderly, so neither she nor he spend very much time in here. Consequently I am Sister, VAD and orderly all in one … and after, quite apart from the nursing, I have stoked the stove all night, done two or three rounds of bed-pans and kept the kettles going and prepared feeds on exceedingly black Beatrice oil-stoves and refilled them from the steam kettles, literally wallowing in paraffin all the time, I feel as if I had been dragged through the gutter! Possibly acute surgical is the heaviest kind of work there is, but acute medical is, I think, more wearing than anything else on earth. You are kept on the go the whole time and in the end there seems nothing definite to show for it – except that one or two people are still alive who might otherwise have been dead …

We have heaps of gassed cases at present who came in a day or two ago; there are 10 in this ward alone. I wish those people who write so glibly about this being a holy war, and the orators who talk so much about going on no matter how long the war lasts and what it may mean, could see a case – to say nothing of 10 cases – of mustard gas in its early stages – could see the poor things burnt and blistered all over with great mustard-coloured suppurating blisters, with blind eyes – sometimes temporally [sic], sometimes permanently – all sticky and stuck together, and always fighting for breath, with voices a mere whisper, saying that their throats are closing and they know they will choke. The only thing one can say is that such severe cases don't last long; either they die soon or else improve – usually the former …

Sister K.E. Luard

Abdomens and Chests Hospital (Casualty Clearing Station No. 32), Brandhoek, Belgium

During May the casualty clearing station at Warlincourt received fewer wounded and there were less operations and deaths. The staff had more time to relax and enjoyed picnics in the woods, and a combined sports day. On 10 May General Allenby inspected the three CCSs and thanked them for looking after 'his Army'. On 3 June the last patient was cleared, the tents were packed, and only the huts were left standing.

After a few weeks resting at St Omer, Sister Luard was sent, with 30 sisters and 30 Medical Officers, to the new abdomens and chests hospital at Brandhoek, only just behind the line in the Ypres sector, in readiness for what was to become the Third Battle of Ypres, which started on 31 July. The hospital had only been on the site for a week and was entirely under canvas. The wards were in huge marquees on both sides of a long, wide central duckboard walk. The theatre was in a long hut. The sisters' quarters were in bell tents, although Sister Luard lived in the same Armstrong canvas hut as before. The mess was in two big marquees.

Friday, 27 July 1917. This venture so close to the Line is of the nature of an experiment in life-saving, to reduce the mortality rate from abdominal and chest wounds. Their chance of life depends (except where the injuries are such as to be beyond any hope of recovery) mainly on the length of time between the injury and the operation.

As modern Field Surgery can now be carried out under conditions of perfect asepsis, the sooner the infection always introduced into every wound with the missile is dealt with, and the internal repairs carried out, the more chance the soldier has of life.

Hence this Advanced Abdominal Centre, to which all abdominal and chest wounds are taken from a large attacking area, instead of going on with the rest to the CCSs 6 miles back.

Our 30 Medical Officers include the largest collection of FRCSs [Fellows of the Royal College of Surgeons] ever collected at any Hospital in France before, at Base or Front, twelve operating Surgeons with theatre teams working on eight tables continuously for the 24 hours, with 16 hours on and 8 off.

Tuesday, 31 July, 4.15am. The All-together began at 5 minutes to 4. We crept out on to the duckboards and saw. It was more wonderful and stupendous than horrible. There was the glare before daylight of the searchlights, star-shells and gun-flashes and the cracking, splitting and thundering of the guns of all calibres at once.

6.30am. We have just begun taking in the first cases. An officer died soon after admission between 4 and 5am. The Air people began streaming over at daylight adding their whirring and droning to the din. The mines have been going off since 5am like earthquakes. Lots of high explosive has been coming over, but nothing so far into this camp. The uproar is almost stupefying.

Same day, 11pm. We have been working in the roar of battle every minute since I last wrote, and it has been rather too exciting. I've not had time to hear any details from any of our poor abdominals, but the news has been good till this evening: thousands of prisoners – and Ypres choked with captured guns and ammunition, and some a few miles of advance. This evening they tell of heavy counter-attacks and some of our advance lost. He is not retreating because he wants to, but is putting up a tremendous fight.

We have a lot of Germans in – all abdominals. Everything has been going at full pitch – with the 12 teams in the theatre only breaking off for hasty meals – the Dressing Hut, the Preparation Ward and Resuscitation and the four huge Acute Wards, which fill up from the theatre; the Officers' Ward, the Moribund and the German Ward. That, and the Preparation and the theatre are the worst places.

Soon after ten o'clock this morning he began putting over high explosive. Everyone had to put on tin-hats and carry on. He kept it up all the morning with vicious screams. They burst on two sides of us, not 50 yards away – no direct hits on to us but streams of shrapnel, which were quite hot when you picked them up. No one was hurt, which was lucky, and they came everywhere, even through our Canvas Huts in our quarters. Bursting shells are an ugly sight – black or yellow smoke and streams of jagged steel flying violently in all directions.

There was a moment about tea-time when I thought the work was going to heap up and get the upper hand of us, but the CO [Colonel Sutcliffe] stopped admitting for an hour and sent them on lower down, which saved the situation. It is going to be a tight fit. Of course a good many die, but a great many seem to be going to do. We get them one hour after injury, which is our *raison d'etre* for being here.

Wednesday, 1 August. Soaking hopeless rain, holding up the advance; the worst luck that could happen. Poor Sir Douglas Haig. It has been so every time. Everything is a swamp and a pond, and tents leaking and dropping. Water in some of the wards is half-way up the legs of the beds.

11.30pm. Just finished my last round. Soaking rain all day still going on, complete hold-up of British Army. Absolute silence of our guns and only an occasional reminder from Fritz. Pétain and his crack Corps have done very well. Our success has varied; one Corps went too far and got caught in the back.

The abdominals coming in are very bad today – both Boche and British. The work thickens as the wards fill up and new wards have to be opened. We are to take chests and femurs too, as soon as No. 44 and the Australian CCSs open, which are alongside getting ready. The staffing of the wards for Night Duty both of Sisters and orderlies is the problem, even with my 33.

It is getting very ghastly; the men all look so appalling when they are brought in, and so many die. I don't see how the Break-the-News Letters are going to be written, because the moment for sitting down literally never comes from 7am to midnight. It is a good thing we are all fresh and fit.

Wednesday, 1 August, 12.15am. It has been a pretty frightful day – 44 funerals yesterday and about as many today.

Thursday, 2 August, 11.45pm. The uproar went on all night – no one slept much. It made one realise how far up we are to have streams of shells crossing over our heads. The rain continues – all night and all day since the Push began on Monday.

The men are brought in with mud over their eyes and mouths, and 126 have died in 3 and a half days. In spite of the awful conditions, a remarkable percentage, especially of the first ones who came in early and dry, are doing brilliantly.

Yesterday morning Capt. C [Captain Noel Godfrey Chavasse], VC, and Bar, DSO, MC, RAMC, was brought in – badly hit in the tummy and arm and had been going about for two days with a scalp wound till he got this. Half the Regiment have been to see him – he is loved by everybody. He was quickly X-rayed, operated on, shrapnel found, holes sewn up, salined and put to bed. He is just on the borderland still; better this afternoon and perhaps going to do, but not so well tonight. He tries hard to live; he was going to be married.

Sunday, 5 August, 11.30pm. Captain C died yesterday; four of us went to his funeral today; and a lot of the MOs; two of them wheeled the stretcher and lowered him. His horse was led in front and then the pipers and masses of kilted officers followed. Our Padre with his one arm, Father E.H. [Eustace Hill], looked like a Prophet towering over everybody and saying it all without book. After the Blessing one piper came to the graveside (which was a large pit full of dead soldiers sewn up in canvas) and played a lament. Then his Colonel [Lieutenant Colonel J.R. Davidson], who particularly loved him, stood and saluted him in his grave. It was fine, but horribly choky.

The weather has cleared and it has been hot and the ground is drying up a bit. They are going over the top tomorrow and we burst into a very 'useful' bombardment this evening – to prepare their way. We are so much in the thick of war up here that no one talks or thinks of anything else on this earth. And how can you with 'Lizzie' splitting her jaws, shells screaming and bursting and bombs dropping. The last are much the worst. He dropped five at dinner-time about 70 yards away, and came over with some more about 10.30 tonight and some more later. There's no sort of cover anywhere and it is purely beastly.

Monday, 13 August. Our 12 Australian Sisters and 10 Australian orderlies rejoin their own Unit tomorrow, so I've had a lot of readjusting of the Staff to arrange. They open tomorrow and we three CCSs take in now in batches of 50 each, abdomens, chests and femurs. We had a big evacuation today.

Wednesday, 15 August, 11.30pm. This has been a horrid day. He bombed a lot of men nearby and all who weren't killed came to us. Some are still alive but about half died here. One of the saddest things I've ever seen is happening tonight. An officer boy is dying with his father (a Colonel) sitting holding his hand. The father happened to meet the ambulance bringing him in, and the boy's servant stopped him and told him his son was inside. He's staying here tonight, and has just been pacing the duckboards with me, saying, 'The other boy is a darling, but this one is the apple of our eye. I knew it must happen.'

12pm. They are still canoodling over, but one learns not to take the smallest notice of them. It's going to be a lively night for tomorrow's Push.

2.45am. Yes, it is.

The Colonel's boy died at 12.30.

Thursday, 12.30am. Not sorry to be crawling to bed, as there was no sleep after the blast began last night and we've had a mighty day today. The two Corps on the left of the Attack have gained their objective and done well. The Corps on the right was held up and it has got to be done again there. It's a big shove and for once it hasn't rained.

I feel dazed with going round the rows of silent or groaning wrecks and arranging for room for more in the night without opening new wards not yet equipped. Many die and their beds are filled instantly. One has got so used to their dying that it conveys no impression beyond a vague sense of medical failure. You forget entirely that they were once civilian, that they were alive and well yesterday, that they have wives and mothers and fathers and children at home; all you realise is that they are dead soldiers, and that there are thousands of others. It is all very like a battlefield.

And between 10 and 11 tonight when I was writing to that boy's mother at his father's request, he dropped bombs on the Field Ambulance alongside of us, and killed an orderly and wounded others, and also on to the Officers' Mess of the Australian CCS alongside of them – not three minutes from us, and killed a Medical Officer and a Corporal.

Friday, 17 August. More dying men all day. The news is bad, parts of it like Gommecourt, 1 July 1916 over again. They let us through and then bobbed up behind and before us and cut us to pieces with machine-guns. Gas-shelling going on heavily too. Officers and men say it is the bloodiest of all the battles.

Saturday, 18 August. We had another beastly night. He played about all night till daylight. There were several of him. He went to CCSs behind us. At one he wounded three Sisters and blew their cook-boy to pieces. The Sisters went to the Base by ambulance train this morning.

At the other he wounded six MOs among other casualties. A dirty trick, because he has maps and knows which are hospitals back there. Here we are in a continuous line of camps, batteries, dumps, etc., and he may not know. A big shell came over about 3am into the Gunners alongside of us and laid out 14 of them.

Tonight we have darkened every glimmer of light everywhere. He is buzzing round already. The Sisters' quarters at the Australians and at No. 44 are sandbagged. I expect ours will be tomorrow. We have been taking-in today, but not so fast. The relatives of died-of-wounds are just reaching 400 in less than three weeks.

Miss McCarthy [Matron-in-Chief] came up today. She was, as always, most helpful and kind. She was much distressed at the conditions and thinks we're too far up. I told her none of the Sisters want to go down. I don't think any of them would.

We've had two dazzling days, but as there is not a blade of grass or a leaf in the camp, only duckboards, trenches and tents, you can only feel it's summer by the sky and the air.

Sunday, 19 August. A Colonel of the Warwicks is arranging an entertainment tomorrow in their lines, to cheer the boys up before going over the top! He asked the Brigadier if he might invite us, and was warmly supported; so the CO and I accepted and we go to their camp tomorrow evening.

Tuesday, 21 August. At 7.30 we were escorted to the Warwicks' camp by one of their officers – about six minutes from here. We had a wonderful evening, and neither they nor we will forget it. There were about 36 officers in the Battalion and they were all ready for their job (St Julien). The party was in their Mess Hut. A palatial supper at one end – lobster mayonnaise, fruit salad, jellies, sandwiches and champagne. Then a very good concert with their own band and their own star turns. The hut was decorated and lighted with candles in biscuit tin reflectors. They fell to entertaining us with unconcealed happiness and soon the room sounded like a huge dinner-party. The Sisters looked charming and enjoyed it all enormously. Some Canadian Sisters also came up in a car from Pop [Poperinghe]. A Major of another Battalion came up and told me what it means to them talking to and seeing people 'clean and fresh' after so many months cut off from their own womankind, and 'just before we go over', he said. There was no rollicking, but a sort of clutch of happiness that everyone could feel.

And at his usual time, about 9.30, Fritz came over. A Lewis gun 10 yards outside barked like a demon and the heavy Archies 100 yards on our other side cracked and roared and 7 bombs dropped on the camps around. It was in a pause between songs (lights were darkened, of course, already) and the conversation never swerved, but the buzz got louder to be heard above the din.

The Hospital [Night Staff] meanwhile was coping with the killed and wounded from the 7 bombs. Some only just lived to get here, and some died here and some are in the wards. What a poisonous business it is. Most damage was done in a Labour Battalion Camp a little to the right of where we were.

22 August, 6pm. This has been a very bad day. Big shells began coming over about 10am – one burst between one of our wards and the Sisters' Quarters of No. 44 CCS, and killed a Night Sister asleep in bed in her tent and knocked three others out with concussion and shell-shock. Another laid out the QM stores in the Australians and many more have had narrow shaves.

Bits came over everywhere, pitching at one's feet as we rushed to the scene of action, and one just missed one of my Night Sisters getting into bed in our Compound. I knew by the crash where it must have gone and found Sister E as white as paper but smiling happily and comforting the terrified patients. Then I came on to the shell-hole and the wrecked tents in the Sisters' Quarters at 44. A group of stricken MOs were standing about and in one tent the Sister was dying. The piece went through her from back to front near her heart. She was only conscious a few minutes and only lived 20 minutes …

Miss Mairi Chisholm

Advanced Dressing Station, Pervyse, Belgium

In August 1914 the eighteen-year-old Mairi Chisholm left her home in Scotland and travelled on her motorcycle to London to find war work. She served for a few weeks as a dispatch rider with the newly formed Women's Emergency Corps where she met Elsie Knocker [qv]. Very soon she was recruited by Sir Hector Munro to serve as an ambulance driver with his flying ambulance service. She was one of the five women, along with Lady Dorothie Feilding, Elsie Knocker, Mrs Helen Gleason and May Sinclair [qv], who were members of his team.

For the first two months they worked day and night collecting wounded Belgian soldiers from the Yser front during the battles of Dixmude and Ypres.

In November 1914 Mairi Chisholm and Elsie Knocker left the ambulance unit and set up a first aid post immediately behind the front line at Pervyse. The line was just being stabilised. The Belgians had let in the sea at Nieuport and the lands of the Yser were flooded. The Germans had crossed the Yser and Pervyse was the scene of a bloody battle. The water swept down and although men and animals were drowned, the line stretching from Nieuport to Ypres was saved. The earthwork trenches were on the railway line at Pervyse and the post was based at first in a cellar of the house next to the level crossing and immediately behind the trenches. Here the two women cared for the wounded, provided general medical assistance and refreshments but soon they realised that it was too difficult to get the wounded up and down the steps of a cellar. They opened a hut at Steenkerke, some way back from Pervyse, and out of range of the German artillery. This was used as an infirmary at the same time as running a new first aid post in a house with only half a roof. They remained here until continuous German shells reduced the house to a ruin, forcing them to move again.

The 3rd Poste was built inside the shell of a house. It was a concrete structure, covered in sandbags and very superior to anything we had previously occupied. For the sake of speed we had an ambulance hidden in its own sandbagged shelter – it was 3 miles in advance of the Army ambulances. In this Poste it was possible for Mrs Knocker, by then Baroness de T'Serclaes, to do some of her finest work, instruments and equipment being A1.

Apart from the steady stream of wounded day and night (we slept in our clothes) we had a surgery. Many of the men in the trenches suffered from boils, sores, foot troubles, etc. VD was prevalent and unattended to in the early stages of the war – all these cases came to our dug-out for attention.

At times the Prisoners Company was in our sector; men could earn total remission of their sentences for an act of extreme bravery – one did not ask why they were in this Company.

One day dealing with a particularly nasty boil the victim said to me 'Mam'zelle, do you never wonder what we have done?' I replied, 'why yes, but I do not ask.' 'Well, Mam'zelle, I killed my wife, she nagged and nagged and I struck her with an axe.' I said 'do you feel sorry about it?' 'No', he said, 'I could not stand her nagging, and what else to do to stop it?' Later he told me that he and nineteen others were going into one of the advanced posts in front of our main line trenches – a German attack was expected. If they lived they could gain remission. I watched the attack – it did not seem possible that any man could survive. But late next night my murderer staggered in, the sole survivor, deeply shocked, but inwardly at peace.

Taking wounded to hospital 15 miles back at night was a very real strain – no lights, shell pocked pavé roads, mud-covered, often under fire, men and guns coming up to relieve the trenches, total darkness, yells to mind oneself and get out of the way, meaning a sickening slide off the pavé into deep mud – screams from the stretchers behind one and thumps in the back through the canvas – then an appeal to passing soldiers to shoulder the ambulance back on to the pavé. Two or three of these journeys at night and ones eyes were on stalks, blood shot and strained. No windscreen, no protection, no self starters or electric lights to switch on when out of range of the lines – climb out to light with a match, if possible, the carbide lamps.

Throughout we worked for and with the Belgians. At no time did we have British orderlies, nor were Tommies in our sector. I cannot speak too highly of the Belgian soldiers and their attitude towards us. Our drivers and orderlies gave us loyal service; they changed from time to time as we were generally allocated men who were temporarily unfit for the trenches.

The Royal Naval Air Service was in continuous action over our lines, and we had the sad work of dealing with their casualties. One of the RNAS pilots took to sending me down boxes of chocolates attached to little parachutes – it was sometimes a moot point where they landed.

In 1917 the 4th British Army took over the Nieuport Sector from the French – the plan being to try to force an advance in co-operation with the British Fleet, along the coastal area of Flanders. Unfortunately the supporting guns were insufficiently camouflaged and the Germans got very accurate range. They attacked the Kings Royal Rifles who held the British Tunnel, the small strip on the east bank of the Yser, and overwhelmed them. The position was extremely critical and Commander Halahan's Naval Siege Guns which had been in position for about two years shot over sights in order to hold the Germans. Three of his guns blew up, killing their crews, but he and the French 75s, which had also been in action for a very long time, saved the situation. He was an outstanding officer and a true friend.

The night of this happening at Nieuport, the British guns, which had moved into action behind us in support of the Belgians, were also the subject of intense fire and spent most of that night on the shell swept road evacuating their wounded. The Baroness had her work cut out in the dug-out i.e. our Poste de Secours. The regimental doctors delighted to work with her and with such good equipment.

Colonel Jennings was an Irishman with a keen sense of adventure. He took me under his wing to give me a few extra thrills and when searching for a suitable observation post in Pervyse from which to direct his gun fire, he took me along. The remaining stock of the church tower seemed fairly robust so his men ran up a pulley rope – I put my foot in a loop and with a pair of binoculars slung on was hauled to the top. The view of the German lines was the best yet but unfortunately they chose that moment to deliver a salvo of shells aimed for Suicide Corner, on which stood the church. The men let me down in a flash, but we had to laugh – it was an anticlimax.

Another time Colonel Jennings had me hauled up on to a three-plank platform fixed in the branches of a tree, which had escaped destruction. It was high up, most unsteady, nothing to hold on to and waving in the breeze.

In our 3rd Poste we had a cook, Gabriel, with a macabre sense of humour who carried an amputated foot in a cake box into the men's dug-out saying 'Madame got this cake for you in Dunkerque'.

Joseph was our driver – his nerve was not always so good; he had been invalided out of the trenches. Octave la Meir was our orderly, and a better man never stepped. He and I had many an adventure and his gaiety in the face of danger was most infectious and infinitely helpful …

1917
Corsica and Italy

Dr Mary Phillips

5th Scottish Women's Hospital Unit, Villa Miot Hospital, Ajaccio, Corsica

In December 1915 a Scottish Women's Hospital unit left Salonika for Corsica, with some 6,000 weak, exhausted and destitute Serbian civilian refugees, two members of the Serbian Relief Fund and two members of the Scottish Women's Hospitals, Dr Mary Blair and Sister Walker. During the sea crossing a baby was born and he was called Abda, after the ship. Another baby born on the day the party arrived was christened Napoleon in memory of the island's celebrity.

When they arrived in Corsica the members of the unit requisitioned Villa Miot, an old white-washed, two-storied building, which looked directly on to the bay, and this was turned into a temporary hospital.

At first they nursed typhoid, appendicitis, pneumonia and maternity cases in one ward under extremely basic conditions – no water, no heating, except Primus stoves, and no sanitary arrangements.

Gradually the hospital facilities were extended – tents, for open-air treatments, were pitched in the garden; an outpatients department was opened, and later more dispensaries were formed in four mountain villages. A fever hospital was established some two miles from Villa Miot, in a beautiful, old building 'on a point jutting out into the gulf, built in the form of a semicircle of small rooms round a central courtyard, with pathways of flags between borders of white roses'.

Soon after the hospital was opened it received over 3,000 worn out, dirty and wounded Serbian soldiers from several decimated regiments, who had escaped across the Albanian and Montenegrin mountains under severe conditions in the snow. Every available bed and corridor space was filled and children were placed on the shelves in the linen cupboard to provide a few more beds. German prisoners in the hospital helped to look after the wounded. After two months' rest the soldiers were sent to Corfu to join the newly re-formed Serbian army.

These soldiers were followed by the schoolboys and students, aged between six and eighteen, who had joined the exodus from Serbia across the Albanian and Montenegrin mountains with the remnants of the army and the thousands of fleeing civilian families. Many of the boys had not changed their clothes for three months, and they had all been desperately short of food during the weeks of escape. Thirty thousand started on the march of which some 7,000 completed the journey. After they reached San Giovanni hundreds more died daily from exhaustion and hunger. After three months at the Villa Miot the boys were divided into two groups and sent to schools in England and France.

In May 1917 a babies' party was held in the grounds of Villa Miot for all the babies who had been born in the hospital over the past eighteen months. Dr Mary Phillips, the chief medical officer, later wrote an account.

It was a lovely day – blue sea, blue sky, and not too hot. A tent was pitched in the garden for refreshments and shade. A few friends, including the Serbian Delegate, were invited to meet the mothers and babies, and the Committee was represented by Mrs Gardner Robertson. Among the guests were Sir Edward and Lady Boyle, Colonel and Mme Pitetitch, and Mme Dedinovatz, the wife of another Colonel at the front. Their joy in seeing these vigorous young Serbians was quite touching, and their thanks profuse.

A few mothers and babies came from the hill villages of Uncciani and Boccagnano, but most were resident in Ajaccio, and about forty infants were present. They varied in age, from Napoleon, the first baby born on the island, to the new baby of 48 hours. Also George and Mary, the first babies christened in the Hospital.

On arrival, the mothers were received at the front door, passed into the consulting-room, and amid much noise the babies were weighed and weights recorded carefully. It was surprising to find that there was no superstition against weighing. From the consulting-room the mothers passed into the garden for refreshment and congratulations and much talk over the respective weights of the infants. As far as I remember, they were of average weight; they were naturally fed, for the most part, and all had made good progress.

The previous winter, 1916, had been very cold. The Corsican houses are not built for cold weather, and many of the children had suffered from broncho-pneumonia, but, true to their race, the Serbian babies have wonderful recuperative powers, even after many weeks of fever. We were very proud of the fact that we didn't lose one, and at the time of the party they were all well again.

Little Slobodanka Cistitch was the most wonderful of them all. She was taken ill with pneumonia up at Piana. First Dr Jackson and then I had to cross the river in spate. The bridge was washed away, and the crossing had to be made in a small boat – after seven attempts, success crowned our efforts. Little Slobodanka was at last brought down to Hospital, and after many weary weeks got well and became the pet of the Unit.

Now a word about baby clothes. The Serbian custom is to bind the child up 'Italian Bambino' fashion, and the straps are most beautifully embroidered, and for peasant babies done in coloured wools. The Jugo-Slavs, of which we had a fair number, used little hair mattresses and pillows German fashion. In hospital the English method was followed, but I fear that, on leaving, the binding was replaced. One particularly fine baby who had never had her legs bound was proudly shown as the English baby.

Writing of them brings them all back to me, dear little people, with their engaging ways and their caresses for 'Doctor' …

Miss Freya Stark

George Trevelyan Ambulance Unit, Villa Trento, Dolegnano, Udine, Italy

In 1914, Freya Stark, who was living in Italy with her mother, decided to train as a nurse at the clinic of St Ursula in Bologna. After an unhappy love affair with a bacteriologist at the clinic she became ill and returned to England in 1916. While she recuperated she worked as a censor. She then went on a six-week training course to become a VAD, before joining George Trevelyan's ambulance unit based in the elegant Villa Trento at Udine. She arrived on 3 September 1917 and shared a dormitory with three other VADs. One, Ruth Trant, an Irish girl, became a close friend. Freya Stark kept a hastily written diary of the two months she was serving with the ambulance unit, from which the following extracts have been taken.

4 September 1917
Last night as I went to bed the heavy sound of the guns – as if something were heaving with great vehemence through a thick surface – came from the way of S. Gabriele. S. Gabriele they say has fallen today; the spurs, Caterina and Daniele, still to take.

Two of our men have been wounded [ambulance drivers]: Sylvester – who already had a medal – has had shrapnel clean through his ankle; Sessions has a fractured thigh and has not yet come; Geoffrey Young is here also, wounded – all on the Gabriele.

The guns this morning came through a haze of sunlight, a short sharp sound unlike last night; now (9.30pm) a terrific bombardment is going on again. Trant and I went up about 8.30 to see: there was still a sullen red glow of sunset over Italy, but night already and pale stars to the east; the guns come in short bursts, like far, reluctant thunder – an angry sound. Over all the line the flashes come; ruddy and quick from the shells, and the long pale star-shells hanging like new planets for some seconds. Most come from the Hermada; a huge red flare suddenly on Gabriele – one could almost see its shape – and from our village Dolegnano a searchlight turns slowly round and upward, inland towards us, in search of aircraft it seems; the church tower on the little hill (whence an 'austriacante' priest was thrown down by the populace early in the war) is caught in the light and stands for a second like a beacon. In the growing darkness the battle seems to come nearer; one feels a part of the great pulse, a tremendous excitement and also a sense of awe at the grandeur of such a tragedy …

I hear our gunners have been badly knocked about. As for the wounded drivers, Sessions has had his leg amputated in Gorizia; the bone was smashed through the knee. A terrible fear that Mr Young will lose his leg also. The three casualties all happened on the same very dangerous stretch of road.

5 September
Monte Gabriele lost again. The men are coming in now, not in great numbers, but I heard Dr Brock say that 20 or 30 daily are promised for the future.

I have been put in the Garibaldi ward – a long granary with only four patients this morning, but ten more have arrived today.

Sister is Scotch and most charming, with a pretty slow way of speaking and a gentle look and manner so that one loves her at once.

It is a comfort to speak Italian and be able to know what these poor boys are thinking and wanting; it is not the language so much as the point of view which is familiar to me and strange to the English nurses – so that they and the patients often seem to be moving in different worlds.

The ten people are:

1. Fractured both legs below the knee; came here in hysterics almost, and seemed quite recovered when I washed and changed him; but in great pain again now
2. A man from Reggio Calabria, wound in the leg
3. Boy from the south; wound in the knee. Problem because he refuses a bedpan and says he will rather die than use it, and he mustn't be moved, so there the matter rests at present
4. A Turinese with cut head; so good and patient; he lights up when I speak to him in Piedmontese. He had a little tin locket which nurse seemed not to realise had value to him … so pleased when I brought it to him with a new silk ribbon
5. A poor man shot through the neck and almost unable to swallow; have been coaxing him to take milk, but he is so weary and sorry for himself
6. A boy shot in the thigh; not seen the wound

The rest came when I was not there.

The work here seems chiefly dressings and not many operations.

Enthralling to watch the traffic along the road, the chaos of lorries, cars, horses, every imaginable vehicle on all kinds of business, trooping to and fro from the front in the white dust between the dusty acacias …

I came back late for Matron, but she was later still. A very energetic, pleasant woman. She has been through Serbian campaign: name Miss Power. The guns are terrific this evening.

6 September
Work from 8 to 6.30; had ward to myself in the afternoon. Sister said I would do very well.

All the men who came yesterday doing well. But a hand and leg are going badly of the earlier arrivals, there is fear the leg may be amputated. Also Geoffrey Young's, I fear.

7 September
Great influx of wounded during the night – all from S. Gabriele. Poor men mostly

asleep exhausted, temperature below normal; they all say they have not eaten for three or four days. Most wounded in the leg, some in the arms; one had eight wounds – little round holes where the lead has lodged. Sister extracted one piece as big as a hazel nut. They are very good and patient, not so stoic as our men but much more appreciative. My poor mouth case with a large hole at the back of his neck asked me if I didn't dislike feeding him! Then he begged to be allowed to stay on here, but he is to go to a special hospital in Udine tomorrow.

It seems a hundred men arrived last night.

Geoffrey Young has had his leg cut off. One hoped to save it to the last.

8 September
Another busy day. The man with the bad neck left before I came in the morning; one is always sorry to lose them. One constant rush till I came off duty at 6 – hardly time to think and I feel so tired still; we just hurry through the meals knowing that whoever is left in the ward is waiting to be relieved.

9 September
We hear from the men from Gorizia that the offensive up here has come to an end, so no more influx of patients. Another 20 arrived today however, and one very bad case was brought into Garibaldi; have been keeping him alive with injections and salines; doubtful if he will pull through.

11 September
I have had a half-day's holiday and spent the afternoon sleeping under a vine … in one of the long rows that stretch in a straight low avenue of tangled sun and shadow: the vintage is just over and the leaves begin to change colour.

Last night the bombardment was so loud the house shook and rattled with it. The night was hot and stuffy, a storm came up, and one could not tell if the almost continuous series of flashes were lightning or the reflection of the explosions on the western bank of clouds. The rain fell in torrents.

Three stretchers brought into my ward today, one fractured thigh, one with both hands, one arm, head and three body wounds. I had to feel his pulse at the temple. But he seemed quite strong, and horrified Sister Brechin by most voluble swearing.

The poor boy brought with fractured thigh on the 9th had to have the leg cut off and died early this morning.

Another death in the next ward. It is horrible to do all one can and find it useless.

Mr Trevelyan spoke to me yesterday. Kind in his keen quick way; a most sensitive face, full of enthusiasm; we spoke of the mountains and poor Geoffrey Young: Mr Trevelyan said that climbing was the one thing G.Y. really cared about.

13 September
The ward this evening seemed full of sighs and moans, most depressing. One of yesterday's patients had been a prisoner that same morning; the Austrian captain leading him to the rear was killed, and he just waited till the Italians came up again.

16 September

Two patients make a terrible noise and drive one distracted – one has both legs fractured and nothing can be done to ease him of the pain, and the other is mad – so Dr Thompson says. I saw him operated upon today and he has now nearly all his leg slit up below the knee and a tube arranged to drip a disinfectant lotion constantly right along inside the wound; his temperature has sunk already, but pulse very bad.

The boy from Mondovi was operated on but the shrapnel is too deep-seated – somewhere between the ribs and kidney, so that it is dangerous to get at.

18 September

No. 72, our madman, has had to have his leg amputated.

Heard today why we are only now getting the serious cases; it seems the advance on the Gabriele was so quick that the stretchers had to be carried a very long way and the men who couldn't walk were only taken very gradually to the rear. Our ward was cleared at once of the light cases so that we were able to fill up with the badly wounded whom we have now.

19 September

I heard this morning that No. 72 died quite suddenly and early. One other patient left, so that we have 15 altogether, of which 7 fractured legs (compound, of course). They are all heavy dressings. One leg has 5 drainage tubes in it, being all riddled with shrapnel.

20 September

Very sad day. Little 94, who has already lost his right arm, had to have the leg taken off at 9 this morning. I was there and held it during the amputation; he was so thin, it was not a long business. And now one wonders if he will live through the night, his pulse is so flickery.

21 September

Comparatively lazy day. No. 94 is better; pulse stronger.

Went up the hill with Mr Glazebrook. From his outstation at Ravna one can sit on the balcony and watch the exposed bit of road, and see the ambulances coming along among the shells, wondering if they will escape … all the crossroads are constantly sprinkled with shells. The bit of road where our three drivers were wounded, 'the rock', is out of sight of the Austrians, but they have the position and it is the only way up Gabriele so they shell it constantly. On the visible bits they seem to try to avoid the Red Cross. It seems that the Austrian side has very bad roads, just mule tracks, so that their lorries have to stop a long way behind the front, and it must cause great difficulties to their transport: such a contrast to the Italian side.

28 September

I am now allowed to put on fomentations by myself; hope to be promoted to dressings soon.

An ambulance just arrived in the moonlight, with some stretchers.

1 October
Four patients left this morning. Three more arrived this evening, wounded in an assault on a fortified gallery of the Gabriele; the major had killed two Austrian officers but the men had not surrendered when our two were wounded.

2 October
Busy day. One new patient early this morning; 23 altogether. We did 14 dressings in the morning, average 15 minutes each.

5 October
Garibaldi is now full again – 35 beds. Most of the new arrivals are light cases, arrived today.

22 October
We hear that the Austrian offensive has begun all along the line from Trentino to the sea. All yesterday, through the night and all today at intervals, they have been shelling our neighbourhood with their heavy long-range guns. Cormons has been hit (two people killed that we know of).

24 October
Since midday the bombardment has continued without a break, one constant indescribable roar. The attack is chiefly south over the Carso. It has been pouring with steady rain all day; the troops march by at a weary plod, with their hoods well drawn over their faces.

25 October
Half-day's holiday – lovely weather. With Gibby [a VAD, Miss Gibson] walked to Brazzano to see the two shell holes; they are about 20 minutes' walk from here. We heard that Cormons was in ruins; walked on, past long trains of big guns drawn by tractors, past whole families plodding away with their belongings. Cormons itself was a desert, and most dreary; soldiers in the streets; the carabinieri at the street corners had their steel helmets on; the visible glass in the windows was broken, but most shutters were closed, many nailed down; the piazza was quite bare. The soldiers were taking last provisions from the shops. The order had been given to evacuate; we wandered about, asking for biscuits and chocolate, quite surprised to find the place suddenly cleared of its stores.

We came back through a red sunset. Heavy guns with their long nozzles covered with leaves, and short double-barrelled howitzers, all trudging on against the orange sky. Staff cars, motor cycles … intense excitement everywhere, but no disorder.

The news that spreads about is rather disquieting. Caporetto they say was taken by the enemy who broke through our first line this morning; but has since been retaken by us. The trenches round here, a few hundred yards away, are being got in order and filling with men. The attack is going to be a very big thing. There are Germans, Bulgarians, Turks against us, as well as the Austrians. Our English batteries that were to leave have not yet gone and are shooting as hard as they can down Carso way.

26 October
This has been a very long, eventful day. We were told at breakfast to have a suitcase ready with all our indispensable property so as to be able to leave at a moment's notice. In the morning an order came to clear the hospital of all patients; we had a great rush to get our fractures into uniforms while ambulance after ambulance drove up to carry them all away. The guns were pounding at slow intervals, nearer than yesterday it seemed.

We got all our beds stripped, the pillows, sheets, and covers tied in a bundle on each bed. About 2pm Braithwaite came to tell us to dismount 25 beds that were to go at once to the rear with some VADs; our stretcher cases were not yet all cleared off. By tea-time they had all gone however and our beds dismounted and carried down, and our dressings, etc., packed – the ward looking like a desert.

The rumours meanwhile were most various. Ravna it seems is really lost; the paper today admits losses on the Bainsizza plateau; Caporetto went and the Austrians reached the Isonzo at Canale. A poor little Alpino, limping along with a shot in his leg, came to us and told us this, and also that we are leaving the guns in the enemy's hands, they come up so quickly with their machine-guns. The road in front here was a sad sight all day – one long dejected stream, soldiers, guns, endless Red Cross ambulances, women and children, carts with household goods, and always more guns and more soldiers – all going towards the rear.

Well, at tea we were told that the order to evacuate had come; we were to take as little as possible – only luggage we could carry ourselves, and leave the rest in the hope of retrieving it later. Then comes the new order – we must stay here and are to prepare for wounded at once. All the beds to make again. We leave the 25 that are dismounted in case of another order, which is quite probable, and lay mattresses along the empty space. A lot of our old patients return; they had wandered from S. Giovanni along the packed roads in all the confusion and instead of getting to Udine arrived here very pleased with themselves. We got them some soup and pudding, all that could be scraped together, as no one expected to have another meal at Villa Trento. Our ward now has 3 bad cases in beds and 20 on the mattresses along the floor; they look very uncomfortable, but we have done all that is possible and they have plenty of covers and a clean pillow – but none are allowed to undress as we may have to leave suddenly. We got them to take their boots off and wash hands and faces; as an aggravation of difficulties the water supply has given up; it comes from near Cividale and a shell must have damaged the aqueduct; so all we have in the house is to be for drinking purposes only.

The news tonight is still bad. Our cars have been carrying refugees today – streams of them, and now Udine is in panic too and people leaving as fast as they can.

One comforting thing is that our new outstation, which had to be given up this morning, is to be re-started tonight; and they say we are going to have a big counter attack.

Am now going to sleep without sheet or pillow-case, with the chance of being called any time in the night to leave, and the Austrians about 9 miles away.

27 October
Today we live in the same uncertainty as to our future. But we are to be the last hospital to move, which is satisfactory so far. Meanwhile a place is found at Conegliano, 80 kilometres west, and our 25 beds are just being loaded and sent on there with all requisites for a start. I hope not to be one of the VADs sent there to open the place. We remain here to collect what wounded there are, but most must have been taken prisoner; we only get stragglers. Cormons hospital is deserted – no one there but a corporal who had not even a drop of iodine to dress a wound which came on to us this morning; Abbazia on the hill behind us I hear is also closed.

Aosta and Garibaldi are the only two wards kept open, and Garibaldi looks a desert with all the mattresses on the floor. We have had all the work there is there; about half a dozen limping soldiers, soiled, ragged, walking with no stockings in their boots – one with a pair of boots picked up by the roadside. We dress the wounds, lay them on the mattresses and find what little food we can get, and the next ambulance takes them along to the rear. Did all the dressings this morning with my own forceps as the ward ones were packed.

This morning's news was that the enemy tried to surround Gorizia and failed. Now Dr Tommy says Santo, Kuk, Gabriele, all is lost to the Isonzo. The train of soldiers coming to the rear is endless, and now there are guns, long lines of them, chiefly field guns; and civilians still with bundles; the roads are almost impracticable – they say everyone seems to have lost his head. We have only our own cars to rely on and they can only crawl along.

Now all the cases are cleared off and we have nothing to do.

The weather continues lovely – a golden autumn day.

28 October. In car No. 88, near Codroipo.
About three o'clock yesterday Matron told Sister Brechin, Trant, Gibby, Murray, Hurley, Bosy and me to be ready at once to start for Conegliano to prepare the new hospital.

We left at 5.15, a wonderful evening. The hospital quite empty, except for two stragglers who had just limped in. Ambler was driving us; Cobby Wood with motor stores followed; Miss Kemball with a new and inexperienced driver left separately and we have seen nothing of her yet.

Through the twilight till the moon came up, a few shells sounding behind us; the road packed with traffic three deep, carabinieri all along to keep order; all talking, shouting, or very tired. One got more and more to feel it as the retreat. Behind us flares went up along the skyline where our men were exploding the stores and munition dumps before the Austrians got them. We got stuck for half-hours at a time, the whole road lined with tired figures, sleeping anywhere, in heaps on the banks; some limping along without their regiments; all so tired. Bivouacs in the fields; big guns with caterpillar tractors; the moon and white villages and cypress hills formed a wonderful background. We saw two lorries overturned – one dead horse lying in the road; and near Udine, where we cross the broad riverbed, the tired men were scattered sleeping on the white stones, and made one realise a battlefield with its dead.

Reached Udine at 9 – 20 kilometres – and as Miss Kemball foolishly had all the rations, went into the station to find some food; so packed with refugees one had to hew a way through them – most pitiful; we got some bread and cheese at last, just a small allowance.

Everyone was turning out of Udine. The flare of the explosions was visible all along the sky; turned to a dull red sunset blaze and it started to rain – with all those poor tired sleepers in the open. The lines of traffic continued three deep. We have now been travelling 20 hours and are only 16 kilometres from Udine. For one stretch the two columns were distinct, one for horses, the other for motors, but then comes a jumble, and we just wait till the thing ahead moves a few yards.

We had sandwich of potted sausage between two sweet biscuits and cold plum pudding at about 2am, all squashed into the ambulance with rain and wind buffetting outside. The men and refugees all come to look in at us and want to have a lift, and we are already overweighted.

Wood caught us up last night and has kept close behind us ever since.

We saw a good deal of fresh cavalry coming out during the night. Pouring rain and wind.

In the morning we saw Braithwaite; he had left his car and hurried up to us walking. The retreat looks like a panic; Udine evacuated; wounded trudge in the rain with the hospital blanket over their shoulders. I saw one man drop it and not have the energy to pick it up. We stayed ages at this village before Codroipo, and found some boiled polenta and made cocoa in a house crammed with soldiers; bread not to be had.

We dressed a man wounded in the head and resting in a stable. We have two women and children in our car.

Our orderlies just arrived from Villa Trento, walking from Udine. They had the order to evacuate as soon as we left yesterday, and the Austrians were in Cividale this morning. It seems that Tagliamento is to make the next stand; the rendezvous is a hill just behind – and we are in the thick of the crush; no one can possibly realise what this means.

29 October. Cross the Tagliamento at 5.30am

The retreat has a rudiment of organisation; some aeroplanes have been flying over the road to set the congestion right; and the soldiers all seem to have been given some hard rations like dog biscuits to eat.

Poor Braithwaite is white as a sheet and so sad; and the men coming down today seem quite cheerful, glad to think that the fighting is over on the heights – only the officers look unhappy about the war – so that we wonder if it is only our own hearts that feel broken. The horror, the horror of it.

30 October, 10am. Hotel Savoia, Padua

About dusk on the 28th, Johnson, a new man, came up to us walking. Had been outside Udine when the alarm of the German arrival was given. A panic spread, all the horses were taken out of their carts and the lorries abandoned, so that it became impossible to get any motors along the road; a lieutenant came up to tell them to leave everything and hurry along on foot if they wished to escape, and the Austrians were now reported 5 or 6 miles from us. We were going at a snail's pace just then, the block ahead being quite impossible: in fact we reached a record by progressing only 2 kilometres in 12 hours on the morning of the 28th. The question was put to us by the men whether we would rather walk on and get across the bridge before they might have to blow it up, or stick to the car and trust to luck; we decided to stay as we were, not having any contrary orders, and also because we thought these were the only two cars that had a chance of escaping so that it was important to save them. Decided to turn down a side road if the Austrians came (NB so as not to be enfiladed). Anyway the probabilities were only of a temporary imprisonment.

Having so decided we dug out the plum cake, tackled our fiasco of wine, put on our brassards conspicuously, and waited for the block ahead to clear away. It was a slow business: in the growing darkness the traffic was being arranged in three columns – motors, carts, and men who were sent by a different side road altogether; the evening cleared and the stars shone; then there was a fire in Udine direction, and shells began landing in the country behind; we saw nothing except the long crowded road throbbing with the impatient motors, but the explosions seemed to come nearer, on either side of the road, in an irregular tentative sort of way. A cheerful artillery man told us that they might be peppering the retrovie with gas shells: but a new bridge was being got ready over the river nearby to hurry us up a bit. At last we crossed the little stream and the pace got better. The first signs of a stand began to show – cavalry, encamped by the road in fields, and a gun emplacement.

We reached Codroipo about 9pm. There the Udine and Gradisca roads across the Tagliamento meet, and the congestion was one solid mass, which a bevy of officers were disentangling. We waited for quite an hour while troops filed by with all their kit, just silhouettes and sudden flashes of light from matches and lanterns; there was a pleasant feeling of order and hurry – one felt they were very anxious to get us along quickly. The shells continued to fall somewhere in the neighbourhood. An officer came and and asked who we were and hoped that the soldiers treated us well along the road – a very kind thought in the midst of all that hurry.

About 10pm who should come along but all the VADs with a Colonel Hailey from the Gradisca artillery. They had taken a southern road and come faster than we, but had left their cars about 5 in the afternoon by Hailey's advice, and were walking to get across the bridge.

We left Codroipo in a deluge of wind and rain again; dead horses on the way, in the desolate shuttered streets with the endless caterpillar of lorries snuffling along them. Wood's car broke down, but he looted an exchange piece from an overturned lorry in the ditch, and rejoined us to our great relief. Percy [Mr Percival, an ambulance driver] also overtook us, with Nino the cook, and Luigia, all tired out.

The slowness of our pace increased, it seemed.

The hours wore on, and yet the pace was as slow as ever – about 20 yards, then a stop of half an hour or more. Towards 4am I could see that our men were getting anxious, and even I knew enough to expect the bridge to be shelled as soon as daylight came. At about 5 Percy said we must get out and walk and wait for the ambulance on the other bank if it could get through. We started at a breathless pace, single file, anxiously kept together by Percy in front and Haston (who turned up in the night, also carless) in the rear: they guided splendidly, in and out of the big wheels, under the noses of the mules, threading the tired files of troops, and all in great haste and well over our ankles in soft mud. We must have gone so about one and half miles; it is confused like a nightmare. At 5.30 the horizon opened; the great width of the Tagliamento spread in front of us, with the long bridge curving across without a parapet, all cold and grey in the first dawn.

Got over about 6am, but Percy still hurried us on through the mud and I was loaded with coat, overcoat, mackintosh and knapsack. At last we reached Casarsa; found a house, all crammed with soldiers where they gave us water to wash and drink; the woman there was very good and quite brave; though expecting to have to leave, she refused any money.

At Casarsa we came upon the others and luckily got a train and two carriages reserved for us to Treviso; no sooner had we crawled out a little way than a German aeroplane flew over the place dropping bombs. I don't know how near to us but the train was rather in a panic, everyone rushing back to the shelter of the carriages, so I didn't like to increase the confusion by getting out to see.

About 6pm we got out of the train and found some of our cars that had got over the bridge waiting in the road. Things were moving better now along the road and we were in Pordenone before 7, and found a whole lot of the Unit there, including – to our great relief – Mr Young and Matron and Trevvy [George Trevelyan] himself. We heard that all except three were safely through with or without their cars.

Our hopes of a night at Pordenone were soon done away with; the place was getting too crowded for anything, and they wanted us to move back before a crush came; so we had a drink of water, a basket of rations, and off we went for Conegliano, all packed the same old way in two ambulances.

Conegliano we saw by moonlight only. We stopped there for food, but were not to spend the night even here. Padua was to be the goal.

The army was being reorganised between Pordenone and Conegliano; no soldier allowed to pass, the carabinieri collected and arrested all the deserters as they came along.

After Conegliano I fell asleep and woke to find all asleep around me, the car standing still in a by-road and the rain still swishing down; a most alarming feeling to have nothing at all moving after the days of tumult. But it turned out to be only a halt for the sake of our poor drivers who had been at it with no rest from 5.15pm on the 27th – about 56 hours; so they had three and a half hours sleep. We could now run along at a fine pace; the roads were clear. We got to Padova towards 9 this morning and are here at the Savoia. The cars are all being ranged up in the station. We have been 64 hours on the way, and shall be glad of a rest.

1 November. Milan

Today the news is very bad; the Tagliamento bridge is blown up, but the Austrians were already across and there is no other decent line of defence.

We heard yesterday that the hospital was to be finished as all our equipment is lost. We have come out extremely well considering, though all the kit and stores worth speaking of have gone and we have lost 20 cars out of 35; but all the men have come through safely …

Miss Amelia (Amy) Nevill

No. 11 General Hospital, Genoa, Italy

From September 1915, Amelia (Amy) Nevill, a thirty-six-year-old VAD, worked at No. 24 General Hospital, Étaples, where her aunt Miss Ann Beadsmore Smith was Matron. Her brother, Wilfred (Billy), fifteen years her junior, was serving as a captain in the 8th Battalion East Surrey Regiment and in March 1916 he visited her at the hospital. Four months later, on 1 July 1916, the first day of the Battle of the Somme, Billy Nevill was in command of one of the leading companies in the attack on Montauban. With Bobby Soames, his second-in-command, Billy led the company in the assault by kicking off two footballs which the men dribbled up to the German front line trench. They were under very heavy fire and both Billy Nevill and Bobby Soames were shot through the head and killed. The footballs were recovered from close to the German trenches the following day.

In November 1917 Amelia Nevill accepted the offer to serve in a hospital further afield. She joined a group of other nurses for a journey in an ambulance train which was expected to last nine days. 'No one knows where we are going, except I hope the engine driver!', she wrote.

15 November 1917. (In the train to Somewhere …?)
When we get there goodness only knows but we have nine days' rations with us. I slept on the top shelf of three layers and 30 of us in the coach. Our supper last night: enamel basins of tea, bread and butter and jam, one knife for the thirty!

That was a treat last night for the rest of the journey we are to have no meal after tea except what we provide for ourselves, so we dashed off to the canteen, ploughing through the mud. I had a flash light thanks be and laid in stores of biscuits and chocolate. We can't deal with masses, it's too close quarters. We can only wash once a day! Of course being in a train like this we are going beautifully smoothly.

Now we have had a good breakfast, have lowered the middle bunk on each side which makes room for three or four to sit on. My lovely pillow and rug are at the moment my two joys in life. We have just had a nice little message through from Miss McCarthy wishing us luck and congratulating us on being the first lot sent on this expeditionary force.

17 November 1917
We are still in the dark as to our movements. All day yesterday we were unable to stir from the train. In the evening we acted charades. First the Sisters, then the VADs, then Australians. It was great fun, we dressed up, and behaved like a heap of children. The real scrum is undressing and dressing in the morning: 30 VADs in the gangway of one coach! We passed a cold and fairly sleepless night, and some of us, those that hadn't washed in the morning, were able to have a wash in a cup full of water. This

morning there was not a drop, so we are all unwashed; can you picture us after a night in the train!

At 9am we stopped for a moment, and were all allowed to get out and stretch our legs for 25 minutes. We did a bolt to the village, and some of us were fortunate in getting a lovely hot drink of coffee, others took cans and got a little water.

We are all in our heart of hearts feeling very depressed as when we got up the first morning one of us was missing, an awfully nice girl from 7 Stationary. Boulter, Aunt Annie will know her well. She evidently got out of the train before it started and we hope she is safely in Abbeville. It's very, very horrible, but we feel sure she is safe, only we can't communicate with anyone to find out. We all got on board about 6. She, Lord and I went to the canteen to lay in provisions. She came back with us and we all saw her undressed and in bed. The train did not start until 5am and she was missing before that, only no one thought anything about it except that she was at Mons. However she is gone and we know nothing. It is too depressing.

When we woke up this morning the country was lovely, only awfully cold, everything covered in a thick frost. We are all too cold to do anything but sit huddled together under our rugs, and our feet on suitcases.

We have just heard letters are being collected 1.30, so with cold hands we are scribbling off letters to catch the post. The OC has just been through and swears he has no idea of our destination.

We have peeps every few minutes up the most lovely valleys, and in between the most beautiful hills looking too lovely for words in the sun.

No more. Crowds of love. Amy

No. 11 General Hospital, Genoa
20 November, 1917
On Monday evening the most bedraggled party arrived. Received by Miss Steenson. None of us having had more than the merest lick of cold water for 5 days!

It was 9.30pm when we sat down dirty to a real good hot meal, soup which we had to drink out of ordinary plates! No spoons – hot meat, beans and potatoes which we all took it in turns to eat as we had about 4 knives and forks for nearly 60 people – and rice pudding. We have the most comfortable beds and fortunately I still have my rug and pillows as we had no bed clothes at all. At last a few blankets were found for the rugless ones. The sun and warmth are delightful and I have found quite a number of Sisters that I know …

24 November
This lovely sun! It makes work so easy. Scrubbing, scrubbing and yet more scrubbing and cleaning again but my hands are almost chapless.

Our luggage has arrived. Hot water is laid on and all is peace – but not quite happiness yet as we have had no news of our missing VAD …

1917
Romania, Russia and Egypt

Miss Margaret Fawcett

Scottish Women's Hospital, Reni, Romania

Margaret Fawcett, Yvonne Fitzroy [qv] and Ellie Rendel [qv], were members of the Scottish Women's Hospital unit that Dr Elsie Inglis took from England in August 1916 to staff two field hospitals for service with the Serbian division in Russia. Margaret Fawcett, an orderly, was with B Hospital at Bulbulmick, under the command of Dr Chesney with Ellie Rendel as her deputy. During the next four months they were constantly on the move. They nursed the wounded in a variety of makeshift hospitals and continued to follow the army in retreat. They reached Ismaila in November where they set up another hospital for a few weeks and were then evacuated to a base hospital in Odessa. By then there was considerable friction amongst the staff of B Hospital and Margaret Fawcett asked to be transferred to A Hospital. On 15 January 1917, 'thankful to get away from Dr C.', she left Odessa 'with thirteen packages of equipment' to join Dr Inglis at Reni, situated at the junction of the Pruth and the Danube rivers. It was an important junction for the evacuation of wounded, the movement of troops and equipment, and became the head-quarters of the Russian Expeditionary Force. Officers had the use of a Turkish-style bath house and Dr Inglis insisted that the women had baths there once a week.

Sunday, 21 January 1917. The train
We left Odessa on Monday for Bolgrad – which in peace times takes about forty hours and took us now about three days. The first part of the journey was the most uncomfortable we have yet struck. We had only one upstairs berth between the two of us and a kit bag, and as the carriage was crowded we had to stay up there all day.

We left Bolgrad in the morning and got to Trianoval at about 11.30. We had to wait the whole day in the station restaurant, as there was no train. Later some Roumanian Naval Officers arrived and the Commandant of the station asked if we might share their train. They said we might – so we are now travelling in style in a first class carriage with a whole compartment to ourselves. It is rather a change after the one top berth. Now that we have actually left the station, I hope we shall arrive at Reni by daylight. I have a wholesome dread of arriving at these places in the dead of night; twice already I have arrived at Reni in the dark, once by train and once by the Danube.

Last Sunday, which was the Russian New Year's Day, we went to a most enjoyable party at the house of some very rich Jews in Odessa.

There is about three inches of snow on the ground this morning, but we are snug and warm in our first class carriage.

Monday, 22 January 1917

We have arrived safely at Reni. We reached the station at about 3.30. I left Turner there with the equipment whilst I went to find the hospital to get carts. As I had no idea of the way and no one seemed to know where the Shotlandskee Gospeetal was, the only thing to do was to go straight along the road and trust that it was in the right direction. It was a pretty beastly walk; there was a blizzard blowing, and the snow was in huge drifts on the road, and I had no idea if I was going towards the hospital or away from it. But as luck would have it I was right, and finally arrived safely at the hospital.

Dr Inglis is here doing splendid work with her staff. They have the serious cases which are sent them from the evacuation hospital at the station.

Today the snow is crisp and freezing hard. When the sheets are hung out to dry they freeze as stiff as boards, and make a most uncanny creaking noise as they swing in the wind. We are cooking under difficulties. The stove is small, the proper cook is away, for fuel we have only wood which is quite green and comes in caked with snow, and the Austrian prisoners who are helping only speak German.

Tuesday, 23 January 1917

Today has been a good day in the kitchen. Yesterday everyone was late for everything – breakfast started at 7am and the last suppers were at 9pm. Today the fire went properly, the lunch was good, and people were more punctual, so we all feel more cheerful.

From our house we can see right across the Danube, across miles of marsh to a gorgeous range of hills. The Bulgars are supposed to be amongst them. The actual Russian first line trenches are at the top of the hill behind the hospital – so that we are really in 'No Man's Land'. I am starting work in the hospital tomorrow.

The guns have been very silent the last few days, and it is possible to go to Galatz, which Dr Inglis left about three weeks ago as they thought the town was going to be bombarded.

We have collected two mascots – one a black cat named Pushkin and the other a black and white Roumanian terrier named Sammy.

Monday, 27 January 1917

Hedges and I went foraging this morning and had a most successful time. The soldier who really did our shopping for us every day said that there was nothing in the town, so we thought we would go and see. We got a whole ham, six pounds of dripping, four pounds of butter, and some leeks.

Most of our carts have been taken off their wheels now and put on to runners. There are several sledges for hire in the village – I must try and have a ride whilst the snow lasts.

Thursday, 15 February1917
We have had some enemy aircraft over today, but they did not worry us. The Russians potted at them for a bit, but they never seem to hit anything.

Bowerman and Brown are going home soon, and when they leave I have volunteered to do the cooking for the Unit. Let us hope they will have enough to eat.

Friday, 16 February 1917
I have started cooking today. The stew will be ready well by eleven o'clock, and as lunch is not till twelve, I hope it will be eatable. The stove we have is a beast, and we only have wood for fuel, with the result that you either have a roaring fire, or no fire at all. Just at 'dishing up time' it is usually the latter, and if you particularly want anything to cook slowly, it will be roaring away like a house on fire.

Today the Danube is frozen solid. For several days there have been ice floes going down, but now they have all become blocked.

Saturday, 17 February 1917
I am having a few days in bed with a bad sprained knee. My horse bolted with me, and after galloping about a mile, finally fell and rolled over on my leg. Matron is supposed to put hot foments on, but as she has only done it once, Dr Inglis now does it herself.

The Danube is frozen across, and it is possible to walk to the other side if you go on planks where the ice is thin. It is frightfully uneven. Icebergs have been floating downstream for three weeks or so, and now we imagine they must have got jammed somewhere, and so the whole lot have come to a standstill and been frozen together.

Sunday, 25 February 1917
The Russian Officers in the district have had an epidemic of giving parties lately; there was one last night, and one again tonight. The one tonight is given by the Black Sea Horse. Isn't it rather a nice name?

We are still nursing Russians. We came out to nurse Serbs, but except at Bulbulmick, where we had about 200, I don't suppose we have nursed more than thirty or forty Serbs at all. Most of our patients have been Russians or Roumanians. We have a case of typhus in now – the first we have had.

All the barges and boats are frozen into the Danube, and the ice has to be blasted away to prevent it pressing too heavily on their sides. The high road, which leads from Roumania into Russia and passes through Reni, is quite passable now.

Tuesday, 27 February 1917
As firewood and bread are very scarce we have only thirty-six patients in the hospital. It is better for them to risk the journey to Odessa than to come here if we cannot feed and warm them properly.

Monday, 19 March 1917
Since the thaw the railway to Galatz is flooded. As we get all our patients from this direction, it will probably mean that we shan't have any in for a bit. Today is the first

day that the Danube has flowed since 16 February. At last the birds are beginning to come back from their winter quarters; ever since they left we have had nothing but otalans and rooks – hundreds and thousands of rooks; I can't imagine where they live, as there are hardly any trees here except willows down by the Danube.

Tuesday, 20 March 1917

This morning before nine o'clock Prince Dolgoroukoff, the General in Command of the Roumanian front, presented us all with the George's Medal of the Fourth Class. They are quite nice little things with orange and black ribbons, and have to be worn always. They are round and silver, with the Tsar's head on one side and an inscription on the other. The inscription is: 'For Valour'.

Monday, 26 March 1917

Yesterday we went to a Revolutionary meeting in Reni Market Square. It was really most impressive – there were about 300 soldiers and just a few civilians, all crowded together outside the church. It was all most orderly, but we were rather disappointed that the two chief speakers were Jews. There was a lot of talk about Anglia and Francia, and we found out afterwards that they said that England and France knew that Russia had been betraying things to the enemy, but that since the Revolution it was up to the soldiers to make them again trust them.

The general opinion seems to be divided between the desire for a constitutional monarchy or a republic. Most of the officers we have spoken to are in favour of the former; they say that Russia is not yet ready for a republic. The chairman of the meeting also explained that a Revolution did not mean that every man could do just as he liked – some of them have been refusing to obey orders – but that they must 'stick to their guns' and back up their officers in everything if they want to win the war.

The local war news is good. The Bulgars are being pushed back the other side of the Danube between here and Braila, and are burning the villages as they go – we can distinctly see the fires from here. We also heard that for the first time two women have been elected for the Duma [Russian Parliament].

We hear that the Tsar and his family are being sent to England. I wonder if it is true.

Wednesday, 25 July 1917

The firing at the front has been going on steadily for the last three days and nights. We can distinctly see the flashing from the bursting shells after dark.

Tuesday, 7 August 1917

I am still on night duty, and am getting rather tired. It is too hot to sleep in my tent this evening, so I am lying outside in my pyjamas trying to get cool. My night duty is nearly over. Matron, who is an awful idiot, will try and persuade me to go on with it as I know the work. That is the sort of reason she gives for everything she does. On the whole I have quite enjoyed my time, although days when they operate at five in the morning – the only cool part of the day, and just at my busiest time – are not nice.

We are still waiting for orders from the Serbs. They may be coming down to this front.

Friday, 17 August 1917
We are in the midst of an immense rush of work – there are 220 cases in hospital, all badly wounded, and every precious minute off duty has to be spent in sleep. Wright and I are in charge of the Dressing Room, a very strenuous but very interesting job. The first day of the rush, the day after I came off night duty, we did sixteen hours, with barely time for meals. Now that things are settling down a bit and people are getting used to working in double quick time, we have arranged to divide our work into shifts so things will not be so strenuous. The cases are by far the worst we have had since we have been here, and we get a huge percentage of deaths. This is very depressing, but is due to the fact that the majority of cases are men who are too ill to be sent on – those who are not so seriously ill are sent on to Odessa. On an average since the rush we have evacuated about twenty slight cases per day and admitted as many serious ones. You can imagine how the number of bad dressings to be done every day accumulates.

Sunday, 26 August 1917
At last there is a lull in the work. For the last fortnight we have been rushed to death with as many as 200 wounded in at a time. This meant that, besides the usual hundred beds in the hospital, we had eight big marquees full. Then we were evacuating every day, so that there were more than 200 dressings to be done every day. Dr Laird and Dr Ward were simply splendid, and ripping to work for; they worked all day and much of the night. For about a week this was their programme:

8am–10am	Dressings
10am–12pm	Operations
12pm–12.30pm	Lunch
12.30pm–4.30pm	Dressings
6pm–7.30pm	Operations

Then after supper they dressed all the new cases that came in.

The new patients hardly ever started to arrive till after supper when we were supposed to have finished work. This meant all the bathing and everything had to be done that night. One night the day sanitars refused to stay on and help with the bathing and stretcher-bearing; and as there were only perhaps half a dozen night sanitars for the whole hospital, we set to and did all the bathing ourselves. For stretcher-bearers we had to rely on an ex-patient named Andrea, who often helped us, a Russian Jew, who was our accountant at the time, and two of the Austrian prisoners who came on without a murmur.

I unfortunately had to take a day off duty in the middle of the rush with malaria, which was particularly unfortunate as all the Sisters were new.

Today and tomorrow we have to evacuate the entire hospital, as we have orders to join the Serbian Division at Hadji Abduli, a place half way between here and Bolgrad. This is very trying – we have been at Reni for eight months with really hardly enough to keep us busy, and now that there is lots of work to be done, we have to leave …

Miss Florence Farmborough

1st Letuchka (Flying Column)

10th Field Surgical Otryad of the Zemstvo of all Russias, Broskautsy, Romania

At the end of August 1916 Florence Farmborough collapsed with a high temperature which was diagnosed as typhoid. She was sent to the base hospital at Podgaytsy and after three weeks she made the long, tiring journey to Yalta in the Crimea to recuperate for a month in a sanatorium at Novy Semeitz. After a few weeks in Moscow she returned to the front in December 1916. By then there was a lull in military operations but the political situation in Russia over the next few months became increasingly confused: Rasputin was murdered, the Tsar abdicated, Alexander Kerensky took control of the provisional government and was followed by Lenin and then Trotsky. The Revolution ceased to be bloodless and unrest spread throughout the country.

In June 1917 Florence Farmborough's flying column was stationed near Podgaytsky, attached to the 23rd Division, waiting for a new Russian offensive. By then there was growing dissension in the army and many troops were reluctant to fight. There were heavy casualties and the column was kept busy tending the wounded and dying. At the end of the month it was transferred to the 8th Army and moved southwards, towards Stanislav and heard rumours of mass desertion in the army. The column reached Grabuvka and was then told to retreat. It continued to nurse the wounded and discovered that the retreating Russian soldiers included many deserters.

At the end of July the flying column was ordered to follow the 8th Army to Romania where, as before, they set up a series of small hospitals and dressing-stations. Here, in a newspaper report, Florence read of Yasha Bachkarova, a Siberian woman soldier who had served in the Russian army since 1915, side by side with her husband. When he was killed she continued to fight. She was wounded twice and three times decorated for valour. When she heard that soldiers were deserting from the army in large numbers Yasha Bachkarova went to Moscow and Petrograd to find recruits for a women's battalion. Many women, from all walks of life, joined the battalion. They were given rifles and uniforms and trained rigorously.

Wednesday, 9 August (Broskautsy, Roumania)

We housed fifteen wounded in our improvised Lazaret. Last Monday, an ambulance-van drove up with three wounded women soldiers. We were told that they belonged to the Bachkarova Women's Death Battalion. We had not heard the full name before, but we instantly guessed that it was the small army of women recruited in Russia by the Siberian woman soldier, Yasha Bachkarova. Naturally, we were all very impatient to have news of this remarkable battalion, but the women were sadly shocked and we refrained from questioning them until they had rested. The van driver was not very helpful, but he did know that the battalion had been cut up by the enemy and had retreated.

Thursday, 10 August, Seret

We were told that we should be leaving that evening for the Front and that our wounded must be despatched without delay.

We left [Broskautsy] about 7pm for the Austrian-Roumanian frontier. At first the roads were very good and there was a pleasant feeling of exhilaration that we were moving towards a new post. An aeroplane had been circling for some minutes over our heads; suddenly a bomb exploded, killing two of our horses.

At 10pm we arrived at Seret, a large town with many fine buildings. Rooms were given to us in the hospital.

Sunday, 13 August

There was much work in the hospital. Each of us Sisters had her own ward. At dinner we heard more of the Women's Death Battalion. It was true; Bachkarova had brought her small battalion down south to the Austrian Front, and they had manned part of the trenches which had been abandoned by the Russian Infantry. The size of the Battalion had considerably decreased since the first weeks of recruitment, when some 2,000 women and girls had rallied to the call of their leader. Many of them, painted and powdered, had joined the Battalion as an exciting and romantic adventure; she loudly condemned their behaviour and demanded iron discipline. Gradually the patriotic enthusiasm had spent itself; the 2,000 slowly dwindled to 250. In honour to those women volunteers, it was recorded that they *did* go into the attack; they *did* go 'over the top'. But not all of them. Some remained in the trenches, fainting and hysterical; others ran or crawled back to the rear. Bachkarova retreated with her decimated battalion; she was wrathful, heartbroken, but she had learnt a great truth: women were quite unfit to be soldiers.

Thursday, 17 August, Illisheyst

A storm blew up, due, probably, to the sultry heat, and we took refuge in the peasant's hut. A woman soldier with a badly contused leg came to us for a dressing. She did not belong to the Women's Death Battalion; she had, however, heard of them and from her curt remarks one could understand that she held them in but little respect …

Miss Dorothy Seymour

Anglo-Russian Hospital, Petrograd, Russia

Immediately after the murder of Rasputin, Dorothy Seymour found it hard to obtain reliable facts about what actually happened, but by New Year's Day 1917 she had managed to gather more information.

1 Jan

Police went and asked Usonpoff where Rasputin's body was. He answered, 'where all dead dogs should lie', so news was instantly circulated by the police that Rasputin has been found, not dead but badly wounded but would recover. Usonpoff then had to show the police to prove his death and the body was found shot in two places on the island just in the Neva.

Now known that at 2.30 four men, Dmitri Pavlovitch, Prince Usonpoff, The Grand Duke Constantine and Pouriskavich, a member of the Duma [Parliament] left the revelry here and went to fetch Rasputin to join it. Instead took him to Usonpoff's Palace and gave him a revolver and told him to shoot himself. He protested that he was divine and couldn't die, but at 6.30 a revolver shot was heard and a body was seen being carried from the Palace to a motor directly after.

Members of the Royal Family cannot be arrested without the Czar's orders and the Duma does not allow any of their members to be arrested without the consent of the Duma, and they had been suspended the day before the murder till 12 Jan, so whole party safe till then – and revolution probable on that date.

2 Jan.

Now known that Rasputin had a shot with the revolver at Dmitri but missed him and wounded Usonpoff. The four then drew lots who should kill him and Usonpoff was the one. But the mesmerism of Rasputin was still so strong that he refused, so they agreed all to shoot together. The Czar has ordered Dmitri and Usonpoff to be under arrest in their own houses. Result: telephone here tapped and all of us shadowed and watched.

6 Jan.

Dmitri Pavlovitch whisked away at 2am this morning to the Caucases under armed guard. Usonpoff sent to the Crimea yesterday. Constantine to his estates and Pouriskavitch to a regiment in the first line of trenches.

Rasputin was buried at 3am at Tsarkoe Selo on 5 Jan by Czar, Czarina and family with great eclat. Metropolitan of Petrograd officiating. Czar pall bearer. Buried under altar in little chapel. His body had been recovered from the Neva. Trepoff has resigned because Protopopoff has been included in the Ministry. Other Ministers all about to do the same. Czar refuses to let them go. Rather an impasse in consequence.

7 Jan.
Went for gorgeous walk on the Neva today. Kronstadt far out in the sky shining like a jewel. A hole opened in the ice and let me through as far as my waist just as I happened to be mentioning Rasputin rather flippantly. Russians justly edified and prophesising an early demise on my part from pneumonia. Hospital Xmas today.

11 Jan.
All Minister's resignations accepted. Prime Minister now Prince Jolitzin.

14 Jan.
Hear Dmitri arrived in Caucases much knocked about and is imprisoned in damp cellar. Grand Duke Nicholas tried to rescue him but failed. New plot talked of in a whisper. Prince Lubanoff came in and was graphic on the subject – 9 Jan. to 12 Jan. Russian date likely to be amusing. Archduke Nicholas Michaelovitch banished to his estate. Has five estates with beautiful houses, but has been sent to only estate without a house of any kind.

Went to opera *Eugene Onegan*.

3 Feb.
Fearfully cold today. We skated yesterday but it was not pleasant. Far too cold, one's nose and lips froze so.

Things have become very quiet lately, quite boring in fact. I've become quite medieval so that I like blood and thunder every day.

28 Feb.
Revolution only a matter of days now.

7 March
Streets full of people. All shops shut. Notices have been put up in all the streets that the troops will fire at any crowd they meet. Also machine guns ready.

15 March
The revolution we've all been expecting daily has come and, we hope, is over, but are doubtful, as even now the Czar is a prisoner. The educated revolutionists want one thing and the mob another. It's been a most wonderfully organised thing, the only blood shed by the Czar's troops or by rioters gone mad and they've really had them wonderfully in hand except for two days, when everything was touch and go for everyone.

We had one or two scary moments, one last night at the Vladimirsky when a drunken mob spent the night in the kitchen and every soul had a rifle or a revolver which he let off at intervals. It was like a shilling shocker night and what gave me fits was that the orderly of our ward thought he'd see if I was safe in the middle of the night, so came and looked into my cubicle, and I could only see a soldier in uniform and thought it was one of the mob with a revolver.

20 March
Things are fairly quiet here for the moment. They say there are rows in the outside towns now, and they are still a little nervous here, as neither the workmen or the soldiers will go back to their job and parade the streets all day long and how they are to be made to, no one can see.

Regiments of Cossacks with red banners, singing as they go, wander about the Nevsky and the infantry don't even keep together …

Sister Burgess

Troopship *Aragon*, en route for Egypt

Sister Burgess left England at the end of November with a group of nurses posted to Egypt. They travelled in groups of thirty via Boulogne, Paris and Lyons and arrived at Marseilles on 3 December. They were sent to a camp outside the port, where they slept in tents in the bitter cold, and waited for the rest of the unit to arrive. They were warned that Marseilles was full of spies and were only allowed out of the camp in 'twos or threes during the day or in fours or sixes after dark'. The day before they left the nurses went up into the hills and picked wild rosemary and lavender.

Sunday, 9 December
Arrived on board the *Aragon* about 6pm. Have a nice little bed in a cabin for two. Warm for the first time for about a week. Have a horrid cold which is not surprising.

Wednesday, 12 December
Throat making me feel a bit dicky. MO says it ought to be painted every day for six weeks when I get to the other side. Life boat drill this am instead of yesterday. Waited from 10am until 12 for a drill which lasted five minutes at most.

Thursday, 13 December
Said at breakfast this am that the 13th of any month generally brought something eventful to me, not particularly evil or good, but eventful. This am Matron asked if I felt equal to work. Said I'd like it, so reported to the MO. Expected to be put on sick Tommies – got two officers.

Sunday, 16 December
Still on duty! From 8.30am till 2.30pm. Nothing much to do. Have mentally been comparing the latter day officer with those of the early days of the war, the majority of the former suffer by comparison. If one stops to think, this war is not really so surprising as it seems at first. Last night I heard something which made me wonder it had not come before. I suppose it is true that evil kills itself and this war is the death

struggle of an evil system of government, it is the killing of a wrong series of thought. If governments had the aim of bettering the community instead of themselves this war couldn't possibly have occurred.

Thursday, 20 December
Forget if I said one of my patients is a doctor (RAMC) and a military cross man. Think he is really going to get well now. I am tired. Alarm just gone for lifeboat drill – everyone dashing in all directions for their belts. After we leave the harbour we have to wear them all day and keep them close to us at night. Revolvers have to be carried by all officers. I asked if they were to shoot periscopes with but I was told they were to 'shoot Sisters who disobeyed orders'. Have decided that this boat ought to be christened *Noah's Ark* as we seem doomed to remain in it so long.

Matron is in bed. Temperature 101 all day. Captain Cook thinks she must have had ptomain poisoning at the camp. She has not been really well since the day we all left. Think Captain Cook is clever. Wish he wasn't so fond of swearing. Spoils him.

Went down the hold today after my kit bag to get my shoes and some soap.

Saturday, 22 December
We left Marseilles harbour 1am yesterday, Friday. Woke at 1.25. Have not slept much since. Inoculated against Cholera on Friday at 5.30pm and wonder if that made me bad. If ever there was anyone who felt sure they couldn't be sick it was me. However I got up on the deck at 8am after nearly fainting. I was so ill because I felt so terribly faint that I would have welcomed a torpedo with open arms. They say the 'swell' was very great and we have no cargo except kits so that we are very buoyant, which makes it worse. Even one of the sailors who has been to sea for years (about 40 years I think) felt bad. This morning I feel as if I have been very ill and need a splint down my back.

I feel that it is good to be human if only to discover how very nice humans can be. Captain Morison was a dear kind brick and looked after me a lot. It seems a long, long time since anyone looked after me; it is nice to be taken care of I think. Most times I have to take care of myself, but I don't like it.

There is one other troopship with us, the *Nile*. It isn't such a good boat and nearly caused us to run into it yesterday. It happened like this: We have three destroyers with us, two Japanese which keep on either side and one of our own which keeps guard all round. We are taking a zigzag course to avoid torpedoes and every four hours the destroyers signal our fresh course. When they did so yesterday, we altered our course, but the *Nile* didn't, and consequently we and they had to stop engines for the time; only a few minutes but the bugler ran up to the Captain's bridge for orders and we thought it must be a torpedo and didn't know exactly what had happened till afterwards.

One of the engineers has suggested taking me down to see the engines at work – hope he won't forget. Of course we have our life belts on all day – no one is allowed on the top deck since we started except some men on submarine guard. There is a rainbow now so will stop and look at it.

Think Captain Cook doesn't want to talk to me any more because I won't flirt with him. I warned him and the engineer officer. Can't be helped. Wish men would be content to tell me interesting things. It's rather too bad, the moment one won't do exactly as they wish, they don't want to talk even sense.

I wonder if I shall ever get used to being lonely. Still one must keep cheerful, there is nothing else to be done and there is always someone to be helped. Curious how fond people are of one when they are in trouble, afterwards one doesn't count. Such is life.

Sunday, 23 December
Arrived Malta.

Monday, 24 December
Still here. Sports for Officers and men. Tables for Christmas dinner arranged.

There are Sisters Shannon, Wilson, McLeod and Burgess with officers, Captain Mitchell, Captain Morison, Captain Somerville and Lieutenant Jones.

Thursday, 27 December
Had quite a jolly Christmas. Menu signed by those at the table. Got a great shock today. Captain Cook brought me a piece of Maltese work in a small basket. Considering the way I've told that man off, I'm more than surprised. Can't quite get over it. Wonder if he really meant it for me.

Friday, 28 December
Left Malta about 4.30pm yesterday. Feeling rather faint in the evening but went to bed and ate dry biscuits and feel much better this am. Premonition!!

Captain Somerville insists on me wearing his pneumatic waistcoat which is easier to carry than the ordinary lifebelt supplied by the ships. He wouldn't accept a refusal.

Sunday, 30 December
We have been torpedoed this am. Cannot write more just now except that we are safe at Alexandria 21st General Hospital.

1918
France

Miss Josephine Pennell

British Red Cross Society Ambulance Convoy, St Omer, France

In January 1918, after six months' training in motor mechanics, twenty-year-old Josephine Pennell, a British Red Cross VAD, joined the St Omer Convoy as an ambulance driver. The convoy had only just been set up and the officers were members of the First Aid Nursing Yeomanry (FANYs). The camp of nissen huts, on the outskirts of the town, was still not finished, but the girls had fun buying material for curtains and a few extra pieces of furniture for their cubicles from the local shops. At first the new recruits acted as 'taxi drivers' taking doctors and nurses from one hospital to another, dentists and oculists on their various hospital rounds, mess orderlies to the market, hospital washing to the army laundry, and coffins to the cemetery for burial. After a few weeks they drove in convoy to the Brickfields by the canal where the Red Cross barges unloaded their wounded, and to the station to meet the hospital trains. Josephine Pennell wrote letters to her mother and father, a surgeon, during the year she served at St Omer.

18 Jan., 1918
We have been acting as 'orderlies' on the FANYs' cars so as to learn our way about, but in a day or two we shall each have our own car.

They are nearly all GMCs, which is practically another name for Buicks for they are nearly identical. They are not really in bad condition either.

The ambulances are pretty basic – they take four stretchers and are supposed to be warmed by the exhaust-pipe which runs along inside. There is a small window for the driver to look through, and a small box-seat to store first aid kits, and accommodate an orderly if necessary.

In front, the driver's seat accommodates three at a pinch, and having no windscreen, is provided with a canvas shield which reaches one's chin.

The engines also are basic. They have four cylinders and a radiator which is liable to freeze up in winter, and so it must be drained in frosty weather, or else must be started up every half-hour during the night if it is to be ready for instant use. They have Bosche magnetoes but no accumulators, so no electric lights, far less self-starters! That means three oil-lamps and on occasions a single headlamp.

The wheels have detachable rims held in place by six screw wedges. There is a spare rim. That makes seven tyres to keep up pressure as there are twin wheels on the back axles. Pumping is by hand!

The oiling consists of the sump and the gear-box and many 'grease-caps' to keep clean and filled.

We are on duty all day till five, and if on night duty – which we do in couples in rotation, we are off from two till five and ten on till ten. Then we go provisionally to bed.

The VADs are – Vera Rose, Marjorie Kerr, Mildred Chichester, Elwes, Dickson, Davidson, Harman, Fabling, Dewhurst, and one other whose name I can't think of, and then of course Fullerton, our senior VAD.

There are about a dozen hospitals to take people to, and we often go to Calais or Boulogne for stores, etc.

All the cars are parked right across the other side of the town out of doors, we get petrol at yet another place, and oil at our camp. We are all very cheerful and fit but for two who are homesick and one with a cold.

The first night was undiluted misery – we were shown our cubicles which had a bedstead and a mattress and nothing else at all. Later in the evening we got a pillow and four blankets, all very damp, and some washing paraphernalia, but our luggage was at the station, so we had nothing dry to lie down on.

I put a leather coat over the mattress, but it was so clammy and beastly, that we all kept our clothes on even to driving gloves and scarves!

The next night, however, we got our luggage and a pillow-case and a towel, so with drier bedclothes and our own rugs and eiderdowns we were very comfortable indeed.

It has poured solidly for one day, one night, and one morning all on end. We were soaked up to knees all day but didn't even feel cold!

22 Jan.

All this time I have only carried one stretcher case. The rest have been taxi jobs. Our real job is to unload the Red Cross barges that bring the worst cases down from the Front, and take them to local hospitals. Then there are the hospital trains which carry far more at a time. These have to be unloaded and sorted out amongst the different hospitals.

The general plan is for the wounded to be taken from the trenches to the nearest Casualty Clearing Station (CCS). There they have their wounds dressed, and very urgent surgery done. These CCSs are usually in tents close behind the Line.

From there they are sent on the next stage of their journey as soon as possible down to the Stationary Hospitals in the Line of Communication, or the General Hospitals which are theoretically further back still. Here they are either operated on and then after convalescence go back to their units, or if they have had an amputation they go back to England.

27 Jan.

A regiment here were having a dance at the YMCA, and asked all of us, but we are not allowed to dance in public, so Miss Thompson, the Commandant, arranged that we should dance over here in our own ante-room, and that half the men should come over from the YMCA next door.

Accordingly the stoves were taken out to make room, and a huge quantity of chalk put down, a piano brought in and a pianist and some drinks, and we had a very jolly time.

Nobody knew anyone, so they just came up and said, 'May I have this dance?' and that was all. In the intervals we walked about our 'mudflat' and drank port wine with soda water.

It was a topping dance. We got to bed about one, with the result that Vera and I had to fly off to roll-call this morning at 8.30 hastily camouflaged in greatcoats and wellingtons, and have been dragging our own weary limbs listlessly about all day.

This evening I am on duty, that is from 5 to 8.30pm so I am sitting in the office, a little hut at the gate, and minding the telephone. I have just been out on a call to take a case from here to a village some kilometres away.

My acetylene headlamp refused to light – reason, I had forgotten the water. Luckily it was a lovely night with a clear moon.

Here is an answer to Father's question about our work. [An incident a few nights previously.]

A train has just been signalled as having started down the line. The news goes up on the board and the last preparations made. Tanks and radiators are filled, tyres are checked for pressure and lamps filled. There's no going out of camp till the train has come and gone. Invitations out to dinner, plans for supper at the 'omelette shop' have to go by the board. By ten o'clock most people have turned into their beds half dressed to sleep soundly till the shrill whistle rouses them and they tumble out of their beds, drag on their gumboots and overcoats and gloves, and run to the cars, winding their mufflers round them as they go. Soon the lights of the camp come to life and the cars respond to the frenzied winding of their drivers and file out into the night, each two lengths behind the one before at the signal of the NCO.

Once at the station they draw up in line waiting for the good news that the train has been signalled and the leading cars drive into the goods yard where the RMC and his sergeant are deep in consultation over their papers.

Great arc-lights spring to life as the long white train slides slowly into position down one side. Then all is movement and work. The first six ambulances are waved up to cars A and B for sitting cases. They draw up at the doors and eight men climb up into the back of the car while one climbs up by the driver and the car moves off.

At the gates stands Sergeant Carr with his lists.

'Nine sitters', calls the driver, and 'Number Fourth Stationary', answers the Sergeant, and the car drives off.

A bit further on the driver pulls up and putting her face to the sliding window she passes through a packet of ration cigarettes, keeping one for her companion in front. Once lighted up she pulls out from the kerb, and dodging the worst of the pot-holes she turns over the canal-bridge and along the quay-side to the Rue Edouard de Vaux. Here the hospital door is locked until 6am and one must go round to the garden door at the back. This house was once the training-college for English priests for the conversion of England.

But now back at the station, and this time it is four stretcher cases, or perhaps one single figure entirely cocooned in bandages like a mummy. He is probably badly burned, and is laid gently on the floor, with his limbs tied up to the stretcher racks. An orderly climbs in beside him, and gives him sips of brandy. (No other sedative.)

This one goes to the nearest hospital. That is No. 58 in the town. He is taken in low gear, along the smoothest parts of the road and given precedence at the door.

Now back again to the station, only to find the train has been emptied. So a round turn, and off at top speed to a bath and blessed bed.

Monday, 19 February

I rose at 6.30am and hied me down to the park to get my car. Two kind souls started it for me. The hoarfrost was standing thick on it. After getting my breakfast I spent a hectic hour with the mechanic helping to cope with a broken throttle.

We got off at last with three other cars on a convoy to carry twenty-two Chinese labourers to Calais.

We had a very nice run but for a burst tyre (mine) and about six stops distributed among the other three cars.

The Chinese invalids are quite useful. They got out to see and one I put to pump and another to jack, and we had it changed in record time.

They are very grubby, but very interesting, especially in their clothes. They wear blue padded denim trousers and jumpers, but their hats and caps are of every description – even toppers!

Arrived at Calais, we deposited them, and then I drove a VAD who was having a joy-ride with me to the Duchess of Sutherland's Hospital. She had a friend there whom she wanted to see, and we were both given dinner.

It's a lovely spot with beautiful woods behind it and the wards are wonderfully fitted up.

They specialise in fractures, and over nearly all of the beds are wonderful overhead railways to which the limbs are slung in all sorts of positions. It looked awfully complicated, and it must take hours to arrange.

Saturday, 23 February

There has been rather a rush of work.

I have had 13 flat tyres since Monday last! Thirteen! Not different tyres each time of course. I burst one two or three times, and found, rather late, that I had a nail sticking through the cover. Then there was one I nipped as I put on the outside cover, and all the rest were valve trouble.

Really to appreciate the humour of the situation you must pump up an oversize Dunlop back-tyre. It takes 500 honest pumps to get one up to 70*lb* pressure off the car, so by a simple calculation 1,000 do two, and when you hear it all sizzelling [sic] out when you have done and you have to take out the valve, and have to 'empesar' all over again. Dios Mio!

27 March
We are very busy at present. There was another convoy of ambulances (ASC) to help us, but they have been moved after being here all the winter, and we and our thirty little cars have to carry on solo.

On Sunday, for instance, we had a big evacuation at 9am to practically clear a hospital. That took till eleven. About two we had a train which lasted till five, and at 6.30 ten ambulances to move some stretcher cases from one hospital to another, and finally at 3am the next morning another train.

It's rather an impressive sight to see 30 ambulances start out by moonlight with no lamps lit. They slink out of the park one after the other like great grey wolves.

We were slack again the next day, but much the same again on Tuesday, and now today we have been pretty busy, and the possibility of another train during the night. We get rather peevish and short-tempered, but otherwise we are cheery enough.

28 March
We have been driving so continuously that we only had one meal and kept going with that and then managed with sandwiches and cocoa which we grabbed from a table set up at the gate. They were handed up by the kitchen staff without our getting down.

I was so tired the second night that I fell asleep as I drove towards the station for the umpteenth time, and starting awake as my front wheel bumped the kerb, only to do the same thing again a few yards further on.

16 April
Many of us were in bed when the sirens began to blow. We shambled across the camp to the hated dug-out with trailing bootlaces. The order was always to come 'ready for the road'. An order that had many interpretations as might be gathered from the glimpses of gaudy pyjama trousers showing below the British warms.

Soon the archies (anti-aircraft guns) began to give tongue, and those standing by the entrances watching the waving searchlight were firmly ordered in. Sometimes in the intervals of firing the sinister 'terrumm terrumm' of the German Taube bombers seemed to come down from right overhead. Then this would be drowned by a new tornado of crashes and screams as our friends out on the hill, the 'Chuck-'em-and-Chance-its', caught another glimpse of the raiders.

A tremendous crash that shook the earth … then another … and another.

'They've got the town', someone volunteered. A voice from the entrance declared that they had fallen by the canal.

The owner of the voice was curtly ordered in, and silence reigned again. Every ear was strained to hear the well-known 'terrumm'.

Soon a new noise forced itself on the attention – 'Rat-tat-tat-tat-tat'. Was that an air duel? Or had the Bosche swooped down to fire on the houses? Not a soul would be abroad in all the cowering, shrinking town. At that moment the telephone rang.

'Ambulances wanted at the Station.'

'How many?'

'Six for a start.'

Twelve names were called out, and quivering with excitement twelve drivers hurriedly gathered up gas masks and tin hats, and ran out into the silvery moonlight into the park across the road.

Two minutes, and we were tearing at full speed up the Rue d'Arras round the corners on two wheels. To the left, to the right and then all out down the straight. Not so much as a cat to be seen in all the wounded and stricken town and at the Station – Silence! Presently a soldier came out. There had been a bomb, but the eleven men who had been hit were all dead. They could wait till the morning.

Presently another figure ran up. 'Come to the Veterinary Hospital, a bomb has fallen through the roof.'

There had been a lull for half an hour or more, but now the inferno broke loose again. The panic in the Salle d'Attente in the Station crammed with terrified refugees was the most awful sight in that awful night.

Though the Station did not receive a direct hit the glass roof had fallen like leaves all onto the heads of the cowering throng.

But there was no time to attend to cuts and we hurried into the Veterinary yard.

One car was directed to a big carriage door where a distracted officer was shouting orders.

Presently as the ambulances stood waiting for the wounded to be brought out and lifted hastily onto the back there was a great crash. A spreading glow rose from the building in the next block.

A boy with a broken arm who had just been helped up onto the front seat gave a scream, and leapt down to the ground and tore back to the shelter of the arch where we heard his hysterical voice refusing to come out again. Soon four stretchers were brought out and lifted hastily into the car, but we found that in the hurry the cross bars had not been locked into place and the stretchers had to be taken out again and fixed before they could slide into the racks. Then the cars pulled slowly out of the yard into the street. I climbed into the back, but except for talking to the men and trying to calm them there was nothing I could do, for out of the moonlight it was too dark to see anything.

I put my arm under one man's head for a pillow and felt his hair soaked with blood, but whether it was bleeding badly it was impossible to say. He lay groaning. Presently he started to mutter, 'Oh Christ! I don't want to die. I don't want to die.'

And then – 'It's no use Sister, both my legs are broken.'

The others lay still and silent. There was nothing to be done, and the car moved along slowly. At the door of the hospital it stopped.

'Sister', came a weak voice from the lower shelf, 'the fellow above and me have always been chums. Can we be put into the same ward do you suppose?' I could only promise to ask. Meanwhile the orderlies had been summoned and one stretcher was being lifted out. I made my request for the two chums that if possible they should not be separated.

The orderly grunted with annoyance. ''Taint nothing to do with me.'

'Well, you can take them in together so that they stand a chance.'

CRASH. Nearer than ever this time.

The building rocked. A man screamed. The terrified orderlies dropped their burdens as one man, and leaving the dead and dying to their fate they dashed into the building and slammed the doors behind them.

Long after the last bricks had clattered down from the new ruin, and the stifling smell of plaster and dust had sunk on the air, the bell clanged unheeded at the great door, till among muttered curses the orderlies came out and began feverishly to drag the stretchers from the cars.

Next to the water-tower.

But only corpses were left of the care-taker and his family.

As we crossed the Grande Place an officer jumped up on the leading car saying there were many casualties at the ammunition dump 2 miles out of the town which had been fired.

Calling at the camp for reinforcements the drivers were replaced by new ones.

At one point they were stopped by a sentry who told them to put on their gas masks. It seemed that gas-shells had been touched off.

After some delay they drew near to the scene of the fire. A great blaze filled the sky where two captive-balloons had caught fire, and as they drew nearer the sound of exploding shells could be distinguished.

They could go no further and must wait there to load up. As one car turned, the driver felt it had run over something in the road. She got down and found the body of a man lying under the car. A dreadful sickness seized her, and she beckoned wildly to a man standing by to help her lift it.

'Don't you take on Miss', he answered. 'It was a shell as caught him in the face.' She turned away as the body of a Chinese labourer was dumped unceremoniously into the ditch.

It was 4am when the last raiders turned for home and by nine the next morning the cars were busy again with the wounded and dead. Bodies had to be taken to mortuaries, civilians to be moved to French hospitals, while the hot sun streamed down on the dusty bloodstained victims, many of them in their night attire with blankets pinned round their shoulders. An orphan baby was passed from arm to arm. No one knew his name. His only covering was a little singlet, stained but not with his own blood. He cried dismally while a vacant-eyed woman held him unnoticingly.

I was sent to take two corpses from a military hospital to a civilian mortuary. I picked them up, and with a young orderly I drove to an Old People's Home in the town. I was directed through a 'portecochere' into a courtyard where a number of old men sat sunning themselves on benches under a vine trellised against a white-washed wall.

A double door led into a tiled hall. On the right another large door gave into what had been turned into a temporary mortuary.

The orderly searched around for help, but there was nothing for it. I must help carry the stretchers. The room was filled with shrouded figures on tressles. There had not been enough grave-diggers to bury the dead for some time, and that, added to the warm weather …

Taking a deep breath we walked in, but it was impossible to hold one's breath long enough to set one stretcher down and get back into the hall.

It took far more courage than being abroad in a bombing raid!

We set them down on the floor and hastened out …

Miss Frances Ivens

Scottish Women's Hospital, Advanced Clearing Station, Villers-Cotterets, France

Frances Ivens qualified as a doctor in 1900. When war broke out she was forty-four years of age and a highly respected consultant in gynaecology at the Liverpool Stanley Hospital. She volunteered for Dr Elsie Inglis's Scottish Women's Hospital and at the end of 1914 was appointed chief medical officer at their first hospital (established in France in the thirteenth-century abbey of Royaumont).

By the spring of 1917 the French medical authorities had gained complete trust and respect for the organisation of the hospital and the surgical and nursing work carried out by the women at Royaumont. Miss Ivens was asked to set up an advance clearing station close to the front line where preparations were being made for an autumn offensive. The site finally chosen, some forty miles north of Royaumont, was a deserted, desolate and muddy evacuation centre in a triangle, formed by the railway to Soissons fourteen miles to the south, the road to Compiègne and the edge of the forest of Villers Cotterets. Dr Leila Henry later wrote that 'there had been a previous camp at this site of nine wooden huts, with oiled paper windows and composition roofs. This was cleaned up and made ready for the expected advance by July. The military authorities allocated to us a number of male stretcher-bearers, men who were medically unfit to return to military action.' The wards in the huts were named after the Allies; the two largest, 'Britain' and 'America', had forty-two beds each. The operating theatre and X-ray installations were in other huts. The staff lived in separate cubicles in huts just large enough to hold a bed and a shelf for a jug and basin. After a quiet period the clearing station received casualties when the French retook the Chemin des Dames in October 1917. The sudden rush brought wounded men, French, Zouaves and Chasseurs, who were operated on and then evacuated. The winter of 1917–1918 was bitterly cold and the camp was under snow for three months. Huge icicles hung from the roofs of the huts and a member of staff wrote: 'Our breath froze to the sheets, our hair to the pillows, our rubber boots to the floor and hot water spilled on the floor would in five minutes be frozen solid.'

In March 1918 there was another big rush of patients when the Germans advanced on the British front. This time the men were severely wounded Canadians, from the Fort Garry Horse, the majority needing immediate operations. On Good Friday morning the staff were still hard at work tending train-loads of casualties. British troops were in the forest and on all the roads round the hospital. As the spring weeks progressed, and the Germans continued their advance, wild flowers grew thick in the woods round Villers-Cotterets and fresh vegetables, planted the previous July, were being enjoyed by the staff and patients. 'Between each hut were growing potatoes, lettuces, peas, cabbages, etc., and in front of the laboratory, office, and kitchen huts there were tiny flower gardens, tended by the staffs of these huts with the greatest care …'

The clearing station was now under army orders and known as 'Hôpital Auxiliaire d'Armée No. 30 (HAA 30)'. On 27 May the Germans made a big advance. Soissons was captured and the enemy troops continued on to the Marne. They then turned towards Paris and marched up to the forest of Villers-Cotterets. German aeroplanes flew over the hospital on their way to bomb Villers-Cotterets, Senlis, Crèpy, Chantilly and Paris. Only the worst cases were received in the hospital as there was no electric light in the camp and the operations were performed by candlelight. Severely wounded men streamed in, the majority had not even received a field dressing. Always retreating in front of an enemy far superior in numbers, they had gone for days without food.

Dr Henry remembered:

> *On the railway at one side of us a train filled with ammunition passed us at 10.30pm. The Germans knew that train, the Gothas were there, bombed it and cut us off from all hope of rail evacuation of our wounded and personnel. There were British troops passing our hospital; a British padré with a small company looked in on us, amazed to find us there. Their tired little fox terrier mascot crept under a bed and was left behind with us. The refugees and tired soldiers streamed past, the traffic of a sad retreat. The Germans were again in the forest …*

On the morning of 27 May, Miss Ivens received orders for the evacuation of the hospital at Villers-Cotterets. She later sent a report to her committee.

At 5pm, 27 May, some badly bombed cases arrived, and at 4.30am on Tuesday morning, 28 May, the stream of wounded began to come in by car. Refugees poured in by every kind of vehicle and on foot, and during the night all the medical staff of a hospital nearer which had been forced to evacuate. We worked practically continuously, and yet the receiving ward was always full. During the few days, more than 3,000 wounded passed through the centre, and we had 127 of the worst, as the big hospital was not yet equipped for work. At midday the Médecin-Principal came to me and said he had very bad news, and that we must be preparing to evacuate. We were dreadfully disappointed but as it was perfectly clear that the wounded could not be kept there, I simply said we should do as we were told, but wished to remain until the last possible moment that we could render service. He said it was inevitable and that we must pack up, and be ready to go and form a hospital on the other side of Paris from Royaumont. I gave orders accordingly, but in the evening he came to me and said that as no other hospital was in a position to work, and as no confirmation of his order had been received, would we stay, as a great many cases were expected during the night. Of course I said we should all be delighted, and the theatre unpacked and the X-rays were put together again in about an hour's time, and work was resumed and went on during the night until the middle of the next morning [Wednesday 29 May]. It was an appalling night. We had to work almost in total darkness for from early in the evening, air fights had been going on and we were a target. Tremendous explosions came from a train of ammunition which had been hit by a bomb, and the whole sky was illuminated. The patients were thick both on the beds and the stretchers in the receiving ward, 'France', and we kept on tackling the worst cases. No one showed the slightest trace of nervousness in spite of the horror of the night. I lay down for half an hour but was soon called up by the arrival of more and we began again on Thursday morning [30 May]. I was in the middle of operating when the Médecin-Principal walked into the theatre and said we must be getting ready to go and must not attempt to do any more operations. A train was expected to evacuate the patients, but did not arrive. When it did only half ours could be put on. The telephone was cut the day before. However, during the morning I had sent down to Royaumont for every available car to come up, sending down at the same time a batch of the younger orderlies, and all the important archives. At lunchtime I told the staff to pack up their valuables to take with them, and the rest of their possessions in their trunks, and to dress to be ready to start at any minute. We then devoted ourselves to getting the patients dressed so that they could be sent off as soon as the opportunity occurred. A train came in, and I was allotted 70 places for the 120, which left me with 50 to dispose of. I accordingly sent off all our three cars with wounded to a little town about 15 miles behind, with instructions to return for more as soon as possible. Then three cars from the American section were placed at my disposal, and I filled them up with wounded. At last our cars from Royaumont began to arrive, very late, owing to the condition of the roads, and we were thankful to pack up the rest of the wounded in them. They were to be taken to S [Senlis] – each car took a Sister. A little before, I had started off a considerable number of the orderlies and doctors to walk as it was quite clear that it would be night before the cars could get back for them, and they would be picked up as opportunity offered. During the afternoon the shells began to whistle overhead, and the American car drivers told me that it was quite time for us to go as the Boche were only 5km away and were coming on very fast. At last all the staff and wounded were off.

We kept the little lorry, and Moore [Miss Evelyn Mercy Moore, a chauffeur] loaded it with petrol, which at that moment was our greatest need, and we started for C [Crèpy]. On the way I met several of our returning cars and sent two or three of them on with orders to help with the evacuation of the big hospital, and if not, to bring any valuables they could. I decided to call at C [Creil] where we had sent some wounded, to see if they had left in a train, or to see what arrangements had been made. It was a station more bombed than any other behind the lines, and a great hole in the station yard greeted us. We looked about and found several of them [the staff] still there, including Mrs Berry and, I think, Tollit [Miss Florence Tollit, an orderly]. We continued our journey to Senlis. The country was illuminated. It was just like gigantic fireworks, for air raids were going on in every direction. As we got into Senlis there was a block – all lights were out. However as we had to pull up, an army doctor came out. We then made for the hotel where I expected to find most of the nurses. Twenty-one were there, and I was very cross on finding them in their beds instead of in the cellars, as the raid was on. We decided to make for R [Royaumont] by a quieter road as we could see the bombs dropping over the one we generally took. It was not a happy selection from that point of view, for we met a continuous stream of Foch's reinforcements and understood that was what the bombs were trying for. It was a most reassuring and impressive sight – silent dark shapes moving slowly along towards us in the night with quantities of guns and cavalry. Not a sound and hardly a light (I saw, I think, 2 cigarettes). After a detour we reached R at 1am and a very short time after, Murray [Miss Elizabeth Margaret Murray, a chauffeur] arrived with four patients from Villers-Cotterets.

The following morning, 31 May, I returned to Senlis to see for myself the Médecin-Principal. I arrived during a conference of all the medical authorities involved. S was to function as a clearing station. We were to fetch and receive our patients from there and HAA 30 was to work at Royaumont. It was all fixed in about 5 minutes. We got a load of wounded and took them back with us. Two extra theatres were arranged. Matron Lindsay took charge of one, and our Theatre Sister (Sister Everingham) was to do the night work.

Miss Katherine Hodges

Section Sanitair Y3 Ambulance Unit, France

Katherine Hodges served as a driver in Romania and Russia with Dr Elsie Inglis's Scottish Women's Hospital between August 1916 and May 1917.

On 27 December 1917 she left Southampton for France with three other female ambulance drivers, driving two Wolseleys and a Ford in the Hackett-Lowther Unit attached to the French army. The unit was divided into canteens for the troops under Miss Hackett, and the ambulance section, destined for front line work, known as the Section Sanitair Y3 and commanded by Miss Toupil Lowther. The members of the Unit ranked as poilus and were paid two sous a day.

The ambulance section initially had seventeen cars, given by private owners and funded from subscriptions, and seventeen drivers. Later they were given six Fords by the Denis Bailey miners. The unit also comprised a maréchal de logee, a brigadier, a fourrier, two mechanics, a cook and a cook's orderly, and Lieutenant Chatenay, who acted as liaison officer between the unit and the French headquarters.

After spending the night in overcrowded Le Havre and going through all the formalities with their papers, the girls started off on a bitterly cold morning through snow and ice. The small Wolseley developed carburetter trouble and they had to tow it on icebound roads. They spent three weeks in Paris and were then sent to Creil for the French authorities to see if they were ready to serve at the front line. Creil was an important railway junction where patients arrived in ambulance trains and were distributed to various hospitals, including Royaumont.

28 January, Creil
We arrived from Paris on the evening of the 25th, started work the next day. I was on duty from 11.30 to 2.30, but hadn't much to do. Work is arranged like this. Three cars have always to be at the station ready, sometimes you're busy and sometimes nothing. We each take three hours duty except when there's a rush on. That night the order came that all cars were to be at the station at 10pm, so at 10pm we all turned up, and we drove backwards and forwards to a hospital 18 miles away until 7.30am. I got into the garage at quarter to eight, oiled the car and then had breakfast and got into bed at 9am. At 9.45am (I was just asleep) a bang at my door. 'Sorry but three hundred wounded are due in soon. All cars wanted at once.' So I staggered up like all the poor

things who'd been working all night too, got to the station and then we drove till about 6pm and I went to bed at once and slept like a log. I was called out on a job then and have been on the go pretty nearly ever since. Had to take some patients to such a beautiful old château lying in the heart of woods and in the woods little primroses. When I came back again, empty, I picked a few. I loved them.

We had an air raid last night, but I don't know if they did any damage.

How sick we got of that station yard, it was so cold and so boring when we were slack, we didn't mind a bit when we were busy. We had a great many air raids at Creil. One night we were all in bed except the two drivers on duty at the station, when a frightfully bad raid took place. We were sent for in a hurry and within fourteen minutes every car was out of the place, not bad when one thinks that all the radiators had to be filled and that we had no self-starters to help us. Most of us were in pyjamas, gumboots and top coats; we didn't stop to dress. I was given two corpses, victims of the raid, to take to the mortuary. It was dark and of course we could use no lights. One of the bodies had the head detached and it was put in as well. I shall not easily forget the horrible sound that head made as it rolled about with the bumping of the car. It gave me a most uncanny feeling.

Two or three days after this raid the victims were given a public funeral and our cars were commandeered to act as hearses. It was a most extraordinary business. First we went to the mortuary and loaded in the coffins, then drove to the church where part of the service was held, then on to the cemetery. A procession of priests led the way, followed by relatives in deep mourning and most of the civilian population of the town, then the ambulances with the coffins. The road to the cemetery was up a steep hill. Half-way up it was the entrance, a right-angle turn and then a narrow drive up through the cemetery as steep as the side of a house. It was terribly difficult crawling behind the slowly moving procession to get the cars up the hill at all. I was with D on her car and going up the steepest part I had to leap out, run behind and push the coffins in, as they were on the verge of sliding out backwards. At last we reached the graveside. A long time elapsed, we thought it was all over and started to drive away when there were agitated shouts and we found to our dismay that we were departing with one coffin still in the car.

We had brought down one of the German planes during this raid and I had to move a German aviator from one hospital to another. He was a tall, finely built man with his head all bandaged, but he was able to walk. His arrogance was immense as he crossed the yard to my ambulance. I had quite a job in keeping some of the French orderlies and people around away from him. They naturally felt very bitter after the destruction and deaths, and his proud swagger didn't tend to conciliate them.

After this bad raid a cordon of yellow saucise balloons was put up round Creil with wires stretched between them, and this helped to keep the enemy planes off.

I was called to a hospital just outside the town to take a civilian victim to the central hospital about 2 miles away. The patient was brought out and put in the ambulance. He was obviously terribly ill, in fact almost in extremis. His poor wife was there, crying quietly and bitterly. She asked me if she could sit inside with him, to which I of course agreed. She had just got in when the Médicin Chef came up and ordered her out, saying that under no circumstances could unwounded civilians ride in the ambulance.

She begged and entreated him, so did I, but to no avail, and to my fury and deep regret she was forced to descend. I started off and she started running behind. I soon lost sight of her and arrived at the other hospital. We unloaded the man, but as we laid the stretcher on the ground, he died. I drove away terribly depressed and, as I crossed the bridge, I saw the pathetic hurrying figure of the poor little wife, sobbing as she ran. I couldn't bear to think of the sad news awaiting her.

I felt so enraged that through ridiculous red tape she had been torn from her dying husband in such an unnecessary and unkind way. It upset me for days afterwards.

We got very tired of all the roads around, for we served hospitals for a radius of about 20–30 miles. In the four months we were working in Creil our seventeen cars carried over 10,000 wounded. One morning the other driver and I moved seventy wounded between us in our three hours of duty.

At last in May we heard with great delight that we were ordered up to the Front and we started off in convoy to Compiègne, where we were to be attached to the 2nd Army Corps of the Third Army commanded by General Humbert.

In Compiègne we were billeted in a villa with a small trench dug-out in the garden at the back.

Things now began to be really exciting, the town had hardly any civilians left in it, they had most of them been evacuated, one or two food shops were still open and a few old cottagers remained. Army Headquarters were in the château.

We had terrific air raids every night regularly from 10pm until 2 or 3am, and a great deal of heavy shelling, as the bridge over the river and the railway station close to it were largely the objective of the enemy, who at this time were only 2 or 3 miles from the town.

Very soon after our arrival all cars were ordered to fetch wounded from a hospital situated in a château near the Front called Offremont. It stood on the top of a very steep hill and it was an amazing place, for leading out of the courtyard was the entrance to vast caves tunnelled in the hill which were being used as hospital wards. It was a brilliant day and as we were waiting in the yard, which was really a huge quarry, suddenly the well known throb of a Gotha was heard. We all had to flatten ourselves against the walls and remain perfectly still until the plane had gone over. This hospital was shortly afterwards given up as the transportation of the wounded to and from it was considered too dangerous.

After a little, things got so hot in Compiègne and the few remaining civilians were ordered out. I was sent to a small cottage to evacuate two old peasants. It was pitiful, I felt simply dreadful. They were old, well over seventy, and heartbroken at leaving their home and possessions. They begged me to allow them to stay, they said they would much rather be killed in their own home than have to leave and go to strange places. Of course I was powerless, I had to make them go, and at last with tears pouring they carefully locked all the windows and doors and sadly got into the car, with bundles containing their most precious treasures. I took them to the station and put them on to the train, but their tragic old tear-stained faces haunted me for a long while.

At the end of June 1918, after a week's leave in England, Katherine Hodges returned to find her unit had moved from Compiègne.

Every day two cars (Fords) were on duty at a Poste de Secours (first field dressing-station) just behind the trenches. The Poste where we were at present working was situated in a brickyard, the actual dressing-station was in large kiln-like places under the main building. It had the usual tall chimney and was about one and a half miles from the German lines.

Our hours of duty were twenty-four hours on and twenty-four hours off, but we didn't always get the twenty-four hours off, certainly not in rush time, and anyhow in the twenty-four hours off you had to get from and to the Poste, clean and overhaul your car, etc., and very often do runs back to base hospitals on the big ambulances which were too heavy to be used for Front Line work. We used to go on duty at twelve midday and be relieved at noon the next day. We all had to wear tin hats and have our gas masks slung over our shoulders.

One day some doctor lit a fire and the smoke went up the chimney. That was enough, instantly every gun was trained on it. Everyone huddled down into the underground 'abri' (dug-out) and there they stayed while shells poured down for hours. Every shell that burst sent a shower of brick dust over them till they could hardly see or breathe. I was told that orders had been sent, but had not arrived, to the effect that the brickyard was too unsafe for a dressing-station and was to be evacuated.

After the brickyard was evacuated the Poste was at a place called Anel in a little cottage at a crossroads. There was a disgusting cellar which served as a dug-out with wire netting stretched along the walls on rough wooden frames, which served as beds when we had time to sleep. The gas curtain hung over the doorway ready to let down in case of gas attacks. The roof of the cellar consisted of corrugated iron and sandbags. There was a garden in which we used to park the cars and sit. We had to pick large branches of trees and put them over the cars as camouflage.

The wounded were carried by hand from trenches to the Poste, where dressings were done and operations, if terribly urgent, and then we took them to a Field Hospital about 10 kilometres back, and from there other ambulances took them to Bases or trains.

The Colonel commanding the 368th Regiment and his staff were at the other end of the village, so most of the shelling was concentrated there. We got a certain amount, but not too bad.

Later on the Colonel and his staff moved up close to us and things got rather more sultry then.

One lovely day he asked us to have a meal with him. We sat out in the ruined garden having a repast which was a definite improvement on our usual rations and he had the Regimental band up to play for us. It was so ironical, there we sat not 2 miles from the German lines with the band playing the waltz from *Coppelia*. Suddenly a violent crash. 'Ne bougez pas', said the Colonel sharply, and we all sat as if we had been struck, rigid as waxworks, with our forks half-way to our mouths, the musicians holding their instruments, and there we remained a frozen group, while a Gotha slowly flew over searching for signs of life. A few more bombs dropped and then the throb of the engine died away. Then 'on with the feast' and on with the *Coppelia* waltz.

One night I had to take the Daimler and fill up with German wounded. They were only slight cases, all sitting. I had eight in the back and one beside me. They were large, strong men. I looked at them and thought, 'Well, if you want to escape I shan't be able to stop you', but I took my largest spanner and kept it beside me in case of accidents. I had to take them about 30 miles, but they were as quiet as mice. I think they were only too delighted to be prisoners and out of it all at last. We carried a good many German wounded about then. One very hot day I took a car load into a hospital yard and found that it was crammed to overflowing, nearly all the yard was covered with wounded waiting to be taken in. People were worked off their feet. One poor man was lying in the blazing sun with a terrible gaping hole in his neck, the bandage had slipped and the hole was full of flies. I managed to clear them out and cover the wound up with a bit of the bandage, but I was severely ticked off for interfering by one of the hospital authorities.

The Allied advance began. We left Anel and moved forward from place to place.

[Letter dated 21 August]
We have been frightfully busy these last days as we have been attacking in our Sector with success. It has been most interesting as each day the Poste has been further forward and we have followed up with it. It is extraordinary going to places the day after the Boche has left them. Terrible devastation everywhere, and the smells! Unburied dead lying in every wood. Horrible! The roads, of course, are unspeakable. Shell holes full of water, large enough to take two or three cars, all over the place. It's pretty harrassing driving over a road of that description that you've never been on before, in the pitch dark. I did 180 miles the other day, never got off the car except for loading in the cases. Most of it at night and a dark night too, lots of gas about. We have to wear our masks often. One thing is you are so occupied and worried with getting the car over the awful roads that you don't notice the shells unless one bursts frightfully near. All the crossroads have been blown up by the Boche on their retreat and it's a chatty job getting over them, I can tell you. We now do twenty-four hours on, twenty-four hours off, forty-eight hours on, twenty-four hours off. Pretty strenuous.

I had the most interesting time the other day. The Poste was at the foot of a hill two and a half miles long, like Harting hill [South Harting, a village near Petersfield, Hampshire], only much steeper and wooded on both sides. I was stationed on the road about a quarter of a mile from the top. The trenches were just over the top and the cases were brought down by hand to me and I took them down to the Poste. I did this for sixteen hours, up and down and up and down. In the darkest time of the night I was sent down to work back, as the hill road was considered impassable at night for a car. It was thrilling as all the batteries were all round me. We put up a heavy barrage for four hours. I had the pleasure of being taken up to a 75 gun by the captain of the battery and watched them for some time, and then he asked me if I would like to fire it, so I did. It's fun to say I fired a 75 in one of the biggest attacks. It was pretty tricky work that day as they were shelling the batteries a lot and also shelling the Poste with gas shells. However, I find I don't care a damn in the day time, but the strain at night makes one's nerve a bit jumpy. One is jolly glad of the arrival of the relief cars when one's duty time finishes.

One man died as I lifted him out of the car the other day and yesterday my cushions, my food basket, my coat were all drenched and saturated with blood, as I'd left them in the well under the stretcher and the poor fellow had a haemorrhage.

You sleep any old where, the other night in a dug-out with about fifty soldiers and half-way through the door opened and a voice yelled: 'Look out. Gas', so we all sat and sweltered in our gas masks for about four hours – perfectly awful.

On one of my ascents [up the precipitous hill described in the letter] as I turned one of the winding corners, crawling up on first gear, I thought what a funny smell of burning metal. Then it flashed on me: gas. I slapped my mask on as quickly as possible, but even that brief sniff left me with a streaming nose, running eyes and a burning sore throat for about three days afterwards.

We carried hundreds of gassed cases at this time, poor things, it was awful to see their suffering. All foliage was shrivelled brown and black where gas had been.

[Letter dated 28 August]
This letter is being brought home by one of the girls. It may interest you to know where we've been working. We started at Clairoix, advanced from there to Longuiel Anel, then to Chevancourt, Melicoq, Ribecourt, Pimprez and I don't know where we are today. At Pimprez the night before last we were gas shelled all night and had to wear our gas masks for five hours. Perfectly awful, you feel you can't breathe in the beastly things. I was standing talking in the evening to a soldier in front of my car and the nightly hymn of hate was going on at the other end of the village when suddenly, Whiz, Crash, and a 210 burst about 600 yards away in an orchard. There was a perfect shower of fragment of shell and a bit the size of a nut hit my shoulder, but only bruised it. I retired to the dug-out quickly, accompanied by my soldier friend. They plunked them over for about two hours. Fortunately there were no wounded to be taken at the moment so one could stay in the dug-out. They are very good about not sending you out under bombardment unless it is very pressing.

I think we're going to have a little rest now, only back work, as our Division is relieved today and goes behind the lines for a rest.

We have changed living quarters fairly frequently. From Clairoix we went to a tiny village called Appilly. We went in the day after the Germans left, most of the wells were poisoned and everything was mined, but the engineers soon put things fairly straight.

I was for a short time now in charge of the Unit and found it a terrific responsibility. In the middle of one night an urgent call came for all cars. There had been a touch of frost so some of the cars were a job to start. There was a terrific air raid going on, our village being the objective, and I can so vividly recall the unpleasant sensation of swinging the cars in the bright moonlight with bombs crashing and shrapnel hurtling everywhere. It was marvellous that no one was hurt.

From Appilly we moved to another village called Villeselve. In all these places we were billeted in bits of ruined cottages which we made as habitable as we could, finding a chair here amongst the debris, and a cooking pot there, all treasures to be salved with joy.

We heard here that four more of us, including myself, were awarded the Croix de Guerre with Star.

[Letter dated 25 September]
Yesterday we were decorated by General de Fonklare, a most nerve-racking performance. We four stood in the middle of a large space (like flies on it!) with crowds of people watching, and had to stand rigidly to attention and not blink an eyelid while the General harangued the multitude about the valour of our deeds (I don't think!). Then he pinned the medals on our chests, thanked us for our services to France, shook us warmly by the hand, and left. I never wanted to giggle so much in my life. It's all nonsense our having them, we've none of us done anything particular to deserve them. Men are doing exactly the same work all the time and it's taken as a matter of course, but because we're women they think they have to decorate us. I think it's awfully nice of them, but I blush every time I see a man ambulance driver who's done a thousand times more than I have and has got nothing.

We wanted to giggle because we really felt terribly self-conscious and nervous. In addition to that I was standing next to Lieutenant Chatenay who was extremely anxious that we should acquit ourselves properly and had given us hours of instruction about the correct behaviour on such an occasion. In the middle of the ceremony a wasp buzzed at my face, I was dying to brush it away, but Lieutenant Chatenay hissed at me so fiercely under his breath through clenched teeth 'Ne bougez pas!', that I didn't dare move. Thank heavens, the wasp turned its attentions elsewhere.

We were working for a Field Hospital at Villeselve. One day when I was there waiting for cases an old French orderly who had become quite a friend of mine, came up to me for his daily chat. He was a little wizened elderly man of about seventy with a thin straggly grey beard. He was, I think, a small peasant farmer in peace time. This particular morning he said to me, 'Mademoiselle, what are you going to do after the war?' 'I really don't know', I replied. 'Well', said he, 'I think you ought to marry.' 'Do you?' I answered, 'Oh, I don't know about that'. 'Yes', he said firmly, 'You ought to marry.' Then he came a step closer and in an ingratiating manner said, 'Now why not marry me?' I was paralised with surprised amusement. I controlled my facial muscles with difficulty and said, 'Really, it's very kind of you, thank you very much, but I'm not very keen on getting married', to which he replied, 'No? Well, to tell you the truth, neither am I. I don't want a woman fussing about the place, but what I do want is two strong boys!' I was so tickled at this amazing proposal that like a fool I told the others, and was I sorry? Yes, I was. Because for weeks afterwards whenever a car passed me a voice yelled: 'How are your two strong boys!'

From Villeselve we moved to Chauny, where our quarters were really more ruined than ever.

[Letter dated 24 October]
It's a weird life, the place we are now in is absolutely gutted. There are about thirty houses with roofs left standing out of a town the size of Petersfield.

This is what happens. You get orders to move to a place, you arrive there and search for quarters, you look at houses that at home you would consider complete ruins, and say 'that's splendid, I'll have that one.' We (I and my room-mate) have got two rooms. The roof is all right in one, but the other has a large hole in it and rain pours through, so appropriately we use it as a bathroom! The other has no windows and had no doors, but today we went on a looting expedition and found, in amongst the ruins, two quite passable doors which we demounted and brought triumphantly home. We fixed them up and feel luxurious. We've put tent cloths over the windows and have to choose between warmth or darkness. We also scoured the country for wood, demolished some German dug-outs and brought the wood thereof back, also a hatchet, very rusty, but still a hatchet, and a large pan for heating water, and a chair and a leaking lamp. So now we've a big wood fire burning and the doors shut and the cloths over the window frames and the leaking lamp lit, and we feel we're in the Ritz at least.

It's rather amusing, very much like Desert Island life, I should think. The excitement at each person's fresh bit of loot is intense. One girl looted a silver teapot the other day. Personally, I think I draw the line at silver, but it's very hard to know where thieving begins and looting ends!

Dinner gong has just gone, in other words the cook, three houses off in the one room standing in the cottage, has beaten a saucepan, so we all rush off to feed. I'll continue this after dinner.

Later. Having fed and put my room-mate to bed with a hot drink, she having a bad cold, I will carry on with this. I really think one's days off duty are almost harder than those on duty. By the time one has cleaned and oiled one's car, etc., got wood for the fire, cleaned the rooms, fetched water from the well (in which, by the way, one can see a Boche helmet, I hope the rest of him isn't there too …), cleaned one's shoes, got one's tea and lit the fire every time it's gone out, you feel glad to come to the end of a perfect day.

We got firewood yesterday in a wood quite recently evacuated by the Boches, and we were so frightened as there were wires everywhere and we knew that they all led to mines, and if we fell over any of them we should probably go to Kingdom Come, so we picked up sticks as if they were red hot, and shrieked 'ware wire' every two minutes, a most nerve-racking afternoon.

I must go to bed now as I'm on duty very early tomorrow. The guns have been going like hell today, so I daresay there'll be a lot of work tomorrow, crowds of wounded, poor things.

The country, where it is not quite destroyed, is so beautiful, very hilly and wooded, and the colour now that the leaves are turning is lovely. I had to tramp all over about six large woods the other day as I was sent to fetch two sick men of the fourth regiment of Engineers, and the directions given to me were that they 'were in a wood off a certain road'. Of course there were dozens of woods, so I had to search each one I came to, and at last, at the sixth, ran them to ground. Rather interesting to see them all in their dug-outs in the woods. From the road you wouldn't dream anyone was there at all, but when you penetrated about 300 yards in, it was just like a beehive, simply swarming with men …

Miss Lesley Smith

No. 50 General Hospital, Rouen, France

After her distressing night duties in the 'Heads' Ward at No. 129 General Hospital near Camiers during the summer of 1916, Lesley Smith continued nursing in various other wards until she went down with mumps in March 1917. After sick leave she went to a hospital at Le Tréport where she remained until she was sent to No. 50 General Hospital at Rouen in the spring of 1918.

When the Armistice was declared the camp buglers sounded the 'Cease fire' and we all stopped work for a few minutes and, with a sort of comic bewilderment, watched the orderlies straggle in procession through the hospital, trying to play *Rule Britannia* on the mess pot lids. They converged upon an equally rag-tag and bobtail file of German prisoners, who were working on the sandbags as a labour gang, and for a moment the rival processions became hopelessly intermixed.

The 'Cease fire' had sounded while I was dressing a man who was covered with painful boils. When the procession had passed and I came back from the door, he looked at me dully and said, 'It's over, then?' I nodded, and he turned on his pillow and I finished the dressing in silence.

The celebrations fizzled out, damped by the wave of depression that overtook us all when we realised that the war was over and our friends were dead.

Sister Brown was off at five o'clock, and she went round to the canteen for some tinned fruit and biscuits and came back to the ward to help Gratton and me to mix the fruit salad in three of the large water buckets. We tried to have a cheerful supper party, but the tension had snapped too suddenly and none of us had regained our balance. Now that we were no longer driven by an overwhelming compulsion to keep step with our friends on a doomed journey, there did not seem to be any very adequate reason for doing any of the things we had unquestioningly accepted as duties till now. The process of our rebirth as individuals had painfully begun, and we were glad, when the night people turned up and we could go back to our rooms and try to make out where we were.

After a day or two of restlessness we found that we were exactly where we had been. Wounded men still poured in and sick men filled the medical side. As the weather got worse the medicals encroached on the surgicals; and then the pneumonia epidemic began and soon filled the whole hospital with dying men …

1918
Russia and Serbia

Miss Margaret H. Barber

Soviet Hospital, Astrakan, Russia

At the end of the nineteenth century, many thousands of Armenians were massacred by the Turkish authorities. In 1914, Turkey, allied to Germany, continued this 'ethnic cleansing' and by September 1915 a million Armenians had been slaughtered. 'The great flight of Armenians, driven from their homeland amid scenes of brutality and terror' continued throughout the early months of 1916.

Margaret Barber, who had served as a VAD in Serbia, went to Russia as a Red Cross nurse with the Armenian Relief Expedition in April 1916 to help these stricken refugees. She worked as a nurse in a hospital in the Van province for three months until her unit was evacuated as the Turkish enemy came closer. She served for a few weeks in the Anglo-Russian Hospital in Petrograd and in October 1916 joined the Friends' War Victims' Committee at a hospital in Samara. She stayed there for eighteen months under the old regime, during the Revolution, and under Bolshevik rule. On 5 August 1918, under the auspices of the Armenian Red Cross, she travelled by train from Moscow to Astrakan, on the north Caspian coast, where many Armenian refugees had gathered after retreating over the Caucasus mountains. Her stores were packed in two railway vans and she was accompanied by an Armenian and three Red Guards.

The streets were gay with fruit, which was being sold at every street corner; grapes, apples, pears, and melons making a wealth of colour. But, better far to the traveller from Moscow, was the sight of beautiful big loaves of white bread for sale. The population was a mixture of three nationalities, Russian, Tartar and Armenian. Mosques abounded, but otherwise the buildings were of Russian pattern, and the town had a fairly up-to-date appearance in the way of tramways, cabs and motor cars. We came to a large, imposing red brick building where we alighted and went up some dirty stairs into a passage. The sight of this I shall never forget, for this passage formed a street, and portions of sheets and strips of gay oriental material formed partitions for eight families of Armenian refugees.

We next entered a large hall, every foot of which was occupied by families of Armenians, without any attempt at privacy, simply sitting on the floor grouped round their few personal effects. Only with great difficulty could one pick one's way among the squatters without treading on a baby or some household god. We then reached a room which boasted seven beds, on five of which were seated five nurses, who sprang up on my arrival, and greeted me, surrounding me, and listening (with amusement at my English accent) to the account of my journey. All assured me there was plenty of work, but said that there was no hospital, and that we had to nurse the people just as they were, on the floor. This sounded quite impossible, but I was all eagerness to begin work; so one of the Sisters said she would be very glad to share her work with me, and promised to take me round her cases in the morning.

We then went into the doctor's bedroom, which did duty for the dining room, and sat down to a dinner of cabbage soup and stew of meat and vegetables, and I was given half a pound of bread and told it must last me the whole day. This seemed to me a huge quantity, as it was four times what I received in Moscow, but I had no difficulty in finishing it; in fact, when I found that small quantities of bread could be purchased from the refugees at two roubles a pound, I very often supplemented it in the morning, as our ration was often not issued until eleven o'clock.

After dinner I helped a nurse to give soup to three or four families of refugees who otherwise lived on melons, as they had no pot or saucepan of any kind in which to do their cooking. The rest prepared their food at the back of the house in all weathers, improvising stoves with bricks and pieces of stick. This yard was an extraordinary sight when the cooking was in progress; the Armenian women in their picturesque attire wearing silk scarves on their heads, draped to cover both forehead and chin, and those from the Caucasus wearing Turkish trousers which showed beneath long coats which were held at the waist by a broad sash. Many of these coats and also the headgear were adorned with silver coins or pendant buttons of wrought silver. They squatted in groups at their work of cleaning fish, baking their curious thin flat bread on concave pieces of iron, or doing the family washing in shallow brass dishes or even washing their children.

As I had feared, it was very difficult to deal with the sick. One was supposed to take the temperature of any sick persons and then make a round with the doctor, pointing them out to him.

He then prescribed medicine or treatment, and one had to pick one's way about administering it. He made another round in the evening, but very often it was quite impossible to carry out all his instructions before they had all turned in for the night. The children nearly all had dysentery, as they practically lived on raw fruit, and there was also much relapsing fever which was extremely infectious, and spread by dirt, which abounded, owing to lack of clothes, and opportunity for obtaining either hot water or a place to wash in.

I was very thankful when we were able to arrange the top floor as a hospital of thirty beds, with wards for men, women and children, and a bath for all on admission. A room at the end of the corridor became the dining-room, with part curtained off for the Sisters' bedroom, while the doctor had a room to himself. The kitchen also was moved upstairs, and the housekeeper now declared that it was much too small to cook extra soup in for the four families whom we had hitherto supplied. I went to the doctor in dismay, but he referred me to the Refugees' Committee, saying that they were responsible, and that his was merely a medical unit. This Committee was reputed to have plenty of funds, and also had, I knew, all the materials I had brought for the refugees. I therefore visited them daily with various needy cases, demanding some form of relief for them. They generally did something for everyone, sometimes giving them a ticket entitling them to fetch a free dinner for their family from some other refugee hostel in the town; but they arranged no organised help and one had to be continually begging on behalf of some case or other to get any help for them at all.

The Russian organisations were arranged more satisfactorily, and I had occasion to visit them with one or two destitute cases of Russian refugees from the Kuban district who had fled on the approach of the White Army.

The Armenian refugees were a greater difficulty. Some were healthy and able to work, and therefore not entitled to assistance if they remained idle, and apart from the difficulty of the language, which restricted possible ways of employment, one had the fact to contend with that the Armenian is essentially a buyer and seller, or speculator, and not a lover of work of any kind. The Turkish Armenian women too were so ignorant and helpless, and are kept, in Turkish fashion, so much in the background in their own homes, that they were often too timid to go out and purchase their own daily food.

The Bolshevik Authorities agreed to give all refugees, as such, second category coupons (which are only intended for workers), whether they worked or not, and all the old people and children received the first category coupons as well as milk tickets, just as the Russian children did. The men soon began to work when they saw the privileges given to workers, and the Armenian boys, true to type, made money by buying fish with their coupons and selling them dearly in the streets. They also walked out to the country or went down to the barges on the Volga and bought nuts or fruit and sold them at the street corners at great profit to workers who had not time or inclination to fetch them themselves. They also went to the town stores, which opened early in the morning and sold fruit and vegetables at low-cost price in small quantities. Here they would buy all they were allowed, and sell them later in the streets to well-paid workers who did not care for early rising or standing in a queue. Grapes they bought at nine roubles the pound and sold at twenty during the day. Of course this petty speculation was against the law, and the Red Guards would sometimes reduce the exorbitant price demanded, and stand by until the goods were sold. But this did not happen every day to wary Armenian boys!

In November, when our hospital had been open for nearly three months, we were suddenly informed that the authorities needed our building, giving us nine days in which to move out. This came as a great shock to us and to the refugees below. As many as possible of the wealthier refugees were induced to hire rooms in which to live, thus leaving more room for the poor ones in the free hostels provided. But the hospital was a difficulty. Our doctor had to obtain official documents and walk into all likely private houses until he found a suitable one to 'commandeer'. But it meant that we were without a hospital for nearly three weeks.

Just at this unfortunate time a thousand fresh refugees arrived from Baku and Petrofsk, in a most deplorable condition of ill-health and starvation. The English had left Baku, and the Turks had returned. At the time of their arrival I had just been visiting our refugees, who had been moved into a large barracks outside the town and were complaining bitterly of the cold. As I left them on that bitterly cold November evening I met the stream of new refugees wending their way to the barracks I had left. There were a few who had hired conveyances for themselves and their possessions, but others were carrying rolls of bedding on their heads, or even in some cases, had unwrapped them, and wore them over their shoulders. Tired women, carrying one child, dragging another, and followed by others carrying various possessions, passed me in a dreary procession. At the sight of the building they uttered ejaculations of thankfulness and eager anticipation of comfort which I, alas, knew they would not find. Indeed, I dreaded to think what their sufferings would be in this town already so closely rationed, so overpopulated and so short of fuel and clothes.

I described what I had seen to our party, and the head doctor decided to go with me next day and distribute clothing and visit any sickness, if necessary. We found that they had been two weeks on board an open barge, that many had had no provision of food during that time, and that over a hundred had died of hunger, illness and exposure on the way.

We distributed the clothing as well as we could but, unfortunately, I had purchased very little warm material in Petrograd, as we then thought our work would be further south, where the cold would not be at all intense. We hoped, however, that by supplying each refugee with a piece of soap and a change of under-linen we were giving them an opportunity for personal cleanliness, but found that, owing to the cold, they merely put on their clean shirts over their dirty ones, and made no attempt at washing. This was the more alarming as we discovered that more than 50 per cent of them were down with typhus. Some had died on arrival and had not yet been removed; some were dying; some delirious, and none had anything to eat. At the sight of doctor and nurse they clamoured for food, for medicine and for the sick to be taken to hospital. We did our best to get the Russian hospital to take them in, to make arrangements for feeding them, for tending the sick, and for burying the dead. The doctor and I returned at four o'clock to our dinner exhausted and overwhelmed with the conditions we had seen.

The doctor now redoubled his energy in endeavouring to secure and open our new hospital with all possible speed, and deputed a lady doctor to visit next day with me, we taking with us a parcel of medicine, chiefly in powder form ready made up into doses, and about ten quarts of milk, which we still received for our hospital although it was closed. The task seemed hopeless. Out of 550 refugees 50 could be said to be in good health. Their diet consisted of half a pound of black bread and raw vegetables, which they had not the means of cooking. All begged for milk, and it was almost impossible to know which cases needed it most when all needed it so much. I finally gave it out in half glasses to those in high fever, and to the motherless infants, to the bitter disappointment of the rest.

The barracks were a good distance away and the weather was very wet and cold. The sick were in the most awful condition of filth and literally alive with lice, so it was almost impossible to prevent these getting into our clothes. From one or other of these causes, or perhaps all combined, after visiting the barracks with milk and medicine six days in succession, I fell ill with relapsing fever, and, after a week, was myself conveyed to our newly-opened hospital. As soon as I was well I took charge of the women's ward. Nearly all the first cases died almost as soon as we could get them into hospital. One poor woman, whose husband had died in the barracks, came in ill, bringing her sick infant and a boy of about six who was suffering from dysentery. On her arrival it was found that the baby had died in her arms on the way to hospital. Her little boy died a week later, which fact we kept from her as long as we could. Ultimately she died also, leaving a young girl of sixteen alone to mourn the loss of her home and father, mother, sister and brother.

Many of the sick died in hospital, but others recovered. Orphans were received into the orphanage, regular food was supplied to the barracks, and a kitchen arranged to cook it in. Those with money enough made every effort to find other lodgings away from this hotbed of disease; others were able to find employment, and thus the winter passed, but not without carrying off a heavy toll of victims from the unfortunate Armenian people …

Dr Isabel Emslie

Scottish Women's Hospital, Ostrovo, Serbia

Scottish Women's Hospital, Vranja, Serbia

At the outbreak of war Dr Emslie, who had qualified as a doctor at the age of twenty-one, offered her services at the War Office in Edinburgh and was told by a RAMC officer that there was 'no use for women doctors in a war'. There was, however a great need by the French army and in August 1915 she went with a Scottish Women's Hospital unit, as medical officer and pathologist, to the first tent hospital on the French front outside Troyes.

Two months later she became a member of the Corps Expeditionnaire d'Orient which was sent by France to Salonika to aid the stricken Serbian army and civilians. She sailed with the Scottish Women's Hospital Girton and Newnham Unit on board the steamer Mossoul. *One of her fellow passangers was Flora Sandes [qv]. Dr Emslie served in a Scottish Women's Hospital in Salonika for three years until the summer of 1918, when, still under the age of thirty, she was appointed to command the SWH at Ostrovo, a mountain town ninety miles west of Salonika. This camp hospital was in arcadian surroundings situated close to a lake and lying in the hollow of the hills which rose on every side.*

After the retreat in November 1915 the remnants of the Serbian army were exiled on the island of Corfu where they waited for almost three years for their chance to reclaim their country. In the middle of September 1918 they mounted a full-scale offensive and although Bulgaria capitulated at the end of the month, the Austrian troops were still fighting and the Serbs were determined to fight until the bitter end. Dr Emslie's unit was ordered to set up a hospital in a vast disused regimental barracks at Vranja, between Skoplje and Nis. This was to be the 'first and foremost hospital in the reoccupied territory'. On 14 October Dr Emslie paid a short visit to Vranja to see the barracks and assess the condition of the road from the hospital at Ostrovo. She took two chauffeurs with her in the little Ford touring car so that the driving could be shared on the journey of over 300km. They were held up on roads riddled with great shell-holes, littered with ammunition and overcrowded with Serbian troops and thousands of sullen Bulgarian prisoners.

After two days they arrived at Vranja.

We entered the great, cobbled courtyard at the back of the barracks, which was crowded with guns and shells and with wounded and sick men lying on the ground. Inside the building, spacious as it was, and although on this sunny day the large French windows were all thrown open, the stench was indescribable. The barrack-rooms were packed with wounded and sick, lying some on the floor, some on straw, and others on bedsteads without mattresses, which were all that the Austrians had left behind. Here and there were bright wool pillows or bed quilts that the villagers had given, otherwise there was no bedding of any sort, and all the patients lay in their uniforms. There were Serbians, French, English, Bulgars, Austrians and Italians, all of them seriously ill, and the Second Drina Dressing Station had been working night and day since Vranja had been taken, sometimes having as many as 1,500 patients in the hospital at one time. The doctors were aching for us to take over, so that they would be free to go on to Nish when it should be taken. There were crowds of peasants in every ward bringing fruit and native foods to the sick men.

The operating theatre was ghastly, and nothing that I had imagined approached it in frightfulness. A trestle table, covered with the refinement of a brown American cloth, stood in the centre of the room, the wooden floor of which was swimming with blood. A few saws and knives were lying about, and pails full of bits of legs and arms lay round the table and were black with greedy flies. The surgeons, with their sleeves rolled up and waterproof aprons black and red with old and new blood, worked steadily and without anaesthetics, while the wounded kept up a heart-rending, soft 'Ku, ku, maika, ku, ku, maika!'. 'Stay with us and save us!' implored the patients as they clung to us. 'Stay and teach us!' cried the women of the village in their appealing accents, sobbing and distraught, for they had no idea whatever of caring for the sick, and there is no system of nursing in Serbia. 'Come back as quickly as you can,' said the doctors and students; 'we'll try to carry on until you return.' These medical men were doing their very best, and it was not their fault that their patients were dying for lack of attention. They had absolutely no equipment, and only as many field-dressings as their pack-mules could carry; these were a mere drop in the ocean of what was required, and each patient needed skilful nursing and treatment in addition.

The road we had come by was the only possible route to Vranja, and also to Nish and Belgrade, and, in addition to the fact that every bridge was down, the road itself was only a track hardly fit for bullock-carts. The railway which runs through Uskub and Vranja northwards to Nish could not possibly be in working order till the spring, as every bridge had been blown up. The rail-head from Macedonia was at Monastir, so that supplies had to come 241 kilometres by road over the precipitous Babuna Pass, which is snow-bound and wolf-infested in winter.

When she returned to Ostrovo Dr Emslie gave her staff the choice of going to Vranja, where they would be working under terrible conditions, and the weather would be harsh, or resigning without dishonour. No one took advantage of the offer to return home. Mrs Green, the administrator, went to Salonika to collect supplies, especially flour and tinned milk, and within a few days the Ostrovo hospital was evacuated and the tents struck. All the equipment was loaded on to goods wagons, taken by rail to Monastir and then by British transport lorries to Vranja.

On 23 October Dr Emslie and her staff set off in a convoy of ambulances and lorries. Two of the lorries carried the sisters and the other vehicles were filled with food for the journey, surgical instruments and the drugs that would be most needed for the first few days at Vranja.

The first night we spent in a field outside Monastir, our camp-beds all in line; all night long troops and prisoners tramped in a steady stream along the road beside us. The next day's journey was difficult, for there were many shell-holes in the road and many rivers to be crossed; there was also a good deal of slow-moving transport blocking the way. The so-called road was deep with churned-up mud and quite unfit for motor transport, so the cars waltzed and skidded most precariously on the edges of the precipices. Dead horses and donkeys lay thick by the roadside. Ammunition lay on all sides, and the traffic became more and more congested as we proceeded. Refugees carrying their bundles of bedding on their backs had now started to go back, and weary old Serbian soldiers who had got detached from their units were wandering along all alone or in twos and threes.

We spent our second night in the open in a desolate valley at the bottom of the Babuna Pass; nearby was a rushing river, in which we washed next morning, and, mud-brown as the water was, we boiled it in a petrol tin and made delicious coffee. Then up the Babuna Pass, which was only a slight climb from this side; then down and down, swirling round thirty-four hairpin bends with dizzy drops, where many cars had already perished and lay far down the ravine. We had a fairly easy run to Veles, where we slept in great luxury in a newly whitewashed and empty school-house. We spent the fourth night in the building that had been Lady Paget's Hospital [qv] during 1914–1915, and where she and her staff had been kept for some time as prisoners. On the fifth day of the trek we started off early feeling that we were almost at our journey's end. The road, however, was a thousand times worse than when I had passed up it before, and the mud was up to our axles; the wheels went racing round at the bottom of deep ruts, and much pushing of the cars had to be done. We made but slow progress along the flat road.

Sleet began to fall for the last few miles of the journey, and by the time we drove into the courtyard of the barracks snow was falling fast and it was bitterly cold. No preparations had been made for us, for, as we discovered on the following day, the town was in the greatest want and confusion, and the existing staff were dead-beat and had to be off on foot the next morning to a dressing-station farther on.

My own staff were cold, tired and hungry, and would have to set to work in the morning. Where were they to sleep? They had lived in tents for the past two or three years, and were hardened to anything but the fearful and awful stench that greeted them that evening as they entered the barracks.

There were neither candles nor oil in the town, and the huge building was in darkness but for an oil-dip or two which glimmered fitfully. We groped our way along the great stone corridors, meeting wild-eyed, delirious patients, some of them moribund, wandering about aimlessly in stained uniforms and moaning 'voda' (water); old, white-haired 'strajas' (guards) tramped about with fixed bayonets, lest some sick Bulgar or Austrian should try to escape.

Two wards were cleared and there each member unfolded her camp-bed. We lit the candle-lamps which we had brought with us, opened wide the windows to try to get rid of the sickening odours.

As soon as daylight came the Second Drina Dressing Station went off, and we became responsible for the patients.

Early next morning we knew the worst. All but the most seriously ill had been 'evacuated', which really meant that they were put on their feet, sent out into the high-road, and staggered along, eating and sleeping where they could, until at length they arrived at their selo (village). There were 450 cases left for us, each one severe and a problem in itself, and among them was a great number of pneumonias, for 'Spanish influenza', a disease new to Serbia, was sweeping over the country.

It was bitterly cold and those of the patients who were not in a raging fever shivered and tried vainly to adjust their tattered uniforms to gain a little warmth. They lay in blood-stained and torn uniforms, and had on their wounds a first dressing which had not been touched since its application in the field; their clothing crawled with maggots and bugs and their bodies with lice. Dying men lay huddled so closely together on the floor that they touched each other. Others sat up gasping and blue in the throes of pneumonia. Blood and pus oozed from the wounds; there was death already on many of the faces, and all showed the ravages of pain, cold and hunger. A few of the patients feebly extended their hands and a flicker of a smile lit their faces, but most of them were too ill to care what happened. None were more pleased to see us than the British Transport men, who were dotted here and there through the barrack-rooms, and I think our sympathy went out most of all to those of our race who were thus fighting for life against such odds.

Late that night as I walked round the building I realised that we had already accomplished something: the patients were no longer roaming the corridors, but were safe in warm wards, for wood had been brought, the stoves were roaring, and the men were warm – the first essential. The night nurses kept on the move all the time and attended to the worst of the cases, each carrying a stable lamp, for it was pitch dark.

That first week was a whirlwind maze of work and affairs for all, and there was no off-duty time for anybody for many weeks to come. All day long from faraway villages came people who had heard that their menfolk were in our hospital. What could be more natural than that they should wish to tend and feed them and remain beside them night and day. It was with great difficulty that they were got out of the wards at night, but they slept just outside the door, ready to steal in from time to time. The hardest of all to refuse were those who came many miles from the towns and villages around, imploring us to come and see their sick; a virulent type of influenza had spread to the villages and people were dying in hundreds of pneumonia.

Tragedy was in the air, and the men often came back to their homes to find that their children or wife had died from Spanish influenza a few days before, or else perhaps they died a few days after the home-coming. Nearly everywhere there was weeping and wailing instead of laughter and gladness. Dysentery and other intestinal troubles broke out too, some of them caused by the black bread, which was vile and full of straws; there was little or no food and much suffering and disillusionment. Even those who came back to happy homes were sad; there was no harvest, no stock, the road and the rail were in ruins, and their treasures and household goods were gone.

The food question was now giving us great anxiety. Although we possessed considerable stores, there were 600 odd people who had to be fed every day. Our army rations, even when they did come through, were scanty, and it was only the British soldiers' rations – which were very liberal – that arrived regularly. The rations for our Serbian patients, which had come in such a business-like manner at Ostrovo, often did not come at all for days on end.

On 31 October a British RAMC Colonel came up from Salonika to see our hospital, and, after inspection, asked us if we would accept officially the responsibility for any of the British Transport drivers who might get ill, for though they had RAMC doctors attached to the companies, they had no hospitals. I had orders from Colonel Vladisavylevitch to receive all nationalities, so I was able to accept them, and reserved as soon as possible two large wards specially for British soldiers. For the whole of the eight months during which they remained in Serbia we undertook the medical and surgical cases of these units. We were all delighted to have them, for at the beginning of the war it was to the British that Dr Elsie Inglis had first offered her services, and had they been accepted we should never have been in Serbia at all. Now it was the British authorities who were begging us to take full charge of their most seriously ill men.

Even with the best of attention and care which we were now able to give our patients, the death-rate during the months of October and November was high. We had usually seven or eight deaths every day, and our small mortuary behind the hospital was never tenantless. The bodies of the men lay there in their uniforms, and it was reported to me that their boots and uniforms were being stolen. Such I found to be the case, and a guard was put on, a poor old chicha, who no doubt often slept; but still the thieving continued. I had an order from the headquarters saying that as soon as a patient died his clothing was to be taken to clothe the living. This was done, and I put the mortuary in charge of a sister, who had the bodies wrapped in old blankets, but the stealing went on as before. We then substituted thin cotton, but in spite of the guard the dead men were again stripped.

And the burials, too, were carried out only with difficulty. The ground was icy, implements were few, and the prisoner orderlies so thin and ill-fed that they had hardly any strength to wield a pick.

On 11 November 1918, we heard it was Armistice Day, but nobody seemed happy about it, and we hardly seemed to realise what it meant. We had now got up nearly all our equipment and our hospital was clean. The whole building had been wired up by Rose West and her assistant, and our Lister engine gave us electric light – a circumstance that gave us far more delight than the Armistice. On the afternoon of this Armistice Day a great convoy of Bulgar prisoners was waiting for treatment at the out-patients' entrance when Jean Lindsay, one of our orderlies, crossed the yard with a large bowl of scraps for some scraggy chickens we had acquired. Suddenly the Bulgarians pounced upon her, knocking her this way and that; they were like hungry wolves and looked scarcely human, fighting, wounding each other, snarling, hissing, swearing and devouring what they could. Then, as they spied the refuse pail in a corner, they overturned it and grovelled on the ground, devouring the potato skins, bones and garbage it contained. What a gruesome sight it was, and this on a day when all should have been happiness and relief …

Biographical Notes

MISS GRACE ALEXANDRA ASHLEY-SMITH (1887–1963)
Born Aberdeen. Daughter of a master grocer and wine merchant. Educated Albyn's School for Girls, Aberdeen and Aberdeen University. Joined FANYs in 1910. Won the Empire Cup for rifle shooting at Bisley in 1911.

In late 1914 she escaped from Ghent, across the border into Holland, helped by Baroness de Crumbrugge. One of twelve who returned to France almost immediately. Worked first in the Lamark hospital outside Calais and then a dressing station at Oostkirke, a mile behind the trenches. In July 1915 she wrote to the War Office on behalf of the FANYs offering a motor ambulance convoy for Calais or any other base. This was refused but she continued to press and eventually the FANY Corps was accepted for service with the British Army. She received nine decorations from the French and Belgians, including the Croix de Guerre (silver star) and was one of the few women to gain a rosette to the Mons star. Her two brothers were killed in action. Married Ronald McDougall in 1915. Three children. Farmed in Southern Rhodesia after the war. Continued to work with the FANYs during the Second World War.

MISS MARGARET H. BARBER
Daughter of a Church of England clergyman. After working in Astrakan for over a year she joined a Red Cross deputation at the beginning of October 1919 to negotiate the repatriation of Armenian refugees. At Port Alexandrovsk the group were treated with suspicion by White Russians and handed over to the British Mission. She was prevented from returning to help the refugees in Astrakan and from sending them a message. After weeks of being sent from one place to another by the British authorities she eventually arrived in England in the middle of December 1919. No further information.

MISS BICKMORE
No information

MISS VERA BRITTAIN (1893–1970)
Born in Newcastle under Lyme, Staffordshire. Family owned a paper mill. Spent most of her childhood in Buxton. Educated at St Monica's, Kingswood, and Somerville College, Oxford.

Left the hospital in Étaples in the spring of 1918 and returned to England because her mother had suffered a breakdown. Brother Edward was killed on Italian Front in June 1918. Returned to Oxford at the end of the war. Became a pacifist and a prolific writer. Married George Catlin, professor of politics at Cornell University in 1925. Two children. Daughter, Shirley Williams, became a politician and was created Baroness Williams of Crosby.

MISS DOROTHY BROOK (1885–1974)

Born in Misson, near Bawtry, Yorkshire. Educated in Retford High School, Nottinghamshire and Dresden, Germany. Married Alexander Cameron McCann, an officer who had been wounded in the fighting.

SISTER BURGESS

One of many rescued, probably by a trawler, before the torpedoed troopship *Aragon* sank. During the rescue operation the destroyer, HMS *Attack* struck a mine and sank. Over 600 sailors and soldiers were drowned. No other information as to her subsequent service or life after the war.

SISTER E. CAMPBELL

Returned to the Dardanelles in September 1915. Hospital ship to India in February 1917 and sailed between Bombay and Persian Gulf with wounded patients for six months. Then to Mesopotamia. Finally returned to Australia in February 1919.

MISS EDITH CAVELL (1865–1915)

Born at Swardeston, Norfolk. Father vicar of Swardeston Church. Educated at home, Norwich High School, schools in Kensington and Clevedon, near Bristol and at Laurel Court, Peterborough, where she trained to become a teacher. She became a governess in England and Brussels. In 1896 started nursing training at the London Hospital. Private nursing for two years and then various hospitals until 1906 when she went to a nursing home in Manchester for a year before returning to Brussels.

Her execution, and that of Philippe Baucq, took place in the early hours of the morning of 12 October 1915 at the Tir Nationale (the National Rifle Range).

Comtesse Jeanne de Belleville, Mlle Louise Thuliez and Louis Severin were reprieved.

In March 1919 Edith Cavell's body was brought back from the rifle range where she was shot. Two months later, after a short service at Westminster Abbey, she was finally laid to rest in a grave in the precincts of Norwich Cathedral.

MISS MAIRI CHISHOLM (1896–1981)

Born in Datchet, Buckinghamshire. Elder daughter of Roderick Chisholm, chief of clan Chisholm. Privately educated. Girlhood in Dorset and Hampshire. Entered into motorcycle trials and rallies.

Gassed in March 1918; returned to Pervyse until hit by another gas shell and the Poste closed. Awarded the Military Medal in October 1917; the Belgian Queen Elizabeth Medal with Red Cross in December 1917; created an Honorary Associate of the Grand Priory of the Order of the Hospital of St John of Jerusalem in England in February 1918.

After the war worked in London motor trade. Drove a Sunbeam sports car well into her eighties. From 1930 lived in Connal, Argyllshire with a group of women friends.

DR HILDA CLARK (1881–1955)
Born into the Quaker shoe manufacturing family in Street, Somerset. Passed her medical examinations in 1908. An ardent suffragist. Qualified as an obstetrician and worked in the Birmingham Maternity Hospital. Continued to work at Châlons and Sermaise until the summer of 1918 when she collapsed from overwork. From July 1919 she organised relief work for destitute babies and children in Vienna; in 1922 she reported on the appalling conditions in Poland; and during 1923 and 1924 continued to investigate the suffering of refugee women and children in Greece, Serbia, Bulgaria and Turkey. She worked for the League of Nations and from 1930 on the International Commission for the Assistance of Child Refugees. She suffered from Parkinson's disease for ten years until her death and is buried under the same headstone as Edith Pye in the Quaker burial ground in Street.

MISS V.C.C. COLLUM (1883–1957)
Freelance journalist. At the outbreak of war was working in the press department of the National Union of Women's Suffrage Societies in London and assisted Dr Elsie Inglis in starting the Scottish Women's Hospitals. Went to the hospital at Royaumont in February 1915 and trained in the X-ray department. Became a skilled technician. Wrote articles during the war for *Blackwood's Magazine* under the pseudonym 'Skia'.

After the war she studied ancient religions and archaeology; wrote on these subjects and went on excavations.

During the Second World War she helped in soil fertility research and encouraged the establishment of canteens in France.

MRS MABEL DEARMER (1872–1915)
Before the war was an established playwright, writer of children's books, and a book illustrator. In 1891 married the Reverend Percy Dearmer, a London clergyman, and well-known hymn writer. Mrs Dearmer died from typhoid and double pneumonia at Kragujevatz on 15 July 1915. She was buried in the local cemetery after Greek Orthodox priests conducted an impressive service in their cathedral.

Percy and Mabel Dearmer's youngest son, Christopher, a pilot in the Royal Naval Air Service, was killed at Suvla Bay three months after his mother's death in Serbia. Their eldest son, Geoffrey, served in Malta, Gallipoli, Egypt and on the Somme. After the war he wrote poetry, plays and novels and between 1939 and 1959 was editor of the BBC's Children's Hour.

MISS OLIVE DENT (1884–1930)
Born in Kelloe, County Durham. Father was a joiner. After the war she became a journalist in London.

DR ISABEL EMSLIE

Dr Emslie remained at the Scottish Women's Hospital at Vranja, Serbia until 1919 when she became CMO of the Girton and Newnham Unit in Belgrade. Later ran a children's hospital in the Crimea. She was awarded Serbia's Order of the White Eagle and the Croix de Guerre avec Palme. She married a young officer (later Lieutenant General Sir Thomas Hutton) she had met in Constantinople. She continued her medical career, wrote several medical books, and became a distinguished psychiatrist.

MISS FLORENCE FARMBOROUGH (1887–1980)

Born in Buckinghamshire. Named after Florence Nightingale, a family friend.

In the Autumn of 1917 the 1st Letuchka (Flying Column) was disbanded. Florence Farmborough returned to Moscow from the Romanian Front. In March 1918 she escaped across Siberia to Vladivostok and was eventually taken by sea to America. (Yasha Bachkarova, of the Women's Death Battalion, having escaped the Red Guards, was also on board.) Returned to England later in 1918 and wrote articles for *The Times*. In 1926 became a university lecturer in Valencia, Spain. Supported General Franco in the Spanish Civil War and made radio propaganda broadcasts to English-speaking countries. Published *Life and People of Spain* in 1938.

She returned to England in 1940. Her First World War diaries contained 400,000 words and were published in 1974. She was made a Fellow of the Royal Geographical Society.

MISS M. FAWCETT (1892–1987)

Educated at Godolphin School, Salisbury. Trained as a Froebel teacher. Recuperated from malaria in Odessa in September 1917 and returned to England in November 1917. During 1918 she served in France in the Women's Army Auxiliary Corps. After the war she taught in Natal. Married Walter Cahill.

MRS ELSIE FENWICK (1874–1948)

Daughter of a banker, Abraham Robarts, senior partner of Robarts, Lubbock & Co. Mother was the younger daughter of the 8th Viscount Barrington. Educated by governesses at home. Married Guy Fenwick in 1895. Served in Hotel de l'Ocean Hospital, La Panne, until November 1917. She started as an untrained VAD and ended as head sister of a ward of eighty surgical patients. Spent last six months of the war nursing in other hospitals near Amiens and Dunkirk. Awarded the Medal of Queen Elizabeth of the Belgians; the French Red Cross Medal; and the General Service Medal.

Returned to her home at North Luffenham Hall, Rutland. During Second World War was head warden in the local ARP and was active in the WVS.

MISS KATE JOHN FINZI (1890–?)

Daughter of a ship broker. Her younger brother was the composer Gerald Finzi. Two other brothers were killed during the war. In May 1917 she married Second Lieutenant Alexander Laidlaw Gilmour of the 7th Northamptonshire Fusiliers.

MISS YVONNE ALICE GERTRUDE FITZROY (1891–1971)
Daughter of Sir Almeric Fitzroy.

After the Scottish Women's Hospital Unit left Galatz, Romania, they were sent to Reni early in 1918. In June Yvonne Fitzroy returned to England as her mother was ill. private secretary to Alice, Marchioness of Reading, Vicereine of India from 1921–6.

MRS KATHARINE FURSE (1875–1952)
Daughter of the writer John Addington Symonds. Lived in Switzerland and Italy. Educated at home. Married the artist, Charles Furse, in 1900. Widowed four years later. Two sons.

At the end of 1914 she returned from France to work at the Red Cross Headquarters in London in charge of the VAD department. In 1916 was appointed commander-in-chief. In 1917 was appointed a Dame Grand Cross and became director of the Women's Royal Naval Service (WRNS).

After the war she worked in Switzerland with Lunn, the travel agents. Became an expert skier and President of the Ladies' Ski Club. In 1920 she formed the Association of Wrens. She was head of the Sea Rangers for ten years and director of the World Association of Girl Guides and Girl Scouts.

MISS DOROTHY HIGGINS (1892–?)
Family were estate agents in Lincolnshire for at least 200 years. Continued to work in the Anglo-Belgian Hospital, Rouen, until 1919. After the war she returned to the small market town of Alford, Lincolnshire, and lived for fifty-two years with Doc Staveley, a woman friend, with whom she had served. She gave the beautiful thatched early seventeenth-century Manor House to Alford; now renovated and restored for art festivals, social functions etc.

MISS KATHERINE HODGES (1888–1982)
Daughter of actor and playwright Horace Hodges. The ambulance unit was disbanded in March 1919. Awarded Russian Medal of St George and Order of St Stanislas and the Croix de Guerre. Married Peter North, an army officer.

In the Second World War she served through the Blitz as a driver with the London Auxiliary Ambulance Service. After the war she worked with the British Red Cross society as a headquarters officer until January 1968.

LADY HOWARD DE WALDEN (1890–1974)
Margherita (Margot) van Raalte was the daughter of a wealthy banker. She inherited her mother's artistic talent and became an accomplished musician. Trained as an opera singer. Spent much of her childhood on Brownsea Island, Dorset, which her family owned. Married Thomas Scott-Ellis, 8th Lord Howard de Walden and 4th Lord Seaford, in 1912. Six children.

She returned to England from Egypt in 1916. Was in charge of a hospital for officers in London. After the war was châtelaine of Chirk Castle; established and presided over the annual Queen Charlotte's Ball and was involved in many charitable organisations. Lord and Lady Howard de Walden's third daughter, Priscilla Scott-Ellis, born in 1916, served in front-line hospitals during the Spanish Civil War.

DR ELSIE INGLIS (1864–1917)
Father served first in the East India Company and then in Indian Civil Service. Between 1875 and 1877 he was chief commissioner of Oude. Elsie born in Naini Tal, a hill-station in the Himalayas.

Father retired and family settled in Edinburgh in 1878. Elsie educated at Edinburgh Institution for the Education of Young Ladies and in Paris. Qualified in medicine in 1892.

In February 1916 Elsie Inglis was told her Unit must leave Krushevatz, Serbia, and they arrived home via Vienna and Zurich at the end of the month. Two months later she was given the Serbian Order of the White Eagle. In August 1916, although she knew she was suffering from cancer, she took a SWH unit of seventy-five women to Russia to serve with two Serbian divisions. Over the following year they were constantly in retreat and nursing under terrible conditions. At the end of September 1917 the Unit was no longer needed as the Serbs returned to Serbia via England and Salonika; by then Elsie Inglis was very ill. After an exhausting journey of four weeks she died a few days after she returned to England in November. She was posthumously awarded the highest decorations from Russia and Serbia, the Gold St George Medal and the Order of the White Eagle with Swords (the first time the latter had been given to a woman). Obituaries and letters flooded the national newspapers; she lay in state in St Giles' Cathedral, Edinburgh. English and Serbian royalty and military, doctors, nurses, old friends and twenty-five Serb boys who had survived the Great Retreat and were at school in Edinburgh, attended her funeral. Her coffin was taken on a gun-carriage drawn by six black horses at the head of a long procession; crowds eight deep lined Princes Street. A few days later there was a memorial service at St Margaret's, Westminster. 'If she were a Serbian we would declare her a saint,' said an Orthodox priest.

MISS FRANCES IVENS (1870–1944)
Brought up in Harborough Parva, Warwickshire. Daughter of a prosperous timber merchant. Mother a descendant of Elias Ashmole, founder of the Ashmolean Museum. Educated at various boarding schools. Entered the London School of Medicine for Women in 1894. Qualified in 1900. Awarded the London University Gold Medal in obstetrics; obtained an honours in medicine and forensic medicine. In 1903 became the third woman to achieve a master of surgery degree. Continued training in Vienna, Dublin and London. Appointed consultant obstetrician and gynaecologist at Liverpool Stanley Hospital, the first woman to hold an honorary position there, followed by an honorary post in the Liverpool Samaritan Hospital. She also held clinics in a rented house for babies from working-class families. She was a protagonist in many feminist struggles in the field of medicine and formed the North of England Medical Women's Society.

Served as the Chief Medical Officer at the SWH at Royaumont from 1914 until the hospital closed in 1919. Awarded Chevalier Legion d'honneur; Croix de Guerre avec Palme; Medaille d'honneur des Epidemies.

She returned to Liverpool Stanley and Samaritan hospitals and became a university lecturer in obstetrics and gynaecology. Involved in planning and founding new hospitals; a member of Liverpool Medical Institution and became vice-president in 1926.

She served on the executive committee of the Medical Women's Federation from 1921 and was president from 1924 until 1926.

In 1929 the University of Liverpool gave her an honorary Master of Surgery degree and the same year she was created a commander of the British Empire.

In 1930, at the age of sixty, she married Charles Matthew Knowles. After her husband retired they lived in his family home at Killagordon, near Truro. Mrs Ivens-Knowles became a dedicated gardener; county medical officer for the Red Cross and head of the women's section of the Truro British Legion. During the Second World War she was chairman of the Cornwall Committee of the Friends of the Fighting French and was active in the Royaumont and Villers-Cotterets Association.

MISS IDA JEFFERSON (later Cliffe) (1889–?)

Childhood spent in 'a Yorkshire town'. After her transfer to India she served in a large Bombay hospital. Became ill with malaria and was sent for a short time to Alexandria on light duties before returning home by sea. Boat slightly damaged by a torpedo and next boat in convoy badly hit.

Private nursing after the war.

LADY KENNARD (d. 1953)

Daughter of Sir George Barclay. Married Sir Coleridge Arthur Fitzroy Kennard, 1st Bt., in April 1911. Two sons.

In November 1916, after a long journey in an overcrowded train, Dorothy Kennard arrived in Jassy, Romania, where there was a severe food shortage. With three other people she was allotted one room – with no bed – in a suburban villa, but was later given a house which she shared with other refugees who were filling the town. She worked in a hospital under chaotic conditions until it was commandeered by the Russians. She continued to work at various Red Cross units and at the English Hospital. The Red Cross stores she had ordered weeks before arrived from England and she planned to 'make of the contents of the cases and the stray English doctors and nurses who turn up at intervals an efficient and well organised unit for the front'. Order was gradually restored in Jassy but there was over-riding uncertainty – acute shortage of food and fuel and lice prevalent in the hospitals where the wounded continued to arrive. As there were no means to combat the lice without serum and disinfectant the doctors resorted to using vinegar. In January 1917 there were over 300 infectious diseases in the English hospital. Her diary ends four months later.

Divorced in 1918. No further information as to when she returned to England or her life from then on.

MRS ELSIE KNOCKER (1884–1978)

Daughter of Lewis Shapter, an Exeter doctor. Orphaned when a child. Educated privately and at a finishing school in Lausanne, Switzerland, and at a cookery school in Trowbridge, Wiltshire. Married Leslie Duke Knocker in 1906 and went to Singapore. One son. Divorced husband. Trained as a nurse and midwife.

Appointed Chevalier of the Order of Leopold in January 1915. In April 1916 Elsie Knocker married Baron Harold de T'Serclaes, a Belgian pilot. He was killed three years later. She was awarded the Military Medal in October 1917 – presented to her in the field by Prince Alexander of Teck. A gas attack during the final German offensive in March 1918 forced the Baroness to evacuate the Cellar House and return to England. She served in the newly formed Women's Royal Air Force for the remainder of the war. Had various jobs until the 1926 general strike when she ran a medical post in the East End of London. At the outbreak of the Second World War she joined the Women's Auxiliary Air Force and became an assistant section officer. She resigned after her son, an RAF wing commander, was killed in action over Holland in July 1942. She then worked for the RAF Association and, between 1949 and 1959, for the RAF Benevolent Fund.

SISTER K.E. LUARD

Sister Luard went home on leave in September 1917. She then spent some months in charge of units at Gottwaersvelt and Estaires. In February 1918 she rejoined Casualty Clearing Station No. 32 with Sir Hugh Gough's 5th Army at Marchelepot, south of Péronne in the Somme area. Evacuated after the Germans advanced on 23 March. Sent to No. 2 Stationary Hospital, then as sister in charge of the CCS at Nampes, south of Amiens. Between May and August 1918 she was with Sir Henry Rawlinson's 4th Army at a CCS on a new camp site at Pernois, between Amiens and Doullens. She went on leave in August and was at a base hospital until the Armistice. She was released from service because of advanced age and the ill-health of her father. Awarded Bar to the Royal Red Cross. No information on Sister Luard's life after the war.

MISS SARAH MACNAUGHTAN (d. 1916)

Scottish descent and daughter of a JP.

Left Hamadan, Persia, accompanied by a 'Tartar Prince', after her car was returned in March 1916. After a terrible, long and hazardous journey she arrived in Tehran. By then she was very ill and was nursed at the British Legation for the next four weeks until it was decided she should continue with her journey home. She eventually arrived in England in May and died two months later. She is buried in the churchyard at Chart Sutton, Kent.

She was made a Chevalier de l'Ordre de Leopold in the summer of 1915, and a month before her death a Lady of Grace of the Order of St John of Jerusalem.

SISTER KATHLEEN MANN (later Barrett) (1882–1975)

Continued nursing on hospital ships. Awarded Royal Red Cross Medal (First Class).

SISTER MARY-ELIZA (JOAN) MARTIN-NICHOLSON (1876–?)

During 1915 she nursed at a CCS 'somewhere near the firing line'. After she returned home she became sister in charge of a large surgical ward at the King's Lancashire Military Hospital in Blackpool. No further information.

DR FLORA MURRAY (1870–1923)

Born in Dumfriesshire, Scotland. Father was a naval officer. Qualified as a physician in 1903. Became a London doctor and founded a children's hospital in 1911.

In November 1914 the Women's Hospital Corps opened a hospital in Château Mauricien in Wimereux, and both this and the hospital in the Hotel Claridge in Paris were 'filled to overflowing'. By January 1915 the latter was closed when it became impossible to heat. *The Times* reported on 19 February 1915 that Sir Alfred Keogh 'had received numbers of unsolicited letters from Paris and Boulogne, which stated that the work of women doctors at the Front was beyond all praise'. He was so impressed that he asked two of the staff to take charge of a hospital in London of 1,000 beds. In May 1915 the Women's Hospital Corps opened a military hospital in Endell Street, Bloomsbury, in the buildings of the old St Giles workhouse. Dr Louisa Garrett Anderson, CBE, was the chief surgeon and Dr Flora Murray, CBE, was the administrator and doctor in charge.

No information on Dr Murray's life after the war.

MISS AMELIA (AMY) NEVILL (1879–?)
Continued to nurse in Genoa, Italy, until February 1919. She was awarded the Royal Red Cross Medal in January 1918. Was the only unmarried daughter in the family and after she returned to England she cared for her mother.

LADY PAGET (1881–1958)
Daughter of General Sir Arthur Paget. Delicate child. Travelled in Europe with her mother. Married Sir Ralph Paget, a diplomat. She accompanied her husband to Belgrade in 1910 where she ran a hospital for the wounded during the First and Second Balkan Wars.

When the Germans arrived in Skoplje, Serbia, in December 1915, life in the Bulgarian Military Hospital became increasingly difficult. In February 1916 Lady Paget and her unit were taken in a convoy of ten Bulgarian motor ambulances on the first stage of their repatriation. When she eventually arrived home in April she was criticised for remaining on good terms with the Bulgarians while she and her staff were prisoners-of-war. She withdrew from the public scene although she continued to help Serbia in many ways for the remainder of her life. A street was named after her – Ledi Pazet Ulica – near the big general hospital in Belgrade. She was awarded the Order of Saint Sava (First Class), the only uncrowned woman to be so honoured and created a dame of the British Empire.

LADY MURIEL PAGET (1876–1938)
Lady Muriel Finch-Hatton was the daughter of the 12th Earl of Winchilsea. Married Richard Paget, who later became Sir Richard Paget, Bart.

She organised soup kitchens in Odessa and Kiev in 1917. Evacuated from Bolshevik Russia early in 1918.

After the war she continued to work with tireless energy in many destitute countries. She founded the Women and Children of Russia Relief Fund in 1919. The following year she organised relief work in Slovakia, Romania, Poland and the Baltic states. In the latter she established a children's hospital in Dvinsk, Latvia, with 100 beds and facilities for treating 500 outpatients. In the 1930s she sent money and food parcels to the last surviving British subjects stranded in Stalin's Russia and eventually succeeded in getting the remaining ones evacuated to Estonia.

Her tremendous philanthropic work in central and eastern Europe was recognised with medals and decorations from the Governments of Imperial Russia, Belgium, Czechoslovakia, Romania, Latvia, Lithuania, Estonia and Japan. (The Japanese medal, with a nightingale and a cross, was given annually to 'one who nurses not only with her head, but with her heart'.) The announcement that she was to be made a Companion of the British Empire came the week before her death. It was given 'in recognition of services rendered in connection with British interests in Russia'.

MISS ELEONORA B. PEMBERTON (1885–1994)
Mentioned in despatches in 1916. On British Red Cross headquarters staff at Grosvenor Gardens from 1919. Lived in Amersham, Buckinghamshire, where she was a well-known figure and gave talks on her experiences during the First World War. Appointed OBE. She died in 1994 aged 109.

MISS JOSEPHINE PENNELL
Born in Buenos Aires. Father was a surgeon. Educated in England.

She was one of twelve members of the British Red Cross Society convoy at St Omer to be awarded the Military Medal for their services during the night raid on the town in May 1918.

Married Roy Tennent, MC, and they went to Singapore where he was a rubber broker. They had four sons.

DR MARY PHILLIPS
Served with Dr Alice Hutchinson in the Scottish Women's Hospitals Unit in Calais from November 1914 and at Valjevo in 1915. No further information

MISS MILDRED REES (1869–1957)
Born in the Waitaki Valley, New Zealand. Educated at Cromwell School and Mrs Tait's School in Timaru. Started nursing training at Blenheim Hospital and completed training, as a staff nurse, at Wellington Hospital in 1894. Private nursing in New Zealand until she arrived in England in February 1910. Served on the staff of the Mayfair and Hampstead Nursing Corps Ltd for three years. Trained as a maternity nurse at Dundee Hospital. At the outbreak of war went with Millicent, Duchess of Sutherland's Ambulance Unit to Namur, Belgium. Returned to England in September 1914 and joined Queen Alexandra's Imperial Military Nursing Service Reserve. She served in France from February 1915. After her five months with No. 4 Ambulance Flotilla, she served in Stationary Hospitals, on barge 366 of the Ambulance Flotilla, at No. 23 CCS and finally at No. 4 General Hospital in Camiers, until peace was declared. She continued to serve in Belgium for the next four months and was fifty years of age when she was demobilised in April 1919. She then returned to New Zealand. She was awarded the 1914 Star, was mentioned in Field Marshall Sir Douglas Haig's despatches on 7 November 1917 'for gallant and distinguished services in the field' and awarded the Associate Royal Red Cross in December 1917.

MISS FRANCES ELEANOR (ELLIE) RENDEL (1885–1942)

Daughter of Lytton Strachey's eldest sister. Studied history and economics at Newnham College, Cambridge, between 1904 and 1908, where she spoke at political debates 'with knowledge, wit, and brilliance'. Founder member of the Charlotte Younge Society. Worked with National Union of Women's Suffrage Societies. Medical student when war broke out. Enlisted as an X-ray operator with SWH Unit but was entrusted with much of the responsibility of a fully qualified doctor. Dr Elsie Inglis praised 'her excellent work'. After serving in Russia and Romania she spent seven months with a SWH Unit in Salonika and Sarajevo.

Finally returned to England in April 1919. Qualified as a doctor after the war and set up as a General Practitioner in London. Became doctor to Virginia Woolf (her cousin) and other members of the 'Bloomsbury' group. Held posts in the 1920s and 1930s at the Hospital for Heart Diseases. At the start of the Second World War she was living with her mother in Surrey.

MISS FLORA SANDES (1876–1956)

Of Irish descent. Daughter of the Reverend Samuel Dickson Sandes, rector of Marlsford Church in Suffolk. Early childhood in Suffolk and later lived with widowed father in St Paul's Road, Thornton Heath, Surrey. Finishing school in Switzerland.

Retreated across the Albanian mountains with the Serbian 2nd Infantry Regiment and reached Corfu at the beginning of 1916. A few days later Serbian Crown Prince Alexander decorated her with the Serbian Order of St Sava. The following year Flora Sandes, by then a sergeant in the 2nd Infantry Regiment, arrived in Salonika with the newly formed Serbian army prepared to fight for their homeland once more. She was badly wounded by a grenade in November 1916 during the battle for Monastir and was nursed at first in the SWH at Ostrovo. Later in the military hospital in Salonika she was awarded the Karadjordj Star for bravery in action – the first time it had been won by a woman. She had many operations and returned to England to recuperate. By September 1918, although exhausted and still weak, she returned to her regiment as a sergeant-major and fought on until the Bulgarians surrendered.

After the war she remained in the Serbian army and became an officer (the commissioning of a woman required a special act of parliament), finally retiring with the rank of captain and the King George Star, Serbia's highest decoration.

In 1927 she married a White Russian émigré Yuri Yudenitch, a retired army colonel. They lived in Paris where she spent some months as wardrobe mistress and chaperone to the girls of the Folies Bergère. Settled in Belgrade. Her husband died in 1941. Defied the German authorities during the Second World War although forced to report regularly to the Gestapo. Returned to Woodbridge, Suffolk, in 1945 with a full army pension for life from the new Yugoslav government.

MISS DOROTHY SEYMOUR (d. 1953)

Daughter of General Lord William Frederick Ernest Seymour. Before the war was Woman of the Bedchamber to HRH Princess Christian.

At the end of March 1917 she managed to get a train from Petrograd to Bergen; then a dangerous and uncomfortable voyage in HMS *Vulture* to Aberdeen. After a few months nursing at the Blake Hall Auxiliary Hospital for Officers in Ongar, Essex, she was sent to run the WAAC Unit 11 at Wimereux. In March 1918 she moved to No. 1 WAAC Camp, Étaples, where the wounded from the German offensive poured in. The hospital was bombed and the nursing staff and patients spent nights in nearby 'caves'. In June 1918 she became VAD area controller in Le Havre. She was involved in the 'Trouville Convoy' – a motor VAD Unit which took wounded from the casualty clearing stations to the hospitals.

In 1919 married Major Jackson. He had been shot by a sniper in the Ypres Salient in April 1916 and sent to No. 14 General Hospital in Wimereux where Dorothy Seymour was nursing. He later became General Sir Henry Jackson.

MISS MAY SINCLAIR (1863–1946)
Born Mary Amelia St Clair in Rock Ferry, Cheshire. Father was a Liverpool shipowner. Educated at Cheltenham Ladies College. Cared for brothers suffering from a fatal congenital heart disease. Wrote novels, short stories and poetry; a significant literary critic and reviewer of modernist poetry and prose. Active suffragist. Member of the Woman Writers' Suffrage League. From 1914 a member of the Society for Psychical Research which influenced much of her later writing.

An established writer by the time she met Ezra Pound, Hilda Doolittle and Richard Aldington in 1911–12. She became a good friend and generous patron to Aldington. He is attributed to be the main protagonist in her 1919 novel *Mary Olivier*.

After she returned from Ghent she remained in England. She continued to write until the onset of Parkinson's disease in the late 1920s. She later lived with a companion in Buckinghamshire.

MISS LESLEY SMITH
Daughter of a middle-class Scottish family opposed to her becoming a VAD. No further information.

MISS FREYA STARK (1893–1993)
Born in Paris. Artist parents, first cousins from an old Devon family, separated when Freya Stark was young. Childhood in Italy (particularly Asolo), France, London and Dartmoor. No formal education but spoke French, German and Italian.

After she returned from the retreat during the battle of Caporetto in Italy in November 1917 she suffered from ill-health, which often troubled her in subsequent years. She learnt Arabic and in 1927 completed a course at the London School of Oriental Studies. Later that year she journeyed through Syria on her first expedition. She lived for a time in Baghdad and between 1929–31 she went on three solo journeys through Iran. She travelled in Arabia during the winters of 1934/5 and 1937/8. During the Second World War she undertook political and publicity work in Aden, Yemen, Cairo and Baghdad. Founded the Brotherhood of Freedom. Returned to Italy in 1943 and worked for the British Embassy. At the end of the war, when she returned to her house in Asolo, which had been used by the Germans as a headquarters, she found everything in order including all her possessions which had been hidden by friends. Married Stewart Perowne, a diplomat and orientalist, in 1947 and accompanied him to Barbados and Cyrenaica.

They separated in 1952. In her sixties she made several arduous journeys, often on horseback, to the remoter parts of Turkey. She travelled in Afghanistan and Nepal and in her late eighties still undertook challenging expeditions. She was the author of many travel books and a three-volume autobiography. She received geographical awards and academic degrees and was appointed CBE in 1953 and created a Dame of the British Empire in 1972.

MRS MABEL STOBART (1862–1954)
Mabel Annie Stobart was the daughter of Sir Samuel Boulton of Copped Hall, Fotherbridge, Hertfordshire, deputy lieutenant of the county. Educated by governesses at home. Well-read, an accomplished pianist, and superb horsewoman. Later became a mystic and an authority on spiritualism. Blessed with extraordinary physical stamina and courage, she was strong-willed, autocratic and rebelled against the conventional constraints of her time.

First husband lost money on stock exchange and in 1903 they farmed and bred horses in a remote corner of the Transvaal. Built their own shanty, lived on tinned food; locusts destroyed their vegetable crop which had taken a year to grow and their land ravaged by veldt fires. Undaunted, Mrs Stobart opened a 'kaffir store' in a corrugated iron shed and sold a range of goods to local people. Loved and respected by the natives she was asked to arbitrate in disputes, give medical advice and assistance, often trekking on her own for many miles across country where tribal wars were prevalent. Her husband died after they returned to England in 1907. That year she was asked to form the Women's Sick and Wounded Convoy Corps, to be used for service between field and base Hospitals in the event of war. In 1911 Mrs Stobart married John Greenhalgh, a retired judge. Part of her 'marriage agreement' was that he would accompany her, in the capacity of an orderly, on all her expeditions and that she should retain her first married name.

In mid-December 1915 Mrs Stobart, her husband and the few remaining members of her First Serbian-English Field Hospital, sailed from San Giovanni de Medua and, accompanied by two torpedo-boats, they reached Brindisi on Christmas Day. They finally reached London on 29 December after nine months service in Serbia. Mrs Stobart was decorated with the Serbian orders of the White Eagle, St Sava and the Red Cross and received many letters of thanks from prominent Serbians. She also received the Order of St John of Jerusalem and the 1914 Star. However, she was shocked and upset by the unfriendly reception she received at the headquarters of the Serbian Relief Fund the day after her return to London. The Chairman reprimanded her for exceeding her instructions and for leading the column into unnecessary risks.

During 1916 Mrs Stobart gave lectures all over England, and in 1917 she and her husband went on an extensive lecture tour throughout Canada and America. She donated the money she received from these lectures to the Serbian Red Cross. One of her two sons and his wife died from the 1918 influenza epidemic.

She became chairman and leader of the Spiritualist Community between 1924 and 1941, and also became a member of the Council of the World Congress of Faiths. She wrote books on her experiences in Serbia and on Spiritualism and psychic research. She lived in Studland, Dorset, until her death. She is buried at St Nicholas Church.

MILLICENT, DUCHESS OF SUTHERLAND (1867–1955)
Daughter of 4th Earl of Rosslyn. Married Marquess of Stafford on her seventeenth birthday. He succeeded his father as 4th Duke of Sutherland in 1892. She combined the roles of a society hostess and a social reformer. Widowed in 1913. Married Percy Desmond Fitzgerald, a serving army officer, in October 1914, a few days before she left for Belgium.

After she was forced to close her ambulance unit in Namur, the German commander arranged for the French Red Cross to drive the Duchess and her staff to Brussels. They left Belgium on 18 September. She then raised enough funds to set up a Red Cross hospital outside Calais where she remained as commandant until the war ended. Marriage annulled.

Married George Ernest Hawes in October 1919. Divorced 1925. After the war she lived in France until her death.

MISS MARJERY A. SWYNNERTON (later Thomas)
Sent to Sick Sisters Hospital No. 41 when ill with dysentary. Recuperation in Simla and leave in Bombay. Caught Spanish influenza and taken off train back to Mesopotamia. After father died she resigned and returned to England with mother and small brother.

Later, spent many years in West Africa.

SISTER VIOLETTA THURSTAN (1879–1978)
Anna Violet Thurstan born in Hastings, Sussex. Cornish father, Scottish mother. Childhood homes in Cornwall and Canary Isles. Spoke several languages. She worked at the East London Hospital for Children and the Fever Hospital in Guernsey before training as a nurse at the London Hospital, Whitechapel, between 1900–5. Various hospital appointments, including matron of a hospital on the Greek island of Spetsia. Returned to England in 1907 and in 1914 she was given an external diploma, the Lady Literate in Arts, from the University of St Andrews, having taken examinations in various subjects in different colleges.

Sent back to England in March 1915 after she suffered a shrapnel injury from a bomb dropped by a German aeroplane and then caught a chill that turned to pleurisy. Worked with the National Union of Trained Nurses and then returned to Russia in 1916 to distribute funds and organise English hospital units helping refugees. On 4 November 1916 she was sent as matron to the thousand-bed Hôpital de l'Ocean at La Panne in Belgium (where Elsie Fenwick was nursing). In July 1917 she went to the Y Corps, main dressing station in France. In August the dressing station was shelled and although she was wounded she continued to assist in the evacuation of the wounded patients. Sent home in October suffering from shell shock. Awarded the Military Medal. In December 1917 went as matron to the Scottish Women's Hospital at Ostrovo, where Dr Agnes Bennett was chief medical officer. She remained until June 1918 (leaving shortly before Dr Isabel Emslie was appointed CMO).

After the war trained in weaving and handicrafts and gained diplomas from Italy, Paris, Berlin and Sweden. Set up a weaving and spinning business in the 1930s. During the Second World War joined the WRNS, after declaring her date of birth as 1890. She recruited all over the country, gave lectures and worked with Naval Intelligence in Falmouth. After the war she was once again active in humanitarian work amongst children and refugees in Cairo, Austria, and Italy etc.

A committed Roman Catholic she had audiences with the Pope during her work in Italy and was made a Companion of the Vatican. From 1946 served in the Department of POWs and Displaced Persons. Returned to live in Cornwall. Continued as a weaver and set up a school of weaving in 1953. Lectured, arranged exhibitions, and wrote books and articles on the subject. Died at Penryn, Cornwall. Her nine medals were buried with her (Military Medal; Russian Order of St George; Belgian Order de la Reine Elizabeth; Mons Star; Allied Medal; Companion of the Vatican; 1914 Star with Clasp and Roses; British War Medal; Victory Medal.)

MISS PAT WADDELL (1892–1972)
Catherine Marguerite Beauchamp was the only daughter of Cranston Waddell, JP, of Warwick Bridge, Cumberland, a woollen manufacturer. Educated at a Dame school in Wetheral village and at Englethwaite, a boarding school at Cotehill. Artistic and musical. Professional violinist.

Remained at the Lamarck Hospital in Calais until January 1916 when she was one of eighteen FANYs to become members of the First British Convoy under the auspices of the BRCS to provide transport for the British sick and wounded at Calais. In May 1917, during an air raid, her ambulance was hit by a train. She was thrown out and dragged along the line. Her left leg was almost severed and had to be amputated.

Units disbanded after the war and Pat Waddell, 'quite undisturbed by having a tin leg', became secretary to the newly formed corps in 1920. Married Captain P. Washington in 1922. In 1940 Pat Washington took a mobile canteen to supply Polish troops with basic necessities at their camp at Coetquidan in Brittany. Continued this canteen work when Polish troops were regrouped in south-west Scotland after the fall of France.

She was awarded the French Croix de Guerre with Silver Star; Belgian Order de la Reine Elizabeth; Belgian King Albert Medal with Bar; three British service medals. Also, the Polish Military gold cross and service medals after the Second World War.

Select Bibliography

The individual autobiographies and biographies from which extracts were taken will be found under Acknowledgements and are not listed again in this section. Place of publication is London unless otherwise stated.

Adam, Ruth. A Woman's Place: 1910–75, Chatto and Windus, 1975 and (Persephone Book No. 20) Persephone Books Ltd, 2000

Bagnold, Enid. A Diary Without Dates, William Heinemann Ltd., 1933

———. The Happy Foreigner, Virago, 1987

Beauman, Nicola. A Very Great Profession: The Woman's Novel 1914–39, Virago Press Limited, 1983 and (Persephone Book No. 78) Persephone Books Ltd., 2008

Billington, Mary Frances. The Red Cross in War: Women's Part in the Relief of Suffering, Hodder and Stoughton, 1914

Borden, Mary. The Forbidden Zone, Heinemann, 1929

———. Sarah Gay, Heinemann, 1931

———. Journey Down A Blind Alley, Heinemann, 1946

Bowser, Thelka. The Story of British VAD Work in the Great War, Melrose c. 1917 and Imperial War Museum (No. 4 in Women in Wartime series), 2003

Brittain, Vera M. Verses of a VAD. Erskine Macdonald, 1918, and Imperial War Museum, Arts and Literature Series Number 8, 1995

———. Testament of Youth: An Autobiographical Study of the Years 1900–1925, Gollancz, 1933

———. Vera Brittain's War Diary 1913–1917. Edited by Alan Bishop, Gollancz, 1981

———. A Life by Paul Berry and Mark Bostridge, Chatto & Windus, 1995

———. Letters from a Lost Generation: First World War Letters of Vera Brittain and Four Friends. Edited by Alan Bishop and Mark Bostridge, Little Brown and Co., 1998

Cadogan, Mary and Craig, Patricia. Women and Children First: The Fiction of Two World Wars, Gollancz, 1978

Cahill, Audrey Fawcett. (Editor) Between the Lines: Letters and Diaries from Elsie Inglis's Russian Unit, The Pentland Press Ltd, Durham, 1999

Cardinal, Agnes, Goldman, Dorothy, and Hattaway, Judith (Editors). Women's Writing on the First World War, Oxford University Press, 1999

Carlyon, L.A. Gallipoli, Doubleday, 2002

Cecil, Hugh and Liddle, Peter H. (Editors). Facing Armageddon: The First World War Experienced, Leo Cooper, Pen and Sword Books Ltd., 1996

Condell, Diane and Liddiard, Jean. Working for Victory? Images of Women in the First World War 1914–18, Routledge and Kegan Paul, 1987

Corbett, Elsie. With the Red Cross in Serbia, Cheney, 1960

Cox, Sydney, MBE. The Red Cross Launch Wessex on the River Tigris – 1916: Being the Diary of Sydney Cox MBE, with notes and explanations, Natula Publications, Christchurch, Dorset, 2002

Creswick, Paul, G. Stanley Pond and P.H. Ashton. Kent's Care for the Wounded, Hodder and Stoughton, 1915

Crofton, Eileen. The Women of Royaumont: A Scottish Women's Hospital on the Western Front, Tuckwell Press Ltd., East Lothian, Scotland, 1997

Cröy, Princess Marie de. War Memories, Macmillan and Co., Limited, 1932

Diary of a Nursing Sister on the Western Front 1914–1915 [K.E. Luard], Diggory Press, 2007

Farmborough, Florence. Nurse at the Russian Front: A Diary 1914–1918, Constable, 1974

Gilbert, Martin. First World War, Weidenfeld and Nicolson, 1994

Grayzel, Susan R. Women and the First World War (Seminar Studies in History), Longman, 2002

Hay, Ian. One Hundred Years of Army Nursing: The Story of the British Army Nursing Services from the time of Florence Nightingale to the present day, Cassell and Company Limited, 1953

Hamilton, Cecily. Senlis, W. Collins Sons and Co., Ltd., 1917

———. Life Errant, Dent 1935

———. William – an Englishman, Skeffington and Son, 1919 and Persephone Books Ltd., 1999 (Persephone Books No. 1)

Harmer, Michael. The Forgotten Hospital [The Anglo-Russian Hospital, Petrograd], Chichester Press Limited in association with Springwood Books, 1982

Harris, Ruth Elwin. Billie: The Nevill Letters 1914–1916, Julia MacRae Books, 1991

Krippner, Monica. The Quality of Mercy: Women in Serbia 1915–18, David and Charles, Newton Abbot, Devon, 1980

Lawrence, Margot. Shadow of Swords: A Biography of Elsie Inglis, Michael Joseph, 1971

Lee, Janet. War Girls: The First Aid Nursing Yeomanry in the First World War, Manchester University Press, 2005

Leneman, Leah. In the Service of Life: The Story of Elsie Inglis and the Scottish Women's Hospitals, Mercat Press, Edinburgh, 1994

———. Elsie Inglis: Founder of battlefield hospitals run entirely by women, NMS Publishing Limited, Edinburgh, 1998

———. Medical women at war, 1914–1918 (article in Medical History, 38, 1994)

Macdonald, Lyn. The Roses of No Man's Land, Michael Joseph, Ltd., 1980 and Penguin Books, 1993

McGann, Susan. The Battle of the Nurses: A Study of Eight Women who Influenced the Development of Professional Nursing, 1880–1930, Scutari Press, 1992

McLaren, Barbara. Women of the War, Hodder and Stoughton, 1917

McLaren, Mrs Eva Shaw. The History of the Scottish Women's Hospitals, Hodder and Stoughton, 1919

Macnaughtan, Sarah. A Woman's Diary of the War, T. Nelson & Sons, 1915

McPhail, Helen. The Long Silence: Civilian Life under the German Occupation of Northern France, 1914–1918, Tauris, 1999

Marlow, Joyce (Editor). The Virago Book of Women and the Great War, Virago Press, 1998

Marwick, Arthur. Women at War 1914–1918, Fontana Paperbacks in Association with the Imperial War Museum, 1977

Mitchell, David. Women on the Warpath: The Story of the Women of the First World War, Cape, 1966

Nicholson, Virginia. Singled Out: How Two Million Women Survived Without Men after the First World War, Viking (Penguin Group), 2007

Oldfield, Sybil. Doers of the Word: A Biographical Dictionary of British Women Humanitarians active between 1900–1950, Continuum, 2001 and Oldfield paperback edition 2006

Oliver, Dame Beryl, GBE., RRC. The British Red Cross in Action, Faber and Faber Ltd., 1966

Ouditt, Sharon. Fighting Forces, Writing Women: Identity and Ideology in the First World War, Routledge, 1994

Plumridge, Lt. Colonel John H., OBE., RAMC. Hospital Ships and Ambulance Trains, Seeley, Service and Co., Ltd., 1975

Popham, Hugh. The FANY in Peace and War: The Story of the First Aid Nursing Yeomanry 1907–2003, New and Revised Edition, Leo Cooper (Pen and Sword Books), 2003

Potter, Jane. Boys in Khaki, Girls in Print: Women's Literary Responses to the Great War 1914–1918, Clarendon Press, Oxford, 2005

Rathbone, Irene. We That Were Young, Chatto and Windus, 1932 and Virago Press, 1988

Reilly, Catherine. Scars Upon my Heart: Women's Poetry and Verse of the First World War, Virago, 1981

Ross, Ishobel. Little Grey Partridge: First World War Diary of Ishobel Ross who served with the Scottish Women's Hospitals unit in Serbia. Introduced by Jess Dixon, Aberdeen University Press, 1988

Sandes, Flora. An English Woman-Sergeant in the Serbian Army, Hodder and Stoughton, 1916

——. The Lovely Sergeant. A Biography by Alan Burgess, Heinemann, 1963

Smith, Angela. Women's Writing of the First World War: An Anthology, Manchester University Press, 2000

Stebbing, E.P. At the Serbian Front in Macedonia, John Lane, 1917

Stuart, Denis. Dear Duchess: Millicent Duchess of Sutherland 1867–1955, Gollancz, 1982

Summers, Anne. Angels and Civilians: British Women as Military Nurses 1854–1914, Routledge and Kegan Paul, 1988

Thurstan, Violetta. The People who Run: Being the Tragedy of the Refugees in Russia, Putnam's, 1916

——. Hounds of War Unleashed: A Nurse's Account of her Life on the Eastern Front during the 1914–18 War, United Writers, Cornwall, 1978

——. A Celebration by Muriel Somerfield and Ann Bellingham, Jamieson Library, Newmill, Penzance, Cornwall, 1993

Wenzel, Marian and John Cornish (Compilers). Auntie Mabel's War [Mabel Jeffery]. An account of her part in the hostilities of 1914–18, Allen Lane, 1980

Whitehead, Ian R. Doctors in the Great War, Leo Cooper, 1999

Wilson, Francesca. In the Margins of Chaos: Recollections of Relief Work in and between Three Wars, Murray 1944

Glossary

ADMS	Assistant Director of Medical Services
Alwyn hut	Small detached cubical apartments of light wooden framework, over which canvas is stretched, with wooden floors and windows of celluloid – and a stove
Arabeah	Also araybier or arabier. Open-fronted, single-horse drawn carriage. The taxi of Cairo
Archies	Anti aircraft guns
Arnaut	Albanian peasant
Armstrong hut	Similar to Alwyn hut. Canvas and wood collapsible hut used by the British in the First World War
ASC	Army Service Corps
Asepsis	Practice of ensuring that bacteria (or other contaminants such as viruses, fungi or parasites) are excluded, to prevent infection during surgery, wound dressing, or other medical procedures
Aubu	Probably a corruption of the French obus – an artillery shell
Beatrice stove	Cast iron stove fuelled by kerosene oil. Used to provide heating or for boiling water or cooking
BEF	British Expeditionary Forces
Blessé	Wounded
Bougez	French for 'move'
Brassards	Badge worn on the arm
Carrel tubes	System consisting of glass syringes and rubber tubing used to irrigate infected wounds with an antiseptic solution, developed by Dr Alexis Carrel
Catwyk	A Dutch ship, carrying a cargo of grain, torpedoed by a German submarine near Flushing on 14 April 1915
CCS	Casualty Clearing Station NB. Depending on the type and extent of his wound a soldier would either struggle on his own, be carried by a comrade, or placed on a stretcher and taken to the regimental aid post situated somewhere on the edge of the battlefield wherever the regimental medical officer could find suitable shelter. Stretcher-bearers, trained in first aid, treated haemorrhages, and gave other immediate help. At the aid post the wound was dressed and then the soldier was taken further back to a field dressing station. After having an anti-tetanus injection he was sent by ambulance to a CCS situated well behind the line. When fit enough he was put on a hospital train which took him to a base hospital. He then either returned to fight again, or was sent back to England to convalesce

Chaldeans	People originating from the 'land of Chaldea' – a territory in southern Babylonia (modern southern Iraq), lying between the Rivers Euphrates and Tigris, at the head of the Persian Gulf
Char	Tea, Chinese (Mandarin) ch'a
Crossley Tender	Vehicle manufactured by Crossley Motors. The 34cwt tender had room for eleven men, three in front with the remainder facing each other on bench seats down each side of the rear. Weather protection was provided by two hoods, one for the front and one for the rear
DMS	Director of Medical Services
DDMS	Deputy Director of Medical Services
DADMS	Deputy Assistant Director of Medical Services
DGMS	Director General Medical Services. (Post held by Sir Arthur Sloggett from October 1914 until June 1918 when he was succeeded by Lt. General C. Burtchaell)
Dixies	Iron pot or kettle for tea/stew etc.
DT	Delirium Tremens. Trembling and delusions resulting from excess of alcohol
Duma	Russian Parliament
Enteric fever	Alternative name for either typhoid fever or paratyphoid fever. See Typhoid fever
Eusol dressing	Dressing soaked in eusol (a disinfecting solution consisting of chlorinated lime and boric acid) used for wounds and ulcers
FANY	Nick-named 'Fanny'. First Aid Nursing Yeomanry
Flavine treatment	Brownish-red crystalline powder used as an antiseptic
Formaline	Also known as formalin. An aqueous solution (in water) of formaldehyde (a pungent gas), used as an antiseptic and disinfectant. Also used for preserving tissues for histological study (the study of tissues under the microscope)
Formamint	Sore throat lozenge manufactured by A. Wulging and Co., and marketed as 'The Germ-killing Throat Tablet'
FRCS	Fellow of the Royal College of Surgeons
Gas gangrene	Severe form of gangrene – tissue infection. The battlefields in France consisted of heavily-manured soil and wounds infected with anaerobic (low oxygen) bacteria became swollen The bacillus in the wound created gas which could be felt in the tissue when the swollen area was pressed with the fingers. If soil and pieces of uniform were present gas gangrene would set in even in a slight wound. There were no antibiotics and no effective disinfectant. Amputations of affected limbs were the only hope, but if the infection spread the men died from the toxic effects of the bacteria NB. Not be be confused with the poison gas in shells first used by the Germans at the Second Battle of Ypres in April 1915
Glaxo	Name of a dried milk product (trade marked in 1906) produced by a heritage company of the pharmaceutical company, GlaxoSmithKline. Derived from galatin, the Greek word for milk. Marketed under the famous slogan 'Glaxo Builds Bonnie Babies', the Glaxo product was an outstanding success and later the trade mark was chosen as the company's name
GS Wagon	General Service Wagon

Gothas	German aeroplanes
Grandmothers	15in guns
Gutta-perche	More commonly known as gutta-percha. A rubbery substance derived from the latex of certain tropical trees, found mainly in Malaysia and the South Pacific. Used in manufacture of orthopaedic splints and in dentistry (e.g. for filling cavities)
Jaconet	Medium weight cotton cloth
Keating	Keating's powder used for killing fleas and other insects (ticks, beetles, mosquitoes, flies, etc.)
Kepis	Military cap
Kvass	Fermented beverage
Laparotomy	Incision and exploration of the stomach
Lazarette	Mobile Field Hospital
L. of C.	Lines of Communication
[Long] liston's	A long splint extending from the axilla (underarm) to the sole of the foot
Macconicie	Special ration of meat and vegetables – a welcome relief from bully-beef
Mealie meal	Ground maize
Monitor	Gunboat specially designed for use in shallow water
Marmite	A metal or earthenware cooking pot with a cover, usually large and often with legs
Mitrailleuse	Many-barrelled breech-loading machine gun
Moribund	The dying
MWF	Medical Women's Federation
Nunc Dimittis	Latin – Permission to depart. [Song of Simeon – Luke ch. 2, v. 29 'Lord now lettest thou thy Servant depart in Peace …']
NUWSS	National Union of Women's Suffrage Societies
OC	Officer Commanding
Otalans [Ortolan]	Any of several new world birds
Paliasse	Straw mattress
PB men	Permanent Base Men
Permanganate of Potash	Also known as potassium permanganate. Forms dark purple solution when dissolved in water, which is used as a disinfectant or antiseptic
Picric acid	More formally known as trinitrophenol. Yellow intensely bitter substance used in dyeing, medicine (as an antiseptic in the early twentieth century, e.g. for burns, smallpox, etc.) and also used in the manufacture of explosives.
PMO	Principal Medical Officer
Poilu	French soldier
Polenta	Pearl barley. Kind of barley meal
QA	Abbreviation for QAIMNS
QAIMNS	Queen Alexandra's Imperial Military Nursing Service
RAMC	Royal Army Medical Corps
RMLI	Royal Marine Light Infantry
RMO	Regimental Medical Officer
RTO	Railway Transport Officer
Sanitar	Hospital attendant or medical orderly [Crimean or Estonian]
Salines	Consisting of, or based on, salts

Sawyer stove	Stove invented by Alexis Sawyer, a French chef who worked at the Reform Club, London, and became an established name. During the Crimean War, when soldiers were dying of malnutrition, Sawyer went to the Crimea, worked with the troops, and invented the stove, still used by the army today
SWH	Scottish Women's Hospitals
Sloughing	Casting off a diseased tissue
Solignum	A preservative treatment for wood/timber
Somnytics	Possibly the brand name for a sleeping drug
Tatars	Muslim people who lived in the Crimea and along the Volga. Annexed by Russia in 1783. (Also known as Tartars)
Taube	A monoplane with a bird-like wing shape. A generic term for this type of aircraft
Trepanned	Trepan, a surgeon's cylindrical saw for removing part of the bone of the skull, to relieve pain
Typhoid fever	An infectious disease contracted by eating food or drinking water contaminated with the bacterium salmonella typhi. See also Enteric fever
Typhus	Acute infectious disease spread by insects or similar animals. In the First World War a typhus epidemic spread between humans by body lice
VAD	Voluntary Aid Detachment
Verst	Russian measure of length – about two-thirds of an English mile
WS and WCC	Women's Sick and Wounded Convoy Corps
Zouave	Member of the French Light Infantry Corps. Originally formed of Algerians and retaining Oriental uniform
Zwicka	A drink

Index